# Urban Health
## Global Perspectives

**DAVID VLAHOV**
**JO IVEY BOUFFORD**
**CLARENCE PEARSON**
**LAURIE NORRIS**

EDITORS

FOREWORD BY MICHAEL R. BLOOMBERG

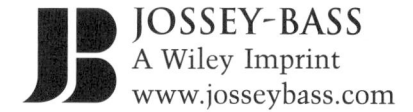

JOSSEY-BASS
A Wiley Imprint
www.josseybass.com

Copyright © 2010 by John Wiley & Sons, Inc. All rights reserved.

Published by Jossey-Bass
A Wiley Imprint
989 Market Street, San Francisco, CA 94103-1741—www.josseybass.com

No part of this publication may be reproduced, stored in a retrieval system, or transmitted in any form or by any means, electronic, mechanical, photocopying, recording, scanning, or otherwise, except as permitted under Section 107 or 108 of the 1976 United States Copyright Act, without either the prior written permission of the publisher, or authorization through payment of the appropriate per-copy fee to the Copyright Clearance Center, Inc., 222 Rosewood Drive, Danvers, MA 01923, 978-750-8400, fax 978-646-8600, or on the Web at www.copyright.com. Requests to the publisher for permission should be addressed to the Permissions Department, John Wiley & Sons, Inc., 111 River Street, Hoboken, NJ 07030, 201-748-6011, fax 201-748-6008, or online at www.wiley.com/go/permissions.

Readers should be aware that Internet Web sites offered as citations and/or sources for further information may have changed or disappeared between the time this was written and when it is read.

Limit of Liability/Disclaimer of Warranty: While the publisher and author have used their best efforts in preparing this book, they make no representations or warranties with respect to the accuracy or completeness of the contents of this book and specifically disclaim any implied warranties of merchantability or fitness for a particular purpose. No warranty may be created or extended by sales representatives or written sales materials. The advice and strategies contained herein may not be suitable for your situation. You should consult with a professional where appropriate. Neither the publisher nor author shall be liable for any loss of profit or any other commercial damages, including but not limited to special, incidental, consequential, or other damages.

Jossey-Bass books and products are available through most bookstores. To contact Jossey-Bass directly call our Customer Care Department within the U.S. at 800-956-7739, outside the U.S. at 317-572-3986, or fax 317-572-4002.

Jossey-Bass also publishes its books in a variety of electronic formats. Some content that appears in print may not be available in electronic books.

**Library of Congress Cataloging-in-Publication Data**

Urban health : global perspectives / David Vlahov ... [et al.], editors. —1st ed.
    p. ; cm.
  Includes bibliographical references and index.
  ISBN 978-0-470-42206-9 (cloth); 9780470880821 (ebk);
  9780470880838 (ebk); 9780470880845 (ebk)
    1. Urban health.   2. Health—Globalization.   I. Vlahov, David.
  [DNLM: 1. Urban Health.   2. Health Status.   3. Urban Health Services—organization & administration.   4. Urbanization. WA 380]
  RA566.7.U744   2011
  362.1'042—dc22

2010028498

Printed in the United States of America

FIRST EDITION

*HB Printing* 10 9 8 7 6 5 4 3 2 1

# CONTENTS

**The New York Academy of Medicine**  vii

**Foreword**  xi
Michael R. Bloomberg

**Preface**  xiii

**Acknowledgments**  xv
David Vlahov

**Introduction**  xvii
Margaret Chan

**The Editors**  xxi

**The Contributors**  xxiii

1. **Urban Health in a Global Perspective**  1
   David Vlahov and Jo Ivey Boufford

2. **Globalization**  13
   Ted Schrecker and Ronald Labonté

3. **The Demographics of Urbanization in Poor Countries**  27
   Mark R. Montgomery

4. **Migration, Health Systems, and Urbanization**  45
   Ndioro Ndiaye, Manuel Carbhallo, and Rougui Ndiaye-Coïc

5. **Immigrant Health in Amsterdam, the Netherlands**  59
   Arnoud P. Verhoeff and Roel A. Coutinho

6. **City Case Studies**
   **Global Climate Change and Cities**  69
   Tord Kjellstrom and Patricia Monge

7. **Age-Friendly New York City**  91
   Ruth Finkelstein and Julie Netherland

8. **Global Infectious Diseases and Urbanization**  105
   Thomas C. Quinn and John G. Bartlett

9. **City Case Studies**
   **Confronting the New Epidemics in Our Cities**  125
   Stephen Leeder, Angela Beaton, Cathie Hull,
   Ruth Colagiuri, and Michael Ward

10. **Chronic Disease Care in Nairobi's Urban Informal Settlements**  139
    Catherine Kyobutungi and Alex Ezeh

11. **Crime, Violence, Public Health, and Urban Life**  157
    Richard H. Schneider

12. **A Global Perspective on Disasters and Their Consequences in the Urban Environment**  175
    Maria Steenland, Godfrey Mbaruku, and Sandro Galea

13. **City Case Studies**
    **Urban Terrorism**  191
    Robert J. Bunker and Pamela L. Bunker

14. **The Culture of Peace Against Violence in Zagreb**  207
    Stipe Oreskovic

15. **Urban Health Services and Health Systems Reform**  221
    Julio Frenk and Octavio Gómez-Dantés

16. **City Case Studies**
    Information Flow and Integrated E-Health Systems   237
    Veronica Olazabal, Ticia Gerber, Beatriz de Faria Leao,
    Claudio Giulliano da Costa, Karl Brown, and
    Ariel Pablos-Méndez

17. **Governance for Health in London: Utilizing the Health Impact Assessment**   253
    Sue Atkinson

18. **Provision of Water and Sanitation Services**   267
    Jonathan Parkinson, Martin Mulenga, and
    Gordon McGranahan

19. **Urban Transportation**   283
    Rae Zimmerman and Carlos E. Restrepo

20. **Informal Settlements: In Search of a Home in the City**   305
    Vanessa Watson

21. **Urban Air Quality**   317
    Jonathan M. Samet

22. **Urban Planning and Aesthetics**   339
    Carola Hein, Kalala Ngalamulume, and
    Kevin J. Robinson

23. **Healthy Urban Governance**   355
    Scott Burris and Danielle Ompad

24. **Global Business at the Local Level**   371
    Nicholas Freudenberg

25. **Citizen Action for Urban Poverty Reduction in Low- and Middle-Income Nations**   389
    David Satterthwaite

26. **City Case Studies**
    **Healthy Cities: Lessons Learned** 405
    Agis Tsouros and Geoff Green

27. **The Healthy City Program in Shanghai** 421
    Fu Hua

28. **Urban Health and Governance Model in Belo Horizonte, Brazil** 437
    Waleska Teixeira Caiaffa, Ana Luiza Nabuco, Amélia Augusta de Lima Friche, and Fernando Augusto Proietti

29. **Improving Population Health in a Rapidly Urbanizing World** 453
    Nicole Volavka-Close and Elliott D. Sclar

30. **Future Directions** 469
    Jacob Kumaresan

**Notes** 483

**Index** 487

# THE NEW YORK ACADEMY OF MEDICINE

The New York Academy of Medicine advances the health of people in cities.

An independent organization since 1847, NYAM addresses the health challenges facing the world's urban populations through interdisciplinary approaches to policy leadership, education, community engagement, and innovative research. Drawing on the expertise of diverse partners worldwide and more than two thousand elected fellows across the professions, our current priorities are:

- To create environments in cities that support healthy aging
- To strengthen systems that prevent disease and promote the public's health
- To implement interventions that eliminate health disparities

## CURRENT AGENDA

America's health system is in crisis with dramatic increases in chronic disease, spiraling health care costs, and unacceptable differences in the health status of our population. At NYAM, we are tackling these health challenges to create a different future. We believe in a future for seniors that promises independent and healthy living; we believe that it is possible to help individuals and communities tackle the avoidable causes of illness, disability, and death; and we believe that by eliminating disparities, vulnerable communities can have equal opportunities for health. Our beliefs are not based upon idealism, but upon NYAM's more than 160-year history of impact and action to accomplish these goals through research, policy advocacy, education, and community engagement. By applying all these strategies to better understand the multiple determinants of health, we can shape programs and policies that give all people the opportunity to be as healthy as they can be.

Each of NYAM's units—Health Policy, the Center for Urban Epidemiologic Studies (CUES), the Social Work Leadership Institute, the Office of School Health Programs, and our nationally and internationally recognized library and rare book collection—work together to address the issues that remain central to the core of NYAM's mission.

A few highlights from this past year provide examples of our work. Our CUES group launched *Project VIVA* in an effort to address the low immunization rates among minorities and people living in poverty. Such vaccination rates have contributed to unacceptably high death rates from influenza and respiratory diseases. By combining community-based research with the provision of immunizations by our partners, NYAM is able to develop a knowledge base that can inform programs to increase access to a variety of such services to these easy-to-miss populations. NYAM's Division of Health Policy, in close collaboration with the New York City Mayor's Office and the City Council, has developed *Age-friendly New York*, a new initiative in which the public and private sector will work together to create the physical and social environment that allow older persons to remain active and contribute their rich experience to the city for as long as they choose. Within NYAM's Office of School Health Programs, we are creating new and earlier points of entry into health professions for under-represented minorities. Our GIRLS program and our Junior Fellows program are important examples of our goal to develop new strategies for increasing the diversity of the health workforce to more effectively engage with our increasingly diverse population. NYAM's Social Work Leadership Institute is a national initiative to transform social work education for the care of older persons and to promote a future health workforce to serve an aging population. It is also working to ensure models for the coordination of health and social care that is critical for America's older adults to live life to the fullest. NYAM's world class library provides students, medical professionals, the media, and the general public with medical library services and access to a unique service that aggregates and disseminates "gray literature" in public health, disaster preparedness, and urban health through web-based portals. The library's rare book, manuscript, and historical collections compose one of the country's finest research libraries in the country in the history of medicine and public health. NYAM's Executive Conference Center is a hub for major conferences, educational programs, and the convening of multiple stakeholders on critical issues in health and health policy.

Building on NYAM's considerable expertise in research, education, community engagement, and policy leadership, along with our special role as convener of different interest groups, we seek to inform the field of urban health, shape its outcomes, and create models that will guide practice and policy in the future.

Jo Ivey Boufford, MD
The New York Academy of Medicine
New York, NY

# FOREWORD

Globalization and urbanization are transforming the way we live. In 2008, for the first time in history, more than half the world's population could be found living in cities—up from only 30 percent in 1950. By the middle of this century, the proportion will likely reach two-thirds. How will the shift affect public health? What risks and challenges should we anticipate? *Urban Health: A Global Perspective* highlights the central role of health in the development and prosperity of cities.

In New York City—where we expect our population to reach 9 million by 2030—we have developed a comprehensive blueprint for accommodating that growth in a sustainable fashion. We call it PlaNYC—our plan for a greener, greater New York.

PlaNYC consists of 127 interconnected initiatives that are designed to help us meet 10 goals that are central to building a healthy and sustainable city. These goals include creating new open space, reducing our carbon footprint by 30 percent, and giving New York the cleanest air of any major city in the United States.

Although public health problems have traditionally been associated with urban areas, the reality is that, on average, urban residents tend to be healthier than their rural counterparts—and for good reasons. Besides providing better access to basic resources, such as food, housing, health care, and education, urban centers can foster active lifestyles. For instance, New York is a walking city, and that exercise helps reduce cardiovascular disease and obesity.

Cities may have inherent advantages, but healthy cities are not just products of luck and circumstance. They are born of collective commitment. Shortly after taking office in 2002, we set out to reduce the number of deaths due to tobacco use. We sharply raised the city's tobacco tax that year, and in 2003 we instituted a smoking ban in all indoor workplaces, including bars and restaurants. Since then, 35 U.S. states and more than a dozen countries have become smoke-free. Through those efforts and a series of hard-hitting marketing and outreach campaigns, we have reduced the number of smokers in New York City by 300,000—a reduction that could save 100,000 lives.

The success we have had reducing tobacco use has led us to expand our fight against the leading cause of preventable death: cardiovascular disease. In 2006, we became the first major city to ban artificial trans fat from restaurant food. And in 2008, we began requiring chain restaurants to prominently display calorie information on their menus and menu boards. Our administration has also implemented programs that improve access to fresh fruits and vegetables in neighborhoods where they are hardest to find. And we have raised the nutritional quality of the 1.5 million meals served daily in city-run schools, hospitals, and senior centers.

These initiatives are all part of our comprehensive public health campaign, Take Care New York, which aims to reduce deaths from preventable diseases and eliminate health disparities among people of different races and ethnicities. We launched Take Care New York in 2004, and it includes 10 key steps that all New Yorkers can take to live longer and healthier lives. The initiative relies on partnerships among individuals, employers, and health care providers, as well as faith-based and community-based organizations. It also relies on data. City agencies closely monitor their efforts and evaluate their impact. By 2007, the Take Care New York initiative had already surpassed four of its goals for 2008. A few examples:

- Smoking prevalence among New York City adults fell from 21.5 percent in 2002 to 16.9 percent in 2007, while teenage smoking fell by more than half.
- In 2002, a quarter of all New Yorkers lacked a regular physician. The proportion has since fallen to 19 percent, meaning that 364,000 additional New Yorkers are now getting better routine health care.
- In 2003, only 42 percent of New Yorkers over 50 had received a colonoscopy within the previous 10 years. By 2007, the proportion had risen to 62 percent—and black New Yorkers were as likely as whites to get screened.

Cities across the globe face many of the same challenges we do here in New York. And as this book demonstrates, major stakeholders—from elected officials and health policy leaders to academics and the public—are increasingly committed to public health as a fundamental part of urban governance. By sharing strategies, and learning from each other's setbacks and successes, we can solve common problems and assure that globalization improves the lives of city residents worldwide.

Michael R. Bloomberg
Mayor of the City of New York
March 1, 2010

# PREFACE

*Urban health* is a term whose meaning has been difficult to communicate. First, *urban* appears to be nearly ubiquitous. Most of us have repeatedly heard that "in 2007, for the first time in history, over half of the world is urban." In North America and Europe, more than three-quarters of the population already live in urban areas. Urban areas are growing and expanding. It would seem that urban covers just about everybody and everything.

Urban areas are determinants of health. They are affecting climate change and are vulnerable to it. They are the seats of globalization through business and economic development, communications, infectious disease transmission, migration, crime, and terrorism. These are all strong forces that can affect the health of urban dwellers. While no specific disease or condition is uniquely urban, the form and composition of urban areas—their size, diversity, density, and complexity—shape health and affect the design of interventions that can have a positive impact on health, but so far, the term *urban health* does not point to a discrete set of interventions developed for other public health challenges, such as tobacco control, road safety, violence prevention, or climate change, leaving the listener unsure of what is to be done.

Urban areas contain hidden disadvantaged cities. Central to understanding and acting on urban health problems is appreciating the health realities of different communities and populations within cities. Earlier reports noted that, on average, health indicators are better in urban than in corresponding rural areas, suggesting an "urban health advantage." The all-too-infrequent disaggregation of urban data has challenged this view by demonstrating pockets (and sometimes wardrobes) of poverty where health indicators are worse than their rural counterparts. The association of poverty with disease is well established, but what is notable is the effect on physical and mental health of widening disparities in such close proximity.

Promoting health within urban areas requires more than single programs and policies, it requires a process of healthy governance. Cities are complex, and achieving urban health requires an appreciation of forces and factors that impact the health of different segments of urban populations and then developing the mechanisms that can bring together the expertise and resources to translate these findings into action. Addressing the wide range of health issues in cities that are affecting a diverse yet interconnected population requires not a program or a policy, but the processes of healthy urban governance that assure inclusive, transparent, and accountable stewardship of public resources by government and robust partnerships with the many non-governmental actors that are critical to making the changes needed to align actions for health. Models exist and more need to be documented.

Support for attention to urban health has gathered momentum. The World Health Organization (WHO) launched the Healthy Cities movement over two decades ago and declared 2010 as the Year of Urban Health, which has included orchestrating events in over 1,400 cities to heighten awareness and encourage problem-solving for the challenges that accompany urbanization. UN-HABITAT started by addressing some of the basic determinants of urban health, such as housing, and has evolved to develop a global set of Urban Observatories that can document and call cities to action on a range of urban issues. More recently, the founding of the International Society for Urban Health has added a more rigorous academic contribution to these efforts. Holding annual conferences, this group has included clinicians, public health researchers, social and physical scientists, urban planners, community activists, and more recently, policy makers and municipal leaders. The purpose has been an exchange of information and networking about best practices for measuring and achieving urban health. What started as an organization to address health disparities in North American inner cities has grown to a concern for urban health inequalities and inequities across the globe. Each learns from the other, but all are part of one global city.

# ACKNOWLEDGMENTS

This book would not be possible without the contribution of others who share this commitment. First, I want to thank my three co-editors—Jo Ivey Boufford, Clarence Pearson, and Laurie Norris—for their support and orchestration of the many details, from selecting authors and reviewing the manuscripts through coordinating the process that produced the final manuscript. Andy Pasternack, public health editor, and Seth Schwartz, associate editor, for Jossey-Bass/John Wiley & Sons Publishers, continue to contribute their support and publishing expertise for this book, the fourth in the global health series. We are also grateful to our production editor, Kelsey McGee; and the copy editors, Barbara Armentrout and Sarah Miller.

The authors of the chapters in this volume provided expert knowledge, and the book benefits from their real global experience. We also recognize Andrew Quinn, who has been coordinator for the International Society for Urban Health and the *Journal of Urban Health*, and Danielle Ompad, as associate director of the Center for Urban Epidemiologic Studies. Colleagues who have provided inspiration and support include Siddarth Agarwal, Hortensia Amaro, Jeremiah Barondess, Eugenia Birch, Kate Bond, Lee Bone, Robert Buckley, Waleska Caiaffa, Tony Capon, Ana Diez Roux, Alex Ezeh, Nick Freudenberg, Jean-Christophe Fotso, Linda Fried, Tom Frieden, Sharon Friel, Howard Frumkin, Sandro Galea, Luiz Galvao, Chris Gibbons, Trevor Hancock, Donna Higgins, Barbara Israel, Ichiro Kawachi, Monica Kerrigan, Anthony Kolb, Dan Kraushaar, Jim Krieger, Jacob Kumaresan, Roderick Lawrence, Suzy Mercado, Mark Montgomery, Pat O'Campo, Anita Palepu, Amit Prasad, Fernando Proietti, Marti Rice, David Satterthwaite, Elliott Sclar, Diana Silimperi, Al Sommer, John Steward, Liz Thomas, Agis Tsouris, Arpana Varma, Arnoud Verhoeff, Fritz Wagner, and Vanessa Watson. To others who have been colleagues but not mentioned here, we owe our apologies along with our thanks. We recognize and honor the leadership role of Trudy Harpham in pioneering this entire area of scholarship.

We also thank Robyn Gershon, who provided immeasurable support throughout the process of generating this volume. Finally, we want to acknowledge all of those at the New York Academy of Medicine, which has been "at the heart of urban health since 1847."

David Vlahov, PhD, RN
New York
May 2010

# INTRODUCTION

All around the world, health in the twenty-first century is being shaped by the same powerful forces. Traditional distinctions between health problems in affluent and developing nations have become blurred. Demographic aging is now a universal trend, as is the globalization of unhealthy lifestyles. Both contribute to another broadly shared trend: the rise of chronic diseases, like heart disease, stroke, cancer, diabetes, and asthma. Previously, these diseases were considered the close companions of affluent societies. Today, around 80 percent of the global burden of chronic diseases is concentrated in low- and middle-income countries, with enormous implications for the accessibility, quality, and costs of long-term care.

These and other health consequences are amplified by yet another global trend: rapid—and often unplanned—urbanization. Cities, with their concentrations of people, infrastructure, institutions, and opportunities, have long boosted the progress of civilization, and these advantages remain magnets drawing migrants from rural areas within countries, or from developing to more affluent countries. But today's pattern of urbanization includes some unique features. In many cases, especially in the developing world, the speed of urbanization has outpaced the ability of governments to build essential infrastructures that make life in cities safe, rewarding, and healthy.

The accelerated pace of urbanization is well-illustrated by a look at historical data on how long it takes a city to grow from one million to eight million inhabitants. For London, this growth took around 130 years. For Bangkok, similar growth took 45 years. For Seoul, it took only 25 years. In the years to come, the World Health Organization (WHO) estimates that the growth of cities with one to ten million inhabitants will outpace the growth of mega-cities. Moreover, most of this growth will occur in low- and middle-income countries.

This volume takes a wide-ranging look at urban health in its multiple dimensions—from the impact of the built and natural environment to the consequences of climate change, from the pressures on vital services to the pleasures of aesthetic improvements and the benefits for health. While urban living continues to offer many opportunities—including opportunities for better health care—these advantages can be extremely uneven in their distribution. As the authors note, today's urban environments all too often concentrate risks for health, magnify the consequences, and introduce new hazards.

Today, nearly all the world's urban centers have pockets of extreme wealth together with pockets of extreme deprivation. They have populations that overconsume health care and populations that forego health care for financial and other reasons. They see malnutrition and obesity side by side.

Many of today's sprawling cities face a triple burden of disease. Infectious diseases thrive when people are crowded together under squalid living conditions, and outbreaks can be explosive, as witnessed by recent epidemics of dengue, urban yellow fever, and sexually transmitted diseases. Chronic diseases are on the rise with the globalization of unhealthy lifestyles, as facilitated by urban life. And urban health is further burdened by waves of accidents, injuries, traffic crashes, violence, and crime.

Rapid unplanned urbanization, especially in the developing world, has been accompanied by a rapid concentration of poverty, often in slums and shantytowns. This trend arises as more and more people move from rural to urban areas within a country, or migrate from a poor country to a more affluent one. Some move looking for opportunities for a better life. Others do so hoping to survive, especially when rural smallholder farming provides a withering livelihood. Many arrive in urban areas impoverished and stay that way. Instead of a better life, they encounter a host of new threats to their health, their mental and physical well-being, and their quality of life. Moreover, as yet another source of pressure, climate change is expected to accelerate urban growth, as destitute "environmental refugees" flee rural areas when crops fail because of drought or fields are inundated by floods.

In general, cities offer more opportunities for better health care, but this is not always the case for poor or marginalized groups, including rapidly growing numbers of the elderly. Once again, conditions in an urban setting can amplify the problems of inequitable access to health care and the great and growing gaps in health outcomes seen both within and between countries.

As the authors note, the risks to health grow when densely packed settlements arise in the absence of adequate health services, adequate systems for social protection, and effective regulatory mechanisms. For example, the population density that characterizes cities can strain municipal capacity to regulate air and water quality, provide sanitation, and safeguard the quality of health care provided by both the public and private sectors.

Rural populations have traditionally enjoyed two healthy assets: high levels of physical activity and healthy diets. Both assets come under threat in an urban setting. Urban lifestyles and the built environment encourage sedentary behavior. Processed foods, usually rich in fats and sugar and low in essential nutrients, frequently become the most convenient—and the cheapest—way to fill the stomachs of the urban poor. Such trends are further supported by the industrialization of food production and the globalization of its distribution and marketing. All of these factors, amplified in an urban setting, contribute to the rise of chronic diseases and the global epidemic of obesity, which affects rich and poor alike.

As documented in this book, the list of other potential ills is long: unhealthy housing, breaches in food and water safety, congested traffic, more accidents and crime, air pollution, stress, increased use of harmful substances, and higher rates of mental illness.

Although the threats to urban health are great, the overall picture is far from bleak. Apart from documenting the problems, chapters in this book offer a collection of real-life success stories, a sourcebook of best practices, and a menu of options for taking protective and corrective action. As the authors convincingly argue, urban health goes beyond the roles and responsibilities of government to include the contributions that civil society, community groups, architects, engineers, and responsible businesses can make. In particular, civil society can create pressure, from the bottom up to make health-promoting and -protecting environments an issue that appeals to the interests of political leaders.

At the same time, many threats to urban health arise in sectors beyond the direct control of public health. Health officials cannot increase taxes on tobacco or alcohol or influence the food items on sale in local markets. Acting alone, they cannot determine where hospitals are sited or how they are built. They cannot stop people from deliberately settling on cheap land close to health hazards or prone to landslides or floods. The health sector has little sway over transportation policies, including regulations and other measures that have a proven ability to reduce traffic-related deaths and injuries.

But the health sector can collect evidence on the hazards to urban health arising in other sectors and exert pressure for change. As experience shows, the social expectations for health care are rising everywhere. People in all countries want care that is fair and efficient as well as affordable. Health problems can be one of the most obvious and socially disturbing examples of urban harm. They can also be a rallying point that unifies public demand and compels political leaders to take action. As I will always argue, these actions should align closely with the values, principles, and approaches of primary health care. I am firmly convinced: primary health care is our best bet and our best buy for improving the efficiency and fairness of health care, in any setting.

Above all, when taken together, the chapters collected in this book provide a compelling call to action. Urban areas can indeed be built, organized, managed, retrofitted, and governed in ways that promote health. Good examples abound. As in so many other areas of urban life, the costs of failing to promote and protect urban health will be amplified, and the price will be high.

Margaret Chan, MD
Director-General
World Health Organization
Geneva, Switzerland

# THE EDITORS

David Vlahov, PhD, is senior vice president for research and director for the Center for Urban Epidemiologic Studies at the New York Academy of Medicine, and professor of clinical epidemiology at the Mailman School of Public Health at Columbia University. He has conducted studies of urban populations in Baltimore, Harlem, and the Bronx, including longitudinal cohort studies, for which he received the NIH MERIT Award. He has led individual- and community-level intervention studies and community-based participatory research to address racial and ethnic disparities through the social determinants of health. Vlahov was the founding president of the International Society for Urban Health (www.isuh.org) and will host the ninth International Conference on Urban Health in New York City. He was a visiting professor at the medical school in Belo Horizonte, Brazil, and is an advisor to the World Health Organization (WHO) as it prepares the 2010 global urban health report. Vlahov is the editor-in-chief of the *Journal of Urban Health*.

Jo Ivey Boufford, MD, is president of the New York Academy of Medicine; professor of Public Service, Health Policy, and Management at the Robert F. Wagner Graduate School of Public Service, where she served as dean (1997–2002); and clinical professor of pediatrics at New York University School of Medicine. She was principal deputy assistant secretary for Health (1993–1997) and acting assistant secretary (1/97–5/97) in the U.S. Department of Health and Human Services (HHS) and served as the U.S. representative on the executive board of the World Health Organization (WHO; 1994–1997). Elected to membership of the Institute of Medicine (IOM) in 1992, Boufford is a member of its executive council and boards on global health and the African Science Academy Development Initiative. She was elected IOM foreign secretary in 2006. She is a fellow of the National Academy of Public Administration. She is board certified in pediatrics.

## THE EDITORS

Clarence Pearson, MPH, is a global health consultant. He is a former senior advisor to the World Health Organization Office at the United Nations and founding president and CEO of the National Center for Health Education. Pearson also served as vice president of the Peter F. Drucker Foundation for Nonprofit Management, and vice president and director of health and safety education for Metropolitan Life. He was a loaned executive for a two-year White House assignment as associate director of a U.S. Presidential Health Commission; a consultant-in-residence in Moscow for the U.S. Department of State, directing a management training program; and a public health consultant in the former Yugoslavia and in Central America. Pearson conceived and serves as executive editor for a series of books on global health, published by Jossey-Bass/John Wiley & Sons. He is an adjunct professor of education at Columbia University.

Laurie Norris, MA, is an interdisciplinary, intercultural communications consultant. She wrote a history of the China Medical Board, an organization that pioneered Western-style medical education in China and Asia, and serves as managing editor for a global health series published by Jossey-Bass/John Wiley & Sons. She has served as director of communications for Catalyst, which builds inclusive workplaces and expands opportunities for women and business, and vice president for communications at the American Heart Association/NYC. Norris serves as an NGO representative at the United Nations for the Gray Panthers, which works for economic and social justice, and as a Friendly Visitor to homebound elders through DOROT. A lifelong New Yorker, she is a Big Apple Greeter, introducing foreign and domestic visitors to New York City through visits she designs and conducts. She earned a bachelor's degree in journalism and a master's degree in intercultural communications from New York University.

# THE CONTRIBUTORS

**Sue Atkinson, CBE, BSc, MB, BChir, MA, FFPH**
Former Regional Director of Public
 Health and Regional Medical Director
National Health Service (NHS)
 Executive London Regional Office
London, United Kingdom

**John G. Bartlett, MD**
Professor of Medicine
The Johns Hopkins University
Baltimore, Maryland
U.S.A.

**Angela Beaton, PhD, MSc (Hons), BSc**
Research Officer
Menzies Centre for Health Policy
University of Sydney
Sydney, Australia

**Jo Ivey Boufford, MD**
President
New York Academy of Medicine
New York, New York
U.S.A.

**Karl Brown, MIA**
Associate Director, Applied
 Technology
The Rockefeller Foundation
New York, New York
U.S.A.

**Pamela L. Bunker, MA**
Senior Analyst
Counter-OPFOR Corporation
Claremont, California
U.S.A.

**Robert J. Bunker, PhD**
CEO
Counter-OPFOR Corporation
Claremont, California
U.S.A.

**Scott Burris, JD**
Professor of Law
James E. Beasley School of Law
Temple University
Philadelphia, Pennsylvania
U.S.A.

**Waleska Teixeira Caiaffa, MD, MPH, PhD**
Professor, Faculty of Medicine
Federal University Mineas Gerais
Belo Horizonte, Brazil

**Manuel Carbhallo, MD**
Executive Director
International Centre for Migration and Health (ICMH)
Geneva, Switzerland

**Ruth Colagiuri, RN, CDE, BEd, Grad Cert Health Policy & Management**
Director and Associate Professor
The Diabetes Unit
Menzies Centre for Health Policy
University of Sydney
Sydney, Australia

**Roel A. Coutinho, MD, PhD**
Director, Netherlands Center for Infectious Disease Control and Professor in Epidemiology and Prevention of Infectious Diseases
Academic Medical Center/University of Amsterdam
Amsterdam, The Netherlands

**Alex Ezeh, MD**
Director
African Population and Health Research Center (APHRC)
Nairobi, Kenya

**Beatriz de Faria Leao, MD, PhD**
Health Standards Architect
Zilics Health Information Systems
São Paulo, Brazil

**Ruth Finkelstein, ScD**
Vice President for Policy
New York Academy of Medicine
New York, New York
U.S.A.

**Julio Frenk, MD, PhD**
Dean
Harvard School of Public Health
Boston, Massachusetts
U.S.A.

**Nicholas Freudenberg, DrPH**
Distinguished Professor
Hunter College, City University of New York (CUNY)
New York, New York
U.S.A.

**Fu Hua, MB, MPH, PhD**
Deputy Dean and Professor
School of Public Health
Fudan University
Shanghai, People's Republic of China

**Sandro Galea, MD, DrPH**
Gelman Professor and Chair of Epidemiology
Mailman School of Public Health
Columbia University
New York, New York
U.S.A.

**Ticia Gerber, MHS/HP**
Senior Program Officer
Health Metrics Network (formerly Manatt Health Solutions, U.S.A.)
Geneva, Switzerland

**Claudio Giulliano da Costa, MD, MSc**
CIO of Bionexo Corporation and President of Brazilian Society for Health Informatics
São Paulo, Brazil

**Octavio Gómez-Dantés, MD, MPH**
Researcher, Center for Health Systems Research
National Institute of Public Health
Cuernavaca, Mexico

**Geoff Green**
Professor of Urban Policy
Sheffield Hallam University
Sheffield, United Kingdom

**Carola Hein, DrIng**
Professor, Growth and Structure of Cities Program
Bryn Mawr College
Bryn Mawr, Pennsylvania
U.S.A.

**Cathie Hull, BA(Hons) Dip Ed (Sydney) BMed(Hons) (Newcastle)**
Associate
Menzies Centre for Health Policy, University of Sydney and Senior Policy Officer, New South Wales Health
Sydney, Australia

**Tord Kjellstrom, BMed, PhD**
Visiting Fellow, Professor
National Centre for Epidemiology and Population Health
Australian National University, Canberra, Australia, and Centre for Global Health Research, Umea University, Umea, Sweden, and University College London
London, United Kingdom

**Jacob Kumaresan, MD**
Director
Kobe Centre
Center for Health Development
World Health Organization (WHO)
Kobe, Japan

**Catherine Kyobutungi, BM, BS, MSc**
Associate Research Scientist
African Population and Health Research Center (APHRC)
Nairobi, Kenya

**Ronald Labonté, PhD**
Canada Research Chair, Globalization/Health Equity
Professor
Faculty of Medicine
University of Ottawa
Institute of Population Health
Ottawa, Ontario
Canada

**Stephen Leeder, MD, PhD**
Director
The Menzies Centre for Health Policy
University of Sydney
Sydney, Australia

**Amélia Augusta de Lima Friche, DrPH**
Assistant Professor
Faculty of Medicine
Federal University Mineas Gerais
Belo Horizonte, Brazil

**Godfrey Mbaruku, PhD**
Deputy Director
Ifakara Health Institute
Dar es Salaam, Tanzania

**Gordon McGranahan, MD**
Head
Human Settlements Group
International Institute for Environment and Development (IIED)
London, United Kingdom

**Patricia Monge, MSc, PhD**
Coordinator, Occupational Health
Central American Institute for Studies on Toxic Substances
Universidad Nacional (UNA)
Heredia, Costa Rica

**Mark R. Montgomery, PhD**
Professor of Economics
State University of New York (SUNY) Stony Brook,
Stony Brook, NY
Senior Associate
Poverty, Gender, and Youth Program
Population Council
New York, New York
U.S.A.

**Martin Mulenga, MBA**
Senior Researcher
Human Settlements Group
International Institute for Environment and Development (IIED)
London, United Kingdom

**Ana Luiza Nabuco**
Secretária Municipal Adjunta de Planejamento
Prefeitura de Belo Horizonte, Brazil

**Julie Netherland, MSW**
Deputy Director
Division of Health Policy
New York Academy of Medicine
New York, New York
U.S.A.

**Ndioro Ndiaye, MD, PhD**
Deputy Director General
International Organization for Migration (IOM)
Geneva, Switzerland

**Rougui Ndiaye-Coïc, M.Geopolitic**
Project Officer
International Organization for Migration (IOM)
Geneva, Switzerland

**Kalala Ngalamulume, PhD**
Associate Professor
Bryn Mawr College
Bryn Mawr, Pennsylvania
U.S.A.

**Veronica Olazabal, MCRS**
Research Associate
The Rockefeller Foundation
New York, New York
U.S.A.

**Danielle Ompad, PhD**
Associate Director
Center for Urban Epidemiologic Studies
New York Academy of Medicine
New York, New York

**Stipe Oreskovic, PhD**
Head
Department of Medical Sociology and Health Economics
Andrija Stampar School of Public Health
Zagreb, Croatia

# THE CONTRIBUTORS

**Ariel Pablos-Méndez, MD, MPH**
Managing Director
The Rockefeller Foundation
New York, New York
Professor of Clinical Medicine and
    Epidemiology
College of Physicians & Surgeons
    and Mailman School of Public
    Health
Columbia University
New York, New York
U.S.A.

**Jonathan Parkinson, PhD**
Programme Coordinator
International Water Association
London, United Kingdom

**Fernando Augusto Proietti, MD, ScD**
Professor
Faculty of Medicine
Federal University Mineas Gerais
Belo Horizonte, Brazil

**Thomas C. Quinn, MD**
Professor of Medicine
Director of Global Health
    Institute
Johns Hopkins University School of
    Medicine
Baltimore, Maryland
U.S.A.

**Carlos E. Restrepo, PhD**
Research Assistant Professor
Robert F. Wagner School of Public
    Service
New York University
New York, New York
U.S.A.

**Kevin J. Robinson, DrPH, MSW**
Assistant Professor
Bryn Mawr College
Bryn Mawr, Pennsylvania
U.S.A.

**Jonathan M. Samet, MD, MS**
Professor and Flora L. Thornton Chair
Department of Preventive Medicine
Keck School of Medicine and Director,
    Institute for Global Health
University of Southern California
Los Angeles, California
U.S.A.

**David Satterthwaite, PhD**
Senior Fellow
International Institute for Environment
    and Development (IIED)
Editor, *The Environment and Urbanization*
The Development Planning Unit
University College
London, United Kingdom

**Richard H. Schneider, PhD**
Professor of Urban and Regional
    Planning
University Research Foundation Professor
College of Design, Construction and
    Planning
University of Florida
Gainesville, Florida
U.S.A.

**Ted Schrecker, MA**
Scientist and Associate Professor
Department of Epidemiology and
    Community Medicine
Institute of Population Health
University of Ottawa
Ottawa, Ontario
Canada

**Elliott D. Sclar, PhD**
Professor of Urban Planning and
 International Affairs
Director, Center for Sustainable Urban
 Development (CSUD)
Earth Institute
Columbia University
Co-coordinator, Taskforce on
 Improving the Lives of Slum
 Dwellers
United Nations Millennium Project
New York, New York
U.S.A.

**Maria Steenland, MPH**
Graduate student
School of Public Health
University of Michigan
Ann Arbor, Michigan
U.S.A.

**Agis Tsouros, MD**
Head
Centre for Healthy Cities and Urban
 Health
World Health Organization (WHO)
 Europe
Copenhagen, Denmark

**David Vlahov, PhD, RN**
Senior Vice President for Research
Director, Center for Urban
 Epidemiologic Studies
New York Academy of Medicine
Professor of Clinical Epidemiology
Columbia University Mailman School of
 Public Health
New York, New York
U.S.A.

**Arnoud P. Verhoeff, PhD**
Head
Department of Epidemiology,
 Documentation, and Health Promotion
Municipal Health Service, Amsterdam
Professor in Urban Health Care
University of Amsterdam
Amsterdam, The Netherlands

**Nicole Volavka-Close, PhD**
Associate Director, Center for Sustainable
 Urban Development (CSUD)
Earth Institute
Columbia University
New York, New York
U.S.A.

**Michael Ward, BSc (Hons), Dip Ed**
Associate
Menzies Centre for Health Policy
University of Sydney
Sydney, Australia

**Vanessa Watson, PhD**
Professor and Director
School of Architecture, Planning, and
 Geomatics
University of Capetown
Rondebosch, South Africa

**Rae Zimmerman, PhD**
Professor of Planning and Public
 Administration
Robert F. Wagner Graduate School of
 Public Service
New York University
New York, New York
U.S.A.

# CHAPTER ONE

# URBAN HEALTH IN A GLOBAL PERSPECTIVE

### DAVID VLAHOV
### JO IVEY BOUFFORD

---

### LEARNING OBJECTIVES

- Identify the megatrends that influence twenty-first century global health
- Describe a conceptual framework for understanding urban health
- Define health inequality and health inequity
- Discuss the role of healthy urban governance

## MEGATRENDS IN TWENTY-FIRST CENTURY HEALTH

The twenty-first century is a time of unprecedented opportunity to improve global health. In recent years, scientific and medical advancements have transformed the field of public health. Health professionals now have considerable knowledge, tools, and resources to promote health, prevent illness, and fight disease. Recent reports, such as the WHO Commission on Social Determinants of Health's "Closing the Gap in a Generation," have promoted recognition of the broader determinants of health, beyond personal medical care and risk behaviors, in the communities where people live that may or may not permit them to exercise healthy choices even if they have the necessary information (WHO 2008). There is increased political visibility and support for action to promote health due to its clear links to economic development, and health is playing a greater role in the global political agenda. The past decade has witnessed a proliferation of global health actors, new partnerships, and financial resources for health problems. The UN Millennium Development Goals are agreed targets for international cooperation to reduce poverty, disease, and death.

Yet, despite these enormous advances, we still face a serious implementation gap between what we know and what we do. Increasingly, the role of governance—the government's ability both to assume its responsibilities as steward of public goods and to work collaboratively with other sectors in society—has emerged as a critical factor in guaranteeing that a country's conditions for policy and program implementation can assure that its people are as healthy as they can be. In addition to country-specific opportunities and challenges for implementation, it is becoming increasingly clear that there are powerful global factors at work affecting health. These "megatrends" are often identified as globalization, demographic shifts, and climate change. What is frequently overlooked in developing global health policy is urbanization—the central role of cities in creating and being subjected to these megatrends—and this is the subject of this book.

### Globalization

Globalization is what transpires across borders. Although the phenomenon is not new, the pace and extent is new. Globalization is driven by advances in and the spread of technology; the unprecedented flows of information; the ability to travel; the migration of people, goods, and services; and the creation or ruin of jobs and economic opportunity. All of these are most apparent earliest in cities and can result in conditions that are positive or negative for health. Cities are also fundamental drivers of national economies, and certain cities host the markets and national and multinational companies that dominate the global economy. If global economic and trade regimes address issues of fairness and equity, and national and urban governance are strong, the effects of globalization can be positive for the social, physical, and economic development of cities, taking advantage of the concentrations of population to provide efficient and accessible educational as well as health and social services. Globalization can also create unique conditions in cities for individuals and families to take advantage of economic development opportunities to increase their income, meet other entrepreneurs, or gain competitive advantage.

However, too often, the early warning signals of the negative effects of globalization can be seen in cities with large immigrant populations who are without employment, appropriate housing, education, or health services. The migrants might join the formal city if the rules were designed to include and benefit them, but where this is not the case, they build an informal economy that creates their own form of advantage. Urban poor immigrants develop or enter an informal economy of microenterprise that can account for up to 40 percent of a country's GDP, including remittances to relatives in depressed rural regions.

Globalization's considerable cultural impact is most profoundly seen in urban settings. As noted in the 2007 United Nations Population Fund Report:

> Since the 1950s, rapid globalization has also been a catalyst of cultural change most strongly felt in cities. Advanced telecommunications and the influx of media from other regions of the world are at the core of the urban transition and have enormous impact on ideas, values and beliefs. Such transformations have not been as uniform or seamless as social scientists predicted. Urbanites may lose contact with traditional norms and values. They may develop new aspirations, but not always the means to realize them. This, in turn, may lead to a sense of deracination and marginalization, accompanied by crises of identity, feelings of frustration and aggressive behavior. Many people in developing countries also associate the processes of modernization and globalization with the imposition of Western values on their own cultures and resent them accordingly. (UNFPA 2007)

How cities are organized and governed will shape how these challenges are managed.

## Demographic Shifts

Demographic shifts involve three elements: migration, fertility, and mortality. Migration involves "push-pull" factors that can be economic, cultural, political, or environmentally based. Examples of "push" include few opportunities, discrimination, political fears, natural disasters, and desertification. Examples of "pull" factors include job opportunities and better living conditions. These movements occur between and within countries, with the predominant pattern being short distances. Daily commuting is a type of migration which has implications for the environment and health. Throughout history, rural-to-urban migration has been a predominant pattern, which became especially salient in 2008, when, for the first time in human history, the majority of the world's population lived in cities. Virtually all population growth over the next thirty years will be in urban areas. By 2030, about 60 percent will be urban dwellers, rising to about 75 percent by 2050 (Montgomery 2008). Urban growth is expected to occur more slowly in mega-cities and faster in mid-sized cities (Satterthwaite 2000), and the growth rate of mega-cities in the developing world will be much higher than in developed world (for example, anticipated growth between 2000 and 2015 in Calcutta is 1.9 percent compared to 0.7 percent in New York City). In 1975, only five cities worldwide had 10 million or more inhabitants; three were in developing countries. The number will increase to twenty-three by 2015, all but four of them in developing countries. Also by 2015, an estimated 564 cities around the world will contain one million or more residents. Of these, 425 will be in developing countries. While large cities of developing countries will account for 20 percent of the increase in the world's population between 2000 and 2015, small cities (less than 5 million) will account for 45 percent of this increase (UN Population Division 2000). These projections highlight the importance of viewing urban health as an international and global issue.

To accommodate population growth, most of the new city growth is through horizontal expansion of small and mid-sized cities. At face value, this might seem to mitigate risks associated with overcrowding, but in fact comes with health challenges as well. For example, horizontal growth requires longer commutes that present sedentary lifestyle and traffic-related health risks. Horizontal growth threatens land needed for food and water supply and, therefore, has implications for sustainability. Creating healthy and sustainable cities represents a complex challenge.

Other demographic shifts include fertility and mortality, which have shown a global decline. Urbanization among the nonpoor is accompanied by lower birth rates and lower death rates. Urban settings provide female literacy and employment that changes valuation of women from sense of status for having and raising children to becoming productive contributors to the family. Contraception and family planning, more available in cities, also contribute to the transition. Declines in mortality have been observed with modernization and availability of preventive and curative care. One net effect of this is the aging of the population. By 2025, the global population of people over 60 will be 1.2 billion, double the number in 2000; it will more than double again by 2050. More prominent now in developed countries, this will become increasingly noticeable in developing countries. This trend will be most pronounced in cities, where most will live. How cities are organized and governed will shape how these challenges are managed.

## Climate Change

A third twenty-first century megatrend is climate change (McMichael, Woodruff, and Hales 2006). Emissions of carbon dioxide and other greenhouse gases are projected to increase temperatures globally in the coming century. Cities generate 80 percent of all carbon dioxide and significant amounts of other greenhouse gases. They contribute to climate change, mainly through energy generation, vehicles, industry, and biomass use. The densely built environment of cities creates a "heat island" effect where temperatures at any time can be 3–4° C higher than geographically adjacent rural areas. Increased temperatures mean less outdoor activity and greater emission of greenhouse gases with air conditioning. Climate change can include temperature-related, extreme weather-related, and air pollution-related health effects. These effects include water, foodborne, vector, and rodent diseases; food and water shortages; and population displacement. Cities are frequently sited on coasts and rivers where they are vulnerable to climate-related changes in the form of rising sea levels, storm surges, and flooding. More recent efforts to make cities "green" address root causes of climate change.

## Urbanization

A fourth megatrend is urbanization. As discussed in the literature, urbanization involves a dynamic process of economic development, population movement and growth, and spatial expansion with issues of sustainability. Certain characteristics of urbanization can have their own impact on the health of the population and require special attention as a context for any change process that may be needed. *Size, density* (with proximity and association), *diversity*, and *complexity* provide an "urban lens" through which to view a variety of influences.

Size provides scalability—presumably the larger the population size, the more scalable a program, although quality is a separate dimension to consider. Density is frequently thought of as synonymous with overcrowding and its related health risks; in fact, density with adequate space per person provides proximity and association that create efficiencies of scale for opportunities and services. The trend toward urban areas with lower density may translate into less overcrowding but comes with other risks, including greater expenditures on utilities, longer commutes, and social isolation.

*Diversity* refers to the mix of populations found in cities; it brings social and cultural richness, but it can also lead to cultural clashes (Massey 1996). Diversity necessitates tailoring interventions to meet the needs of different subpopulations. *Diversity* also refers to the rich variety of services within urban settings that can provide both specialization and multiple service options.

Finally, cities can be characterized by their complexity. Multiple systems interact; pluralistic political structures create competing stakeholders. Cities are inextricably linked to other sociopolitical levels, such as neighborhoods, metropolitan regions, and nation-states, each making demands and offering resources to the other levels, and local political and social forces create wide variations in the contexts of program delivery.

The implications of varying size, density, diversity, and complexity between cities and urban areas mean that simple interventions are rarely sufficient to solve problems, programs may have unintended as well as intended outcomes, and generalization from one setting to another can be problematic. This contextual complexity requires a similar level of intervention complexity—an intersectoral governance approach that integrates different sectors within government and with business and community participation. This complexity also requires special attention to the level of analysis and data gathering to understand the realities of the health of urban populations and their determinants.

## Health Inequalities and Inequities in Cities

Health inequalities and inequities within the urban setting are by their nature concentrated and factors that require more refined levels of analysis than aggregate statistics for the geographic city. Urban health action not only improves the average level of health in a city but addresses the inequities that preserve inequalities in environment and health status. *Health inequalities* refers to differences or disparities between groups. A related term is *health inequities*, which refers to inequalities that can be corrected but are allowed to stand, due to distorted power and decision-making arrangements.

Although it is generally understood that city dwellers, on average, enjoy better health than their rural counterparts, this may reflect the practice of aggregating data that provide an average of all urban residents—rich and poor—rather than disaggregating population groups by income or other measures of socioeconomic status. For example, in developing countries, slums without legal status are often officially unrecognized and, therefore, their populations frequently uncounted, distorting the urban average. As a result, the different worlds of city dwellers and the substantial health challenges of the urban poor are overlooked. These differences in health outcomes within urban areas, disaggregated by absolute or relative poverty, are seen around the world and for a wide variety of health outcomes.

Differences in health outcomes are also seen by geographic area-specific levels of infrastructure and services within cities. A child who lives in a slum in Kenya is far more likely to die before the age of five than his or her compatriot living in another part of the city (APHRC 2002). In 1990, life expectancy for black males in Harlem, an urban area of concentrated disadvantage in New York City, was lower than for men in Bangladesh (McCord and Freeman 1990). A frequently quoted study from Glasgow shows dramatic differences in life expectancy by neighborhoods, with the lower-income neighborhoods approaching rates in the cities of developing countries (Macintyre, McKay, and Ellaway 2005).

As these four megatrends—globalization, demographic shifts, climate change, and urbanization—play out in cities, they create complex environments both to understand and to govern. It is important to have a framework for approaching urban health action.

# CONCEPTUAL FRAMEWORK FOR URBAN HEALTH

Several frameworks for organizing thinking on urban health have been published. These frameworks overlap in noting that urbanization is not inherently positive or negative. Underlying drivers—also referred to as *social determinants*—converge in urban settings, which strongly influence health status and other outcomes. For simplicity, we start with the model proposed by Galea, Freudenberg, and Vlahov (2006), shown in Figure 1.1.

The framework notes that health (and nonhealth) outcomes are influenced by "living conditions," which includes physical and social environments as well as health and social services. These, in turn, are influenced by municipal factors that include government, markets, and civil society. These, in turn, are influenced by national and international trends. Enduring structures refer to the fact that cities reside in different contextual settings that shape the dynamics of these other influences. Taken together, urban settings can be a determinant of health.

## Urban Physical Environment

The urban physical environment includes geological and climate conditions of the site where the city is located, the air city dwellers breathe, the water they drink

**FIGURE 1.1  Conceptual Framework for Urban Health**

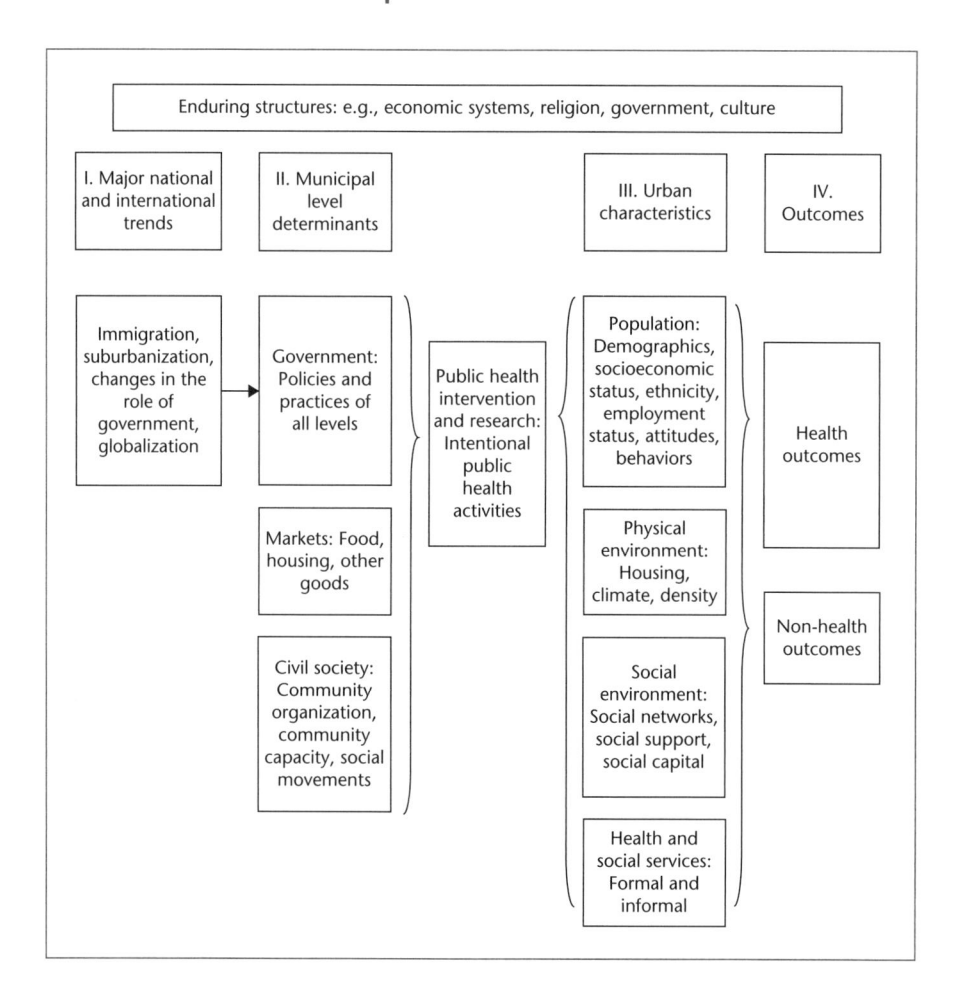

| Enduring structures: e.g., economic systems, religion, government, culture |

| I. Major national and international trends | II. Municipal level determinants | III. Urban characteristics | IV. Outcomes |
|---|---|---|---|
| Immigration, suburbanization, changes in the role of government, globalization | Government: Policies and practices of all levels → Public health intervention and research: Intentional public health activities | Population: Demographics, socioeconomic status, ethnicity, employment status, attitudes, behaviors | Health outcomes |
| | Markets: Food, housing, other goods | Physical environment: Housing, climate, density | Non-health outcomes |
| | Civil society: Community organization, community capacity, social movements | Social environment: Social networks, social support, social capital | |
| | | Health and social services: Formal and informal | |

and bathe in, the indoor and outdoor noise they hear, the park land inside and surrounding the city, and the built environment. The human built environment includes housing, highways, and streets, and other transportation infrastructure as well as parks and other uses of open space. The urban sanitation infrastructure is also part of the physical environment and determines how a city provides water and disposes of garbage. Choices on energy sources have implications for the built and natural environment (Melosi 2000). Because most of the new city growth is through horizontal expansion of small and mid-sized cities, it may create health challenges by threatening land needed for food and water supply.

### Social Environment

The social environment is the structure and characteristics of relationships among people within a community. Components of the social environment include social networks, social capital, segregation, and the social support that interpersonal interactions provide. A city's social environment can both support or damage health through a variety of pathways (Leviton, Snell, and McGinnis 2000; Freudenberg 2000; Geronimus 2000). For example, social norms in densely populated urban areas can support individual or group behaviors that affect health (for example, smoking, diet, exercise, sexual behavior) (King and others 2003). Social supports can buffer the impact of daily stressors and provide access to goods and services that influence health (for example, housing, food, informal health care; Berkman and others 2000).

### Health and Social Services

Cities are characterized by a rich array of health and social services (Casey, Thiede Call, and Kingner 2001; Felt-Lisk, McHugh, and Howell 2002). Even the poorest urban neighborhood often has dozens of social agencies, each with a distinct mission and service package. Services vary by type, mix, quantity, and quality.

The conceptual framework (Figure 1.1) permits us to isolate and measure seemingly discrete factors that affect urban populations. In reality, the effects of the physical, social, and service environments are more difficult to separate. For example, decent shelter that comes with land security and tenure provides people a home, security for their belongings, safety for their families, a place to strengthen their social relations and networks, a place for local trading and service provision, and a means to access basic services (UNFPA 2007). The conceptual framework is not an analytic tool but can help to organize our thinking about urban health challenges.

## MEETING THE CHALLENGES AND OPPORTUNITIES IN URBAN HEALTH

Each of the sections of this book was selected to provide a global perspective on the health risks and opportunities for urban dwellers. After delving into more detail about the megatrends of the twenty-first century, we move to the infectious and chronic disease threats, how they manifest themselves in urban settings, and the opportunities for positive action. Then we move on to explore issues of crime, manmade and natural disasters, and terrorism that exert a toll on the physical and mental well-being of city dwellers. Next, we examine the challenges of creating systems in cities that can effectively provide health care and the information needed about the health of the population to plan services and provide the public with much needed health information. Because the determinants of health are much broader than those under the direct control of the health sector and go beyond health care and traditional public health services, it is important to look in depth at the critical elements of urban infrastructure that affect health: provision of water and sanitation, housing, transportation, urban planning, and air quality.

To meet these challenges and optimize health in cities, governance is a critical factor. The form of government in cities, especially mega-cities and national capitals, is often defined by national policy and practice; the degree of decentralization within a country from the center to more peripheral governmental bodies in regions and districts sometimes fails to consider the special needs of cities. The relationship between national or regional government and city government can be critical to the ability of cities to innovate and create systems to manage for health. Such innovation is needed, because although governments have the ultimate responsibility for assuring the conditions in which their people can be as healthy as they can be, government cannot do the job alone.

This requires new forms of "governance"—"the alignment of multiple interests to achieve a shared goal" or "joined up" governance (Harpham 2009)—models that allow governmental health leaders to work effectively with their relevant colleagues across governmental sectors that influence health and with nongovernmental sectors in civil society, including NGOs, advocacy groups, business, academia, and the media, among others. Good urban governance responds to local needs in a participatory, transparent, and accountable manner in treating current issues and planning horizons that extend beyond current needs. A number of cities have taken steps to create specific mechanisms for participatory governance, enabling communities and local governments to partner in building healthier and safer cities (Montgomery 2009; Caiaffa 2010). The World Health Organization has facilitated this process through the Healthy Cities programs, which has included the process of Health Impact Assessments and Health in All Policies.

Interspersed in each section of the book are case studies of cities that tell how they have taken on the challenges of the detection and management of direct health threats—traditional and new; how they have tackled the challenges of creating healthy urban infrastructure; and, for each, the governance arrangements that have made effective change possible. This volume concludes with a look to the future of urban health from a global perspective.

## SUMMARY

Cities are traditionally the economic engines for a country and, increasingly, are shaping the world. Urbanization must be considered as a megatrend, affecting global health along with globalization, demographic shifts, and climate change. Cities offer advantages and opportunities as well as threats to health for their residents. Although individual behavior shapes health and illness, the urban environment shaped by upstream influences can impact both behavior and health. Inequities in decision making can preserve and maintain inequalities that impact all urban dwellers. The size, density, diversity, and especially the complexity of cities present tough challenges for addressing the health of urban populations. Good urban governance that brings together the health sector and other sectors with authentic community participation is essential to meet these challenges and achieve urban health.

## REFERENCES

African Population and Health Research Center (APHRC). 2002. *Population and health dynamics in Nairobi's informal settlements: Report of the Nairobi Cross-Sectional Slums Survey (NCSS)*. Nairobi: APHRC.

Berkman, L. F., T. Glass, I. Brissette, and T. E Seeman. 2000. From social integration to health: Durkheim in the new millennium. *Social Science and Medicine* 51(6):843–857.

Caiaffa, W. T., A. L. Nabuco, A. A. de Lima Friche, and F. A. Proietti. 2010. Urban health and governance model in Belo Horizonte, Brazil: A case study. In *Urban health: Global perspectives*, ed. D. Vlahov and J. I. Boufford. San Francisco: Jossey Bass.

Casey, M. M., K. Thiede Call, and J. M. Klingner. 2001. Are rural residents less likely to obtain recommended preventive healthcare services? *American Journal of Preventive Medicine* 21(3):182–188.

Felt-Lisk, S., M. McHugh, and E. Howell. 2002. Monitoring local safety-net providers: Do they have adequate capacity? *Health Affairs* (Millwood) 21(5):277–283.

Freudenberg, N. 2000. Health promotion in the city: A structured review of the literature on interventions to prevent heart disease, substance abuse, violence and HIV infection in U.S. metropolitan areas 1980–1995. *Journal of Urban Health* 77(3):443–457.

Galea, S., N. Freudenberg, and D. Vlahov. 2005. Cities and population health. *Social Science and Medicine* 60(5):1017–1033.

Geronimus, A. T. 2000. To mitigate, resist, or undo: Addressing structural influences on the health of urban populations. *American Journal of Public Health* 90(6):867–872.

Harpham, T. 2009. Urban health in developing countries: What do we know and where do we go? *Health and Place* 15:107–116.

King, G., A. J. Flisher, R. Mallett, J. Graham, C. Lombard, T. Rawson and others. 2003. Smoking in Cape Town: Community influences on adolescent tobacco use. *Preventive Medicine* 36(1):114–123.

Leviton, L. C., E. Snell, and M. McGinnis. 2000. Urban issues in health promotion strategies. *American Journal of Public Health* 90:863–866.

Massey, D. S. 1996. The age of extremes: Concentrated affluence and poverty in the twenty-first century. *Demography* 33(4):395–412.

Macintyre, S., L. McKay, and A. Ellaway. 2005. Are rich people or poor people more likely to be ill? Lay perceptions, by social class and neighbourhood, of inequalities in health. *Social Science and Medicine* 60(2):313–317.

McCord, C., and H. P. Freeman. 1990. Excess mortality in Harlem. *New England Journal of Medicine* 322(3):173–177.

McMichael, A. J., R. E. Woodruff, and S. Hales. 2006. Climate change and human health. *Lancet* 367(9513):859–869.

Melosi, M. 2000. The sanitary city: Urban infrastructure in America from colonial times to the present. Baltimore: Johns Hopkins Press.

Montgomery, M. R. 2008. The urban transformation of the developing world. *Science* 319(5864):761–764.

Montgomery, M. R. 2009. Urban poverty and health in developing countries. Population Reference Bureau 64(2):1–15.

Montgomery, M. R., et al., Panel on Urban Dynamics, National Research Council, eds. 2003. *Cities transformed: Demographic change and its implications in the developing world*. Washington, DC: National Academies Press.

Satterthwaite, D. 2000. Will most people live in cities? *British Medical Journal* 321(7269):1143–1145.

United Nations Population Division. 2000. *World urbanization prospects: The 1999 revision*. New York: United Nations Population Division.

United Nations Population Fund (UNFPA). 2007. *State of the world population: Unleashing the potential for urban growth*. Washington, DC: UNFPA.

WHO, Commission on Social Determinants of Health (CSDH). 2008. *Closing the gap in a generation: Health equity through action on the social determinants of health: Final report of the Commission on Social Determinants of Health*. Geneva: World Health Organization.

Yen, I. H., and S. L. Syme. 1999. The social environment and health: A discussion of the epidemiologic literature. *Annual Review of Public Health* 20:287–308.

# CHAPTER TWO

# GLOBALIZATION

## TED SCHRECKER
## RONALD LABONTÉ

### LEARNING OBJECTIVES

- Understand and be able to illustrate with examples the relation between globalization and the use of urban space, especially its implications for social determinants of health

- Critically analyze the connections among globalization, the distribution of domestic sources of political influence, and the changing role of the state in contests over urban priority-setting

- Identify the significance of the policies of local/metropolitan and higher levels of governments for social determinants of health in metropolitan areas

- Use this body of knowledge in professional practice to propose effective strategies for improving public health in metropolitan areas in the face of constraints that globalization may impose

THE financial crisis that swept the world, starting in summer 2008, dispelled any doubts about the reality of globalization as a phenomenon and about its importance to the well-being of much of the world's population. For some, the definition of globalization itself remains contested. A text on globalization and health published in 2003 highlighted the extent of this disagreement and characterized globalization as a process as having spatial, temporal, and cognitive dimensions. However, the author's discussion repeatedly returns to the economic underpinnings of each of these dimensions, whether she is addressing the global reorganization of production and its effects on working conditions; the profitable promotion of unhealthy lifestyles by transnational tobacco and fast food corporations; or the role of the World Bank in promoting a market-oriented shift in health policy "from Health for All [the theme of the landmark 1978 Alma Ata declaration] to pay your own way" (Lee 2003).

This fundamentally economic nature of globalization is evident, with special clarity in its influence on metropolitan areas and the health of those who live and work in them. In this chapter, we draw on a large, multidisciplinary literature to make this point, but we cite it only selectively for reasons of space. The most important sources for those new to the study of globalization and cities appear in boldface type in the reference list. A similarly extensive literature addresses social determinants of health (SDH): the conditions of life and work that make it relatively easy for some individuals to lead long and healthy lives, and all but impossible for others. The importance of SDH was underscored by the report of the multinational WHO Commission on Social Determinants of Health, published in 2008 (Commission on Social Determinants of Health 2008); for updates on post-Commission activities go to http://www.who.int/social_determinants/en). Presuming the importance of SDH, in this chapter we first describe main pathways that lead from globalization to social conditions in metropolitan areas that are arguably most relevant as influences on health and then, more briefly, identify obstacles to policy interventions that would be effective in reducing the negative consequences for health.

## "DISEQUALIZING" GLOBALIZATION

Economist Nancy Birdsall has described globalization as "inherently disequalizing" in several respects (Birdsall 2006). Global markets favor the well-prepared

---

Research for this chapter funded in part by Canadian Institutes of Health Research grants 79153 and 80070.

and well-endowed (individuals and countries). Their negative effects are felt first, and worst, by the poor and otherwise vulnerable; the effects of the financial crisis are a prime example, as the effects of climate change will be in the future. The world economy's most powerful actors, such as transnational corporations and the G7 countries, are able to shape the rules that govern the world economy to their benefit. This ability is evident, for instance, in the multiple asymmetries of resources and bargaining power that characterize trade negotiations and in the dominance of decisionmaking at the World Bank and International Monetary Fund (IMF) by the G7 countries. In future, this dominance may be somewhat tempered by reforms to provide greater voice within these institutions from the larger developing economies, such as China, India, and Brazil. This has not yet happened; if and when it does, the question will remain: whether the governments of such countries will take policy positions that are conducive to widely shared improvements in SDH within their borders or internationally. This cannot be assumed.

The most familiar aspects of globalization's disequalizing effects involve the global labor market that has gradually emerged as production and service provision have been reorganized across multiple national borders (Dicken 2007). This reorganization began more than thirty years ago but has now accelerated because much of the population of India, China, and the transition economies has been added to the global labor force, roughly doubling its size. Well before this happened, deindustrialization wiped out over half the manufacturing jobs in U.S. cities, such as Chicago, Philadelphia, and Detroit, starting in the 1960s (Abu-Lughod 1999, 323–4; Hodos 2002, 365); *total* employment among residents of Detroit fell by 41 percent between 1970 and 2000; in the "steel city" of Gary, Indiana, by 43 percent; and in Cleveland by 37 percent (Savitch 2003, 592). The loss of relatively well paid, often unionized manufacturing jobs accessible to those with limited formal credentials was characteristic of most high-income countries (Nickell and Bell 1995; Wood 1998). In the United States, it led to the emergence of ultra-low-wage, precarious urban labor markets; the virtual abandonment of some downtown areas; and, sometimes, to the drug economy as an urban survival strategy (Tourigny 2001; Bourgois 2003).

Deindustrialization is sometimes attributed to technological change rather than to global reorganization of production, but it is difficult and probably unnecessary to disentangle the two influences. A *Business Week* article noted, "A global economy . . . demands such change; rapidly evolving technology allows it" (Hammonds, Kelly, and Thurston 1994, p. 77). It is more important when studying urban health to recognize that deindustrialization was not confined to high-income countries. In Mumbai, unemployment "more than doubled" between 1981 and 1996, while informal employment and self-employment increased substantially—a consequence, in part, of the decline of labor-intensive textile production in the face of international competition (Patel 2007) and a long strike during which the national government sided with employers. In São Paulo, Brazil's largest metropolitan area and the center of its manufacturing industry, 23 percent of manufacturing jobs disappeared between 1985 and 2003, as the country's economy was opened to international markets and casual or precarious labor became the norm (Buechler 2006). In Johannesburg, informal employment increased as a percentage of total employment from 9.6 percent to 16 percent in just three years (1996–1999); in 2001, the city's official unemployment rate was 37 percent (Mabin 2007). The World Bank, normally a reliable cheerleader for globalization, concedes that labor market outcomes will increase economic inequality in countries accounting for 86 percent of the developing world's population over the next two decades, with the so-called unskilled poor left even further behind (World Bank 2007, 67–100)—as they already have been in most high-income countries.

The disequalizing effects of globalization operate not only by decreasing the earning power of those at the bottom of the income scale but by concentrating income at the top in countries as diverse as the United States, where the share of national income going to the top one percent of households more than doubled between 1979 and 2006, and India, where a similarly dramatic increase was observed during the 1990s alone (United Nations Human Settlements Programme 2008, 60; Sherman 2009). Such trends reflect not only divergences in labor market income but also a shift, sometimes quite substantial, of national income shares from labor to capital.

An extensive body of research has sought to identify "global" or "world" cities: the physical locations of activities and institutions that control worldwide flows of capital and choices about the location of production. Although this category is useful for many purposes, the location of a city or metropolitan area within a ranking structure, such as the hierarchy of world cities defined by the Globalization and World Cities study group (http://www.lut.ac.uk/gawc/), does not reflect the extent to which a city's population is or is not influenced by globalization: some of the most devastating effects can be observed in cities too small even to rate a mention in discussions of world cities. However, world-city status is associated with high concentrations of producer services that constitute essential infrastructure for the management of global production and finance, such as accounting, management consulting, law, information technology, and advertising. The highly paid professional and managerial providers of these services generate a parallel demand for an expanding stratum of low-paid and insecure service-sector workers who drive taxis, clean buildings, and provide a variety of personal services, contributing to an increasingly polarized income distribution within cities. In many high-income countries, these jobs are the end point of global "survival circuits" and are filled by (authorized or unauthorized) immigrants fleeing even worse conditions that globalization has generated in their home countries (Sassen 2002).

## ECONOMIC INEQUALITY AND THE METROPOLIS

In cities rich and poor alike, whether or not they are world cities, the excluded must survive in the increasingly inhospitable interstices of the metropolitan economy, sometimes literally in the shadows of the glittering towers where globalization's winners live, work, and play. It is estimated, for instance, that "more than half" of Mumbai's 12–16 million people live "in slums and on pavements or under bridges and near railway tracks," occupying only a small fraction of Mumbai's land area (Patel 2007, 76), and that the homeless constitute almost half the population of Central Los Angeles (Soja 2006).

At least two bitter ironies exist here. First, the poor and marginalized who are not yet homeless often constitute an attractive and vulnerable market for landlords (both small- and large-scale). They offer minimal accommodation at exploitative prices to those who have few other options, given their need to be close to their sources of livelihood in either the formal or informal economies. The problems are compounded by the commodification and commercialization of basic services like water and sanitation, where these exist at all (see, for example, Huchzermeyer 2008 on Nairobi). Second, the poor are at constant risk of displacement to peripheral locations or to those that are undesirable because of exposure to environmental hazards (like Manila's infamous garbage dumps, where 150,000 of the city's poor scavenge as their only source of livelihood) in favor of higher-value land uses. This risk is magnified by the growing importance of real estate investment as a basis for capital accumulation, which—like other aspects of the changed economic environment associated with globalization—creates new and powerful domestic constituencies. Even in some of the world's poorest cities, like Dhaka, real estate markets are booming and speculation is rampant. At least before the financial crisis of 2008, that speculation was fuelled, in part, by remittances that constituted a substantial element of total financial inflows to the low-income countries in question, even while they also were sometimes used for private financing of health care and education.

Contests over urban space often involve fortification, which is especially widespread in situations where globalization's winners and losers continue to live in close proximity. Teresa Caldeira (2000) describes São Paulo, a metropolitan area in which this pattern is especially conspicuous, as a "city of walls" built not only by the ultra-rich but also by the so-called middle class. Similar observations have been made (for instance) about "revitalized" enclaves in the similarly polarized metropolitan area of Johannesburg. Private fortification is also evident in high-income cities (see, for example, Abu-Lughod 1999, 425), the general points here being that (a) public and private protection from theft or assault exist in an unstable and asymmetrical relationship, with the latter often being more important for those who can afford it, and (b) in low- and high-income metropolitan areas alike, the poor and otherwise marginalized are the most frequent victims of violence while having the fewest resources to protect themselves.

Labor historian Kim Moody correctly observes that "space is a class issue" (Moody 2007, 241). A 2003 UN-HABITAT report, *The Challenge of Slums*, drew on twenty-nine city case studies to conclude that "the prime resources of the city are increasingly appropriated by the affluent. And globalization is inflationary as the new rich are able to pay more for a range of key goods, especially land" (United Nations Human Settlements Programme 2003, 43). In the high-income countries, this process takes the form of gentrification of downtowns, usually involving conversions in tenure and types of occupancy with associated losses of affordable housing. Variations include the displacement of residential uses altogether in favor of highly subsidized convention, cultural, and sports facilities to reinvent the city as a site for consumption (often with high-income visitors as the intended audience) and brand it as "world class" for those with the price of admission, while creating new opportunities for profitable investment. Although most frequent in high-income countries, the process is spreading: for instance, consider Beijing's preparations for the 2008 Olympic Games and South Africa's for the 2010 World Cup.

Operating in parallel with contests for space at the city center is the process that a former U.S. Cabinet secretary called "secession of the successful" (Reich 1991): migration to suburbs or exurbs with abundant amenities and, at least in the U.S. context, where social provision creates fewer demands on the local tax base. The extreme variant is gated communities, which are a variant of fortification. Suburbanization is also conspicuous in many developing world cities and is of special concern because the transportation systems demanded by the affluent (high-speed roads) are fundamentally different from the affordable public transportation needed by the less affluent, and both groups are competitors for scarce resources and imply fundamentally different settlement patterns. Giving priority to roads has direct health consequences in the form of rising air pollution and road deaths among nondrivers (see, for example, Rodgers 2007 on Managua) and leads to social exclusion that is literally cast in concrete. Urban segregation is becoming multidimensional, involving not only geographical location and physical separation but also economically mediated access or lack of access to a variety of essential networks.

## THE STATE AND THE GLOBAL ECONOMY

The 2003 UN-HABITAT report concluded that "the main single cause of increases in poverty and inequality during the 1980s and 1990s was the retreat of the state" from a variety of redistributive policies (United Nations Human Settlements Programme 2003, 43) that had at least the potential to compensate for globalization's disequalizing effects. Perhaps most notably, in many developing countries, national government policies were shaped by structural adjustment programs (SAPs) mandated by the World Bank and IMF as the price of loans designed to reschedule debts to foreign creditors. Debt crises that drove governments to seek this assistance reflected both the increasing interconnectedness of the world's economies and the asymmetrical character of the connections: the need to find profitable outlets for oil revenues "recycled" from the Middle East through Western financial institutions, declining prices for the developing world's exports on glutted world commodity markets, and capital flight (the wealthy shift their assets to safer and more lucrative jurisdictions) were among the major causes.

Domestic austerity policies that were part of the structural adjustment recipe included cutbacks in public expenditure on health and education and the introduction of cost recovery measures such as user fees—promoted with particular zeal as health sector "reform" by the World Bank (Lister 2005). These pressures were compounded in many low- and middle-income countries by revenue losses associated with import liberalization that was supposed to improve the efficiency of national economies but had the effect of seriously reducing governments' fiscal capacity. The destructive effects of SAPs were documented in a multicountry UNICEF study as early as 1987 (Cornia, Jolly, and Stewart 1987) but with little effect on policy makers, and they were later highlighted in the 2003 UN-HABITAT report (United Nations Human Settlement Programme 2003, 43–46) and elsewhere (Davis 2006, chapter 7).

For many researchers, SAPs are best understood as part of a political strategy where "an alliance of the international financial institutions, the private banks, and the Thatcher-Reagan-Kohl governments was willing to use its political and economic power to back its ideological predilections" (Przeworski and others 1995, 5). Although not all observers would agree, the history of structural adjustment situates the activity of the international financial institutions within a larger pattern where the integration of global markets creates pressure for convergence on a model that political scientist Philip Cerny describes as the "competition state": domestic social and economic policy alike emphasize "promotion of economic activities, whether at home or abroad, which will make firms and sectors located within the territory of the state competitive in international markets" (2000).

That competitive environment "mercilessly weeds out those centers with below-par macroeconomic environments, services, and labor-market flexibility" (World Bank 1999, 50). For example, despite two decades of aggressive embrace of the global marketplace, notably as a leader in establishing export processing zones (EPZs) designed to attract foreign investment, Mexico is losing hundreds of thousands of low-wage manufacturing jobs to China, and Vietnam is being considered as an alternative site for production as a precaution against the possible rise of labor costs in China.

## WHEN THE STATE BECOMES PART OF THE PROBLEM

Integrating national economies and societies into the global marketplace involves many losers, but it also creates highly lucrative opportunities for those within and outside a country's borders well placed to take advantage, for instance, of deregulation, privatization of state assets at fire-sale prices, and opportunities to drive up urban property values. These new constituencies quickly parlay their wealth into political influence, compounding external pressures for market-oriented policy reform and helping to explain why, as Mike Davis has put it, "Regardless of their political complexions . . . most Third World city governments are permanently locked in conflict with the poor in core areas" (2006, 99). For example, Indian governments have been actively clearing out shantytowns in favor of commercial offices and techno parks. An official of the Maharashtra state government has been quoted as saying, "With the slum demolitions, we showed political courage for the first time and sent a strong signal that you cannot expect free space in this city anymore" (Lakshmi 2005). This is just one case among many of state-supported displacement of urban populations in favor of higher-value uses; Beijing displaced 1.5 million people to construct facilities for the Olympic Games (Fowler 2008). Forced evictions, often justified with reference to the "public interest," are widespread enough to be recognized as an important human rights issue (see, for example, du Plessis 2005; Ocheje 2007; and the websites of the United Nations Special Rapporteur on adequate housing as a component of the right to an adequate standard of living, http://www2.ohchr.org/english/issues/housing, and of the Centre on Housing Rights and Evictions, http://www.cohre.org).

Such evictions, whether conducted by the state or merely permitted by it, are instances of a larger pattern where governments no longer attempt to compensate for the negative effects of market distributions of income and economic opportunity. Rather, they actively intervene to accelerate the marketization of their economies and societies. In other words, the lure of the global marketplace has often led the state to become part of the problem rather than an institution for developing and implementing equitable solutions. In other examples, post-1994, both the Johannesburg city government and the South African national government adopted urban policies "essentially similar" to those of Reagan and Thatcher (Mabin 2007, 58), crucially including the reorganizing of water and electricity provision on cost-recovery lines, not only as a way of avoiding redistribution but also as a means of social control, a way of inculcating a politics of expectations geared to income (Ruiters 2006; Ruiters 2009). A further dimension of state action in support of marketization involves criminalization of urban poverty, exemplified by police violence against the poor in Brazil; drastic growth in the numbers of poor, mainly nonwhite residents incarcerated in the United States; and the proliferation of U.S. state and local laws targeting the homeless. Even when they are well intentioned and less coercive than the examples just cited, efforts at urban "revitalization" that rely on private investment and attracting affluent households usually require either removing the poor and unsightly or rendering them invisible.

The state can become part of the problem at a national level as well, through policies that magnify economic inequalities in ways that have a disproportionate impact on metropolitan areas. For example, post-1995 social policy in Canada reduced by more than half the proportion of unemployed workers who were eligible for unemployment insurance, contributing to a general pattern of social policy now failing to compensate for more than a fraction of the increasing inequality in market incomes—entirely congruent with advice provided to the Canadian government by the IMF in 1994 and 1995. Welfare "reforms" enacted in the United States in 1996 eliminated a decades-old guarantee of at least minimal economic support for families with children and had the effect, if not the intent, of dramatically expanding the low-wage urban labor force. In each case, the policies in question were implemented in the context of growing intrametropolitan economic polarization that they almost certainly contributed to, although disentangling the various causal influences is difficult. The point cannot be explored further here, but it is important to situate political support for such policies within an ideological framework that embraces commodification and reduces citizenship to "responsible" participation in the marketplace (for a valuable critique, see Somers 2008)—a theme that is evident in such diverse contexts as the cost-recovery policies of South African utilities and the codification of U.S. welfare retrenchment as the Personal Responsibility and Work Opportunity Reconciliation Act.

# PUBLIC HEALTH AND THE POLITICS OF TRIAGE

In multiple ways, globalization deepens economic, spatial, and juridical divisions between the included and the excluded; often these divisions are mutually reinforcing. In the first instance, negative health effects arise from multiple material deprivations, normally compounded and reinforced by cumulative biological effects of high levels of stress and by the powerlessness that accompanies social exclusion. Many of these effects are addressed elsewhere in the book.

How to address the underlying processes in ways that are relevant to SDH? One of the knowledge networks that supported the work of the Commission on Social Determinants of Health called for "rights, regulation and redistribution" as a generic response to the global marketplace (Labonté and others 2007). An urbanist not specifically concerned with health, David Harvey counterposes the "right to the city" against property rights and access to global-scale concentrations of capital that provide the basis for what he calls colonization of urban space by the affluent (2008). These positions and others all repudiate the market-oriented policy directions that governments have followed over the past few decades, defying current conventional wisdom as well as formidable concentrations of economic and political power.

Even if we leave aside this difficulty, the challenge is institutionally complicated because most large metropolitan areas comprise a patchwork of local government jurisdictions; when coordinating structures exist, their mandates tend to be limited. The effect is to fragment decision making, and sometimes to create incentives for destructive competition among jurisdictions. If these issues could be remedied, for instance, by way of elected metropolitan-level governments with an institutional structure that did not privilege particular interests or intra-metropolitan regions, it would often remain the case that many policy choices that are most important for the life of cities are made by provincial/state or national governments. Such choices have been described in the U.S. context as "stealth urban policies" by Dreier, Mollenkopf, and Swanstrom (2005), who refer in particular to national government subsidies for home mortgages and expressway construction and to military spending that favors suburban industries. However, a larger range of social protection and economic development policies qualify as stealth urban policies when they have substantial, distinctive, and disproportionate impacts (positive or negative) on metropolitan areas.

The analysis in this chapter further suggests a basic problem that arises from the interaction of domestic politics with the distribution of economic opportunities and political allegiances associated with globalization. Public health policy and practice normally operate on the implicit presumption that at least a rudimentary social contract exists between rulers and subjects: in other words, that governments care about the welfare of people within their national borders, even when no opportunities for mutually advantageous exchanges between rulers and ruled exist over the short term. Today's patterns of urban life and policy in much of the world make it hard to escape the conclusion that many governments have made a conscious choice to pursue integration with the global marketplace, while accepting major health and economic losses on behalf of a substantial, if relatively powerless segment of their populations. Davis's reference to "the late-capitalist triage of humanity" at the conclusion of his book *Planet of Slums* (2006) is singularly appropriate, and must be taken seriously by all those working in urban health.

At a higher level, the international community appears to have accepted the inevitability of this triage at least in some forms, despite its commitment to the Millennium Development Goals (MDGs) based on a UN General Assembly resolution passed in 2000. Three of the MDGs (involving child mortality, maternal health, and communicable diseases) refer directly to health, and all the others have substantial implications for social determinants of health. However, it is now widely acknowledged that several of the MDGs and associated targets will not be met by the specified date, usually 2015, especially in sub-Saharan Africa (United Nations 2008). A target under MDG 7, which addresses environmental sustainability, refers to making a significant improvement in the lives of at least 100 million slum dwellers between 2000 and 2020. However, the number of people living in slums in low- and middle-income countries is anticipated to rise from more than 850 million circa 2003 to 1.4 billion in 2020 in the absence of decisive policy intervention (Garau, Sclar, and Carolini 2005). The arithmetic is clear and brutal. Adverse impacts of climate change, which will be felt disproportionately by the poor and vulnerable in the developing world's urban areas (McGranahan, Balk, and Anderson 2007; Douglas and others 2008; Hardoy and Pandiella 2009) and were not addressed at all by the MDGs, add a further dimension of inequity, one with which the global health research community as a whole is only beginning to come to grips.

Ethical analysis would require a separate chapter, but to us it is clear that the world's cities and their inhabitants deserve better.

# SUMMARY

Globalization is best understood with reference to the integration of national economies and societies with the global marketplace and their "disequalizing" effects on income, wealth, and the social determinants of health. The most familiar dimension involves labor markets, within and across national borders, as production is reorganized across multiple national borders. Labor market outcomes are only one of several channels through which globalization affects metropolitan areas, leading to a situation where "space is a class issue," as disparities between globalization's winners and losers magnify the intensity of conflicts over urban space. Rapid urbanization in the developing world is expected to dramatically increase the number of slum dwellers, creating formidable public health challenges. A further dimension is added by commodification and commercialization of basic services in metropolitan environments, which magnifies both economic and health inequalities.

These problems are compounded by the retreat of the state from redistributive policies, which itself reflects not only external constraints associated with globalization (notably in the form of structural adjustment programs demanded by the international financial institutions during the debt crises of the 1980s and thereafter) but also the way that globalization changes the distribution of resources and economic opportunities within national borders. This latter consideration may be the most important explanation for government policies that have magnified the disequalizing effects of globalization within metropolitan areas—a form of state complicity that urbanist Mike Davis describes as part of "the late-capitalist triage of humanity." Although the international community appears to have accepted the inevitability of this triage at least in some contexts, an ethical argument can be made that the world's cities and their inhabitants deserve better.

# REFERENCES

Abu-Lughod, J. 1999. *New York, Chicago, Los Angeles: America's global cities.* Minneapolis: University of Minnesota Press.

Birdsall, N. 2006. The world is not flat: Inequality and injustice in our global economy. WIDER Annual Lectures. Helsinki: World Institute for Development Economics Research. http://www.wider.unu.edu/publications/annual-lectures/en_GB/AL9/_files/78121127186268214/default/annual-lecture-2005.pdf.

Bourgois, P. 2003. *In search of respect: Selling crack in El Barrio.* 2nd ed. New York: Cambridge University Press.

Buechler, S. 2006. São Paulo: Outsourcing and downgrading of labour in a globalizing city. In *The global cities reader*, ed. N. Brenner and R. Keil, 238–245. London: Routledge.

Caldeira, T. P. 2000. *City of walls: Crime, Segregation and Citizenship in São Paulo.* Berkeley: University of California Press.

Cerny, P. G. 2000. Restructuring the political arena: Globalization and the paradoxes of the competition state. In *Globalization and its critics: Perspectives from political economy*, ed. R. D. Germain, 117–138. Houndmills, UK: Macmillan.

Cornia, G. A., R. Jolly, and F. Stewart, eds. 1987. *Adjustment with a human face.* Vol.1 of *Protecting the vulnerable and promoting growth.* Oxford: Clarendon Press.

Davis, M. 2006. *Planet of slums.* London: Verso.

Dicken, P. 2007. *Global shift: Reshaping the global economic map in the 21st century.* 5th ed. New York: Guilford Press.

Douglas, I., K. Alam, M. Maghenda, Y. Mcdonnell, L. Mclean, and J. Campbell. 2008. Unjust waters: Climate change, flooding and the urban poor in Africa. *Environment and Urbanization* 20:187–205.

Dreier, P., J. Mollenkopf, and T. Swanstrom. 2005. *Place matters: Metropolitics for the twenty-first century*. 2nd ed. Lawrence, KS: University Press of Kansas.

du Plessis, J. 2005. The growing problem of forced evictions and the crucial importance of community-based, locally appropriate alternatives. *Environment and Urbanization* 17:123–134.

Fowler, D. 2008. One world, whose dream? Housing rights violations and the Beijing Olympic Games. Geneva: Centre on Housing Rights and Evictions. http://www.cohre.org/store/attachments/One_World_Whose_Dream_July08.pdf.

Garau, P., E. D. Sclar, and G. Y. Carolini. 2005. A home in the city: UN Millennium Project Task Force on Improving the Lives of Slum Dwellers. London: Earthscan. http://www.millenniumproject.org.

Hammonds, K., K. Kelly, and K. Thurston. 1994. The new world of work. *Business Week*, October 17: 76–86.

Hardoy, J., and G. Pandiella. 2009. Urban poverty and vulnerability to climate change in Latin America. *Environment and Urbanization*, 21:203–224.

Harvey, D. 2008. The right to the city. *New Left Review*, new series no. 53:23–40.

Hodos, J. 2002. Globalization, regionalism, and urban restructuring: The case of Philadelphia. *Urban Affairs Review* 37:358–379.

Huchzermeyer, M. 2008. Slum upgrading in Nairobi within the housing and basic services market: A housing rights concern. *Journal of Asian and African Studies* 43:19–39.

Labonté, R., C. Blouin, M. Chopra, K. Lee, C. Packer, M. Rowson and others. 2007. Towards health-equitable globalization: Rights, regulation and redistribution. Globalization Knowledge Network final report to the Commission on Social Determinants of Health. Ottawa: Institute of Population Health, University of Ottawa. http://www.who.int/social_determinants/resources/gkn_final_report_042008.pdf.

Lakshmi, R. 2005. Bombay moves to push out the poor: Slums are razed as plans envisage reinvented city. *Washington Post*, August 5.

Lee, K. 2003. *Globalization and health: An introduction*. Houndmills, UK: Palgrave Macmillan.

Lister, J. 2005. *Health policy reform: Driving the wrong way? A critical guide to the global "health reform" industry*. London: Middlesex University Press.

Mabin, A. 2007. Johannesburg: (South) Africa's aspirant global city. In *The making of global city regions: Johannesburg, Mumbai/Bombay, São Paulo, and Shanghai*, ed. K. Segbers, 32–63. Baltimore: Johns Hopkins University Press.

McGranahan, G., D. Balk, and B. Anderson. 2007. The rising tide: Assessing the risks of climate change and human settlements in low elevation coastal zones. *Environment and Urbanization* 19:17–37.

Moody, K. 2007. *From welfare state to real estate: Regime change in New York City, 1974 to the present*. New York: New Press.

Nickell, S., and B. Bell. 1995. The collapse in demand for the unskilled and unemployment across the OECD. *Oxford Review of Economic Policy* 11:40–62.

Ocheje, P. D. 2007. "In the public interest": Forced evictions, land rights and human development in Africa. *Journal of African Law* 51:173–214.

Patel, S. 2007. Mumbai: The mega-city of a poor country. In *The making of global city regions: Johannesburg, Mumbai/Bombay, São Paulo, and Shanghai*, ed. K. Segbers, 64–84. Baltimore: Johns Hopkins University Press.

Przeworski, A., P. Bardhan, L. C. Bresser Pereira, L. Bruszt, J. J. Choi, E. T. Comisso and others. 1995. *Sustainable democracy*. Cambridge: Cambridge University Press.

Reich, R. 1991. Secession of the successful. *New York Times Magazine*, January 20: 16+.

Rodgers, D. 2007. "Nueva Managua": The disembedded city. In *Evil paradises: Dreamworlds of neoliberalism*, ed. M. Davis and B. Monk, 127–139. New York: New Press.

Ruiters, G. 2006. Social control and social welfare under neoliberalism in South Africa cities: Contradictions in free basic water services. In *Cities in contemporary Africa*, ed. M. J. Murray and G. A. Myers, 289–308. Houndmills, UK: Palgrave Macmillan.

Ruiters, G. 2009. Free basic electricity in South Africa: A strategy for helping or containing the poor? In *Electric capitalism: Recolonising Africa on the power grid*, ed. D. A. McDonald, 248–263. London: Earthscan.

Sassen, S. 2002. Global cities and survival circuits. In *Global woman: Nannies, maids, and sex workers in the economy*, ed. B. Ehrenreich and A. Hochschild, 254–274. New York: Metropolitan Books.

Savitch, H. 2003. How suburban sprawl shapes human well-being. *Journal of Urban Health* 80:590–607.

Sherman, A. 2009. *Income gaps hit record levels in 2006, new data show*. Washington, DC: Center for Budget and Policy Priorities. http://www.cbpp.org/files/4-17-09inc.pdf.

Soja, E. W. 2006. The stimulus of a little confusion: A contemporary comparison of Amsterdam and Los Angeles. In *The global cities reader*, ed. N. Brenner and R. Keil, 179–186. London: Routledge.

Somers, M. 2008. *Genealogies of citizenship: Markets, statelessness, and the right to have rights*. Cambridge: Cambridge University Press.

Tourigny, S. C. 2001. Some new killing trick: Welfare reform and drug markets in a U.S. urban ghetto. *Social Justice* 28:49–71.

United Nations. 2008. The millennium development goals report 2008. New York: United Nations. http://www.un.org/millenniumgoals/pdf/The%20Millennium%20Development%20Goals%20Report%202008.pdf.

United Nations Centre for Human Settlements. 2001. Cities in a globalizing world: Global report on human settlements 2001. London: Earthscan. http://www.unhabitat.org/pmss/getPage.asp?page=bookView&book=1618.

United Nations Human Settlements Programme. 2003. The challenge of slums. London: Earthscan. http://www.unhabitat.org/pmss/getPage.asp?page=bookView&book=1156.

United Nations Human Settlements Programme. 2008. Harmonious cities: State of the world's cities 2008/2009. London: Earthscan. http://www.unhabitat.org/pmss/getElectronicVersion.asp?nr=2562&alt=1.

WHO Commission on Social Determinants of Health. 2008. Closing the gap in a generation: Health equity through action on the social determinants of health (final report). Geneva: World Health Organization. http://whqlibdoc.who.int/publications/2008/9789241563703_eng.pdf.

Wood, A. 1998. Globalisation and the rise in labour market inequalities. *The Economic Journal* 108:1463–1482.

World Bank 1999. World development report 1999/2000: Entering the 21st century. New York: Oxford University Press. http://go.worldbank.org/YH54DW4WS0.

World Bank. 2007. *Global economic prospects 2007: Managing the next wave of globalization*. Washington, DC: World Bank.

# CHAPTER THREE

# THE DEMOGRAPHICS OF URBANIZATION IN POOR COUNTRIES

## MARK R. MONTGOMERY

### LEARNING OBJECTIVES

- Characterize population trends related to urbanization in the developed and developing world and the distinction in trends between mega-cities and smaller cities
- Provide a rationale for spatially disaggregated information on urban populations and levels of health, especially for the smaller cities and towns
- Distinguish slum dwellers from the urban poor who live outside slums

As poor countries continue to urbanize, the health systems and risks characteristic of their cities and towns will begin to feature more prominently in national health strategies than they do today. This chapter describes the demographic elements of the urban transformation that will warrant consideration. Its principal theme is the need to disaggregate urban populations—separating the poor and slum dwellers from the mass of better-off urbanites—so that the large within-city variations in health risks can be documented and addressed. The health circumstances of small cities and towns likewise need to be distinguished from those of larger cities.

When a disaggregated approach is applied to urban health, it brings to light gross inadequacies in the basic population and health information that ought to provide much of the evidence base for policy. At present, few developing countries can supply data on health determinants and outcomes with sufficient spatial detail to depict inequities within and across cities. Yet as urbanization proceeds, and greater percentages of national populations come to reside in geographically small, dense units, a way will need to be found to organize and map data at the level of city neighborhoods, wards, and other within-city jurisdictions.

This is more than a matter of complete accounting. While the urban demographic transformation is underway, many countries are also transforming their political and administrative systems via decentralization, placing more responsibilities for health programs and service delivery in the hands of municipal and even lower-level tiers of government (Panel on Urban Population Dynamics 2003). These governments are being tasked with new roles in health despite their general lack of experience in the sector, deficiencies in technical expertise, and pervasive difficulties in revenue-raising. At a minimum, to understand how many of their constituents will need health services, and to identify the neediest groups among them, municipal and other local governments will require spatially disaggregated data.

From where will such disaggregated data come? One source is, or at least should be, readily accessible. Most poor countries have managed to conduct a national census over the past decade or so, and most will participate in the new census round going into the field beginning in 2010. Unfortunately, the governments that have mounted censuses, and the international agencies supporting them, have not often given priority to spatially disaggregated analysis of these essential, geographically detailed data. Nor has the international demographic research community lent a hand: since the early 1980s, population researchers have tended to neglect population censuses in favor of national sample surveys. Where health data are concerned, it is less clear how the urban populations can be studied in the necessary depth. In poor countries, all but a few of which lack vital registration systems, there has been little alternative but to rely on national-level surveys—principally those in the Demographic and Health Surveys and the Multiple

Indicators Cluster Survey programs. These surveys have been the main source of information on urban infant, child, and reproductive health. Although extremely valuable in providing scientifically justified, nationally representative portraits of selected health conditions, such surveys cannot reliably portray health conditions in any given city, to say nothing of the variations in health across the neighborhoods of a city. In looking ahead to what will be an increasingly urban demographic landscape, it is apparent that substantial investments will be required in new methods of urban-sensitive population and health data collection and analysis.

In the first section of the chapter, we examine the urbanization trends that are underway in poor countries, with attention to features that are commonly misunderstood. The second section explores the demographic features that bear directly on urban health: the age and sex structure of urban populations, links between urban living standards and health, and the distinction between slum dwellers and the urban poor. The third section is the conclusion.

# THE URBAN DEMOGRAPHIC TRANSFORMATION

The process of urbanization is complex and even its broadest features are often misperceived. Journalistic accounts tend to conjure up a future of grim mega-cities choked with slums, flooded by streams of rural migrants, and teetering on the brink of chaos—and views not unlike these are echoed in much of the research literature. To be sure, the scale of urban change underway is impressive, and some of the developments are historically unprecedented. No one doubts that urbanization will present most poor countries with daunting challenges in governance and management. Even so, a review of the trends does not support the more alarmist interpretations that have tended to dominate the literature. Some of the features of today's urban transition are not far from the historical norm—they were also seen in the West in comparable periods of development (World Bank 2009). In concentrating attention on the largest cities and the presumed role of migrants, the popular and scientific literature have overlooked the continuing significance of small and medium-sized cities in the urban scene and the important role played by urban natural increase in city growth, which in quantitative terms rivals and often outstrips migration (UNFPA 2007).

## A Sketch of Urban Growth

The anticipated scale of the urban transition is depicted in Figure 3.1, which shows the urban and rural population growth that has been experienced since 1950 as well as the further growth forecast by the United Nations (United

**FIGURE 3.1 Estimates and Forecasts of Urban and Rural Population Growth from 1950 to 2050, More Developed (MDC) and Less Developed (LDC) Countries**

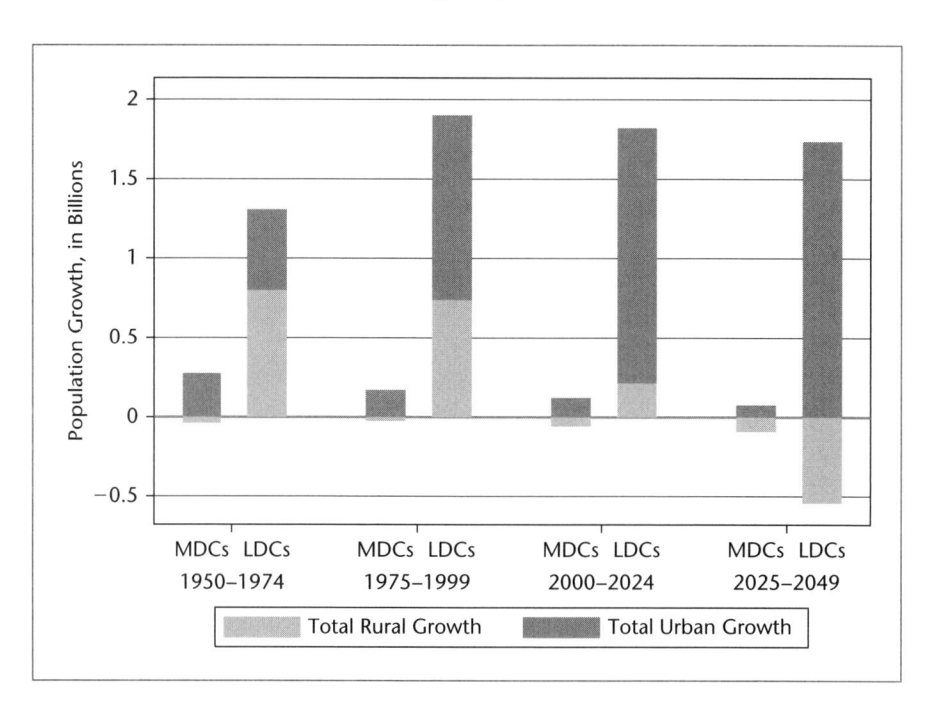

Source: United Nations (2008).

Nations 2008). By 2025, the world's total population is projected to be larger by some 1.9 billion persons than what it was at the turn of this century, with the greatest share of this increase—about 85 percent—expected to take place in the cities and towns of developing countries. The UN forecasts that 3.6 billion urbanites will live in these countries, up from 2 billion in 2000; and by 2050 the expected number of urban dwellers is forecast to reach 5.3 billion. After 2025, the forecasts suggest that the rural populations of poor countries will begin to decline, as they have for some decades now in the higher-income countries.

The percentage of urban dwellers in each country's national total is rising steadily with time, and in Asia and Africa, urban dwellers are likely to account for the majority of the regional population by 2030; in Latin America, this halfway point was passed decades ago. Not surprisingly, given its dominance in terms of population overall, Asia now contains the largest total number of urban dwellers among the major regions of developing countries, and will continue to do so

**FIGURE 3.2** Total Urban Population by Region, Developing Countries

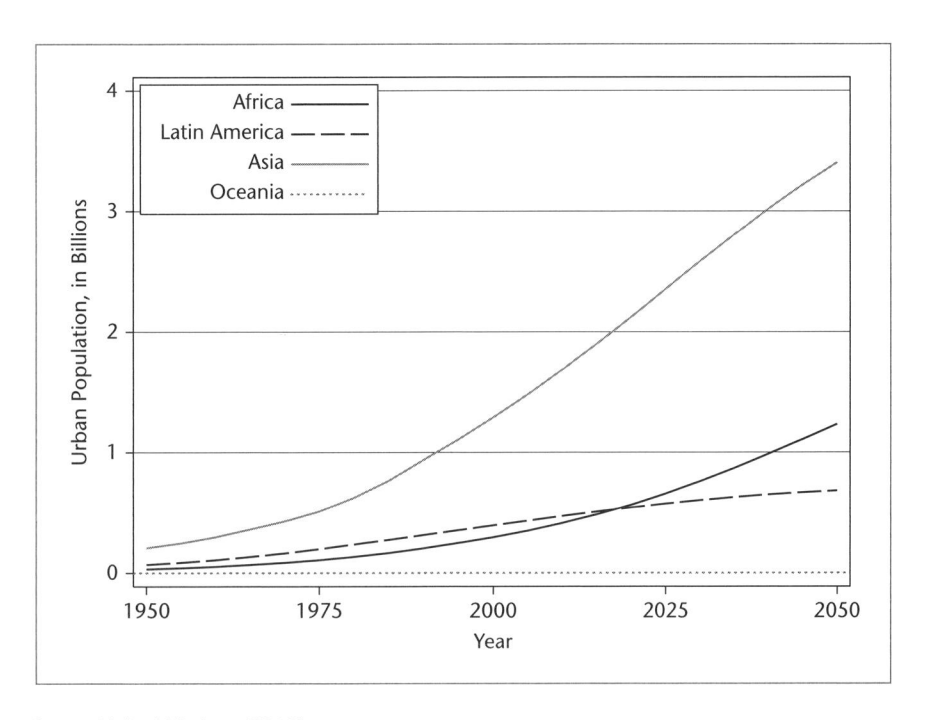

*Source:* United Nations (2008).

(Figure 3.2). By 2025, Africa will likely have overtaken Latin America in terms of urban totals, moving into second place among the regions. The urban population of developing Oceania is shown in the figure, but the numbers for this region are small by comparison with the other three regions, with only 1.9 million urban residents as of 2000 and about 6 million projected for 2050.

Figure 3.3 re-expresses these regional trends in terms of population growth rates. In the 1950s, 1960s, and well into the 1970s, regional urban growth rates were in the neighborhood of 4 percent, although declines were already making an appearance in Latin America. (Growth rates for the small urban populations of Oceania are shown in the figure for completeness.) Had the growth rates of this early era been sustained, the urban populations of the three major regions would have doubled roughly every seventeen years. By 2000, however, the rates had fallen considerably. As the figure indicates, further growth rate declines are thought to be in store for the first few decades of the twenty-first century, with urban Latin America projected to approach a state of zero growth.

**32   URBAN HEALTH**

FIGURE 3.3   Growth Rates of Total Urban Population
by Region, Developing Countries

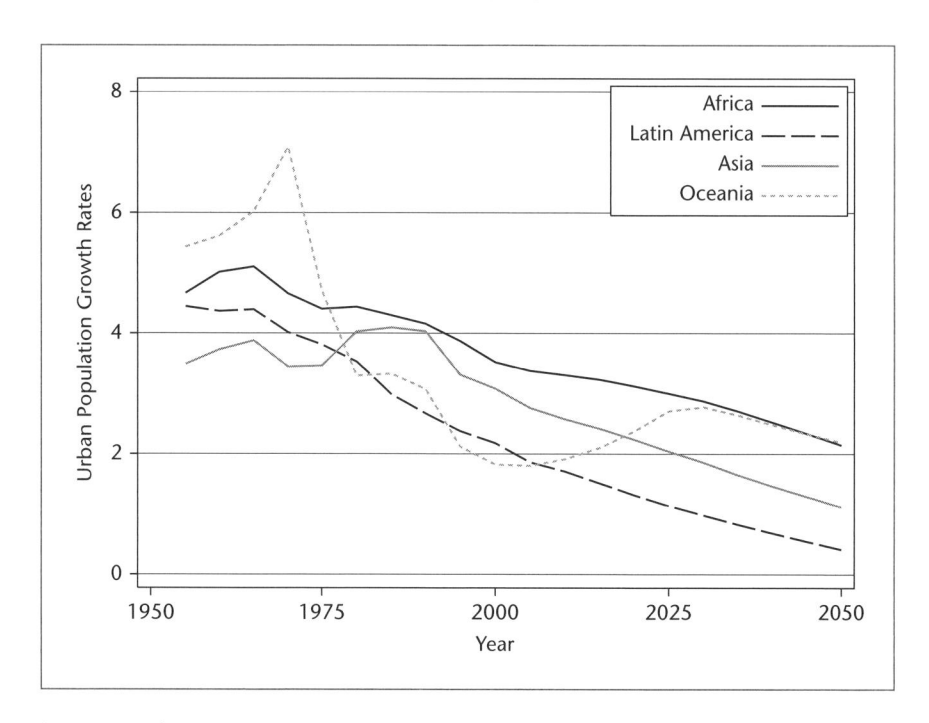

*Source:* United Nations (2008).

Much as with population growth rates overall in developing countries, the urban growth rates in force before 2000 were substantially higher than the rates seen during comparable historical periods in the West: the difference is due to lower urban mortality in present-day populations and stubbornly high urban fertility in some cases, as well as the in-built momentum in urban population growth that stems from the age and sex structures bequeathed by past growth (Panel on Urban Population Dynamics 2003). Even if the projected downward trends in growth rates come to pass, by 2050, urban growth rates in Africa will remain about 2 percent per annum, a rate that would double the urban population of that region in thirty-five years.

One feature of today's urban transition has no historical precedent: the emergence of hundreds of large cities. In 1950, only two metropolitan areas in the world—the Tokyo and the New York–Newark agglomerations—had populations of 10 million or more. (Cities of this size are commonly called *mega-cities*.) By 2025, according to the UN forecasts, the developing countries alone will contain 21 cities of this size. Even more striking is the number of cities in the 1–5 million range. In 1950, only thirty-four such cities were found in the developing world, though by 2025 there will be a projected total of 421 cities in this size range. Most of the large cities in developing countries are in Asia, in keeping with its large urban totals, but both Africa and Latin America have a number of cities in the 1–5 million size category.

This remarkable aspect of the urban transition has attracted a great deal of attention; it seems to have fostered the impression that most urban residents of the developing world live in mega-cities or the near equivalent. This is simply not the case. As United Nations (2008)-shows, among all developing-country urban dwellers in 2005, only 8 percent lived in mega-cities. By contrast, over half (52 percent) resided in small cities and towns with populations under half a million. Smaller cities are generally less well-provisioned than large cities with basic services, such as improved sanitation and adequate supplies of drinking water (Panel on Urban Population Dynamics 2003). In these cities, rates of fertility and infant and child mortality can be not much different from the rates prevailing in the countryside. Their municipal governments seldom possess the range of expertise and the managerial talent found in governments of large cities. Yet in an era of political decentralization, smaller cities are increasingly being required to shoulder substantial burdens in service delivery and take on a larger share of revenue-raising responsibilities (Panel on Urban Population Dynamics 2003, chapter 9). Given all this, it is surprising how often small cities have been neglected in policy discussions—but see UN-HABITAT (2006) for a treatment of the issues.

## Migration versus Natural Increase

A common perception is that city growth is largely the product of rural-to-urban migration. The evidence bearing on this view, although limited, is either weak or flatly contradicts it. When urban population growth rates for developing countries are divided into a natural urban growth component—the difference between urban birth and death rates—and a residual that combines net migration with spatial expansion, the results indicate that natural growth accounts for the larger share (Chen, Valente, and Zlotnik 1998). In poor countries, about 60 percent of the urban growth rate is due to natural growth (the 60-40 division reflects the situation of the median country in the UN's sample). For India, a similar rule has prevailed over the four decades from 1961 to 2001, with urban natural growth again accounting for about 60 percent of the total (Sivaramakrishnan, Kundu, and Singh 2005, 32). Even in China, where the migration share is larger, natural growth is responsible for some 40 percent of the urban population growth rate.

As discussed in *State of World Population 2007* (UNFPA 2007), many developing country policy makers have been apprehensive about rates of city growth in their countries and have not infrequently acted aggressively to discourage growth, mainly by razing the slums and expelling their residents. Such brutal measures have probably caused more poverty than they have eliminated—and yet have proven themselves to be ineffective in stemming growth over the long term. More enlightened regional development policies seldom generate rapid changes in the pace and spatial distribution of city growth that policy makers would hope to achieve.

It is therefore surprising how little attention has been paid to a growth-rate policy of a very different character: voluntary urban family planning programs. Over the past half century, these programs have compiled an impressive record of effectiveness across the developing world in facilitating fertility declines and reducing unwanted fertility. Even if the reproductive health benefits of family planning are set to the side by policy makers fixated on the need to slow city growth, these programs deserve much more attention than they have received. Voluntary family planning offers an effective and humane alternative to the punitive but ineffective measures that have been applied all too often to the urban poor.

## Forecasting Urban and City Growth

The UN Population Division prepares medium-term forecasts of both total urban and city-specific population growth. The record of these forecasts has been mixed at best. For reasons that are not yet well understood, the UN forecasts have consistently projected urban and city growth rates (and thus population sizes) that are too high. To take two examples: the twenty-year-ahead urban forecast for Latin America that was made in 1980 proved to be 20 percentage points too high when the region's 2000 urban population was counted; the forecast for South Asia was 27 percentage points above the mark. The tendency to overproject is not evident in the UN's forecasts of total population at the national level. The Panel on Urban Population Dynamics (2003) explains the UN's forecasting method and provides a critical review of the issues, as does Bocquier (2005). While the UN investigates the causes of the problem, users of its forecasts would be advised to interpret them cautiously.

## Mapping Urban Data

A notable development of the past decade is the outpouring of new, spatially specific, mappable urban data. Especially rapid growth has been underway in the compilation of remotely sensed images of the built-up area of cities across the developing world. Google Earth can now provide the nontechnical user with a glimpse of an enormous range of cities from small to large; and a vast storehouse of LANDSAT imagery is about to come into the public domain in 2009–2010, which will give technical analysts a basis for constructing a time series of such images dating from the 1970s to the present.

This remarkable expansion of information will soon enable national and local planners to give closer scrutiny to the areas on the peripheries of large cities, where much urban population growth is believed to take place, and will provide them with a view of the communities situated between large cities that are likely to fuse with their neighbors. Geo-coded data also open a window on the smaller cities and towns, where as we have seen, a large percentage of urban residents live. To be sure, remote images alone cannot supply estimates of population as such, and much remains to be learned about whether such images can be reliably processed to uncover characteristics of housing that could serve as spatial proxies for poverty.

To illustrate the potential that a combination of spatial and census data holds for studies of urban health, consider one climate-related health risk that faces the residents of coastal cities: exposure to hurricanes and typhoons, storm surges, and coastal flooding. McGranahan, Balk, and Anderson (2007) were able to map these risks on a global basis by defining the low-elevation coastal zone, the coastal area lying within 10 meters of sea level. An example is shown in Figure 3.4, which

FIGURE 3.4 Population Exposed to Seaward Hazards in the Low-elevation Coastal Zone of Medan, Indonesia

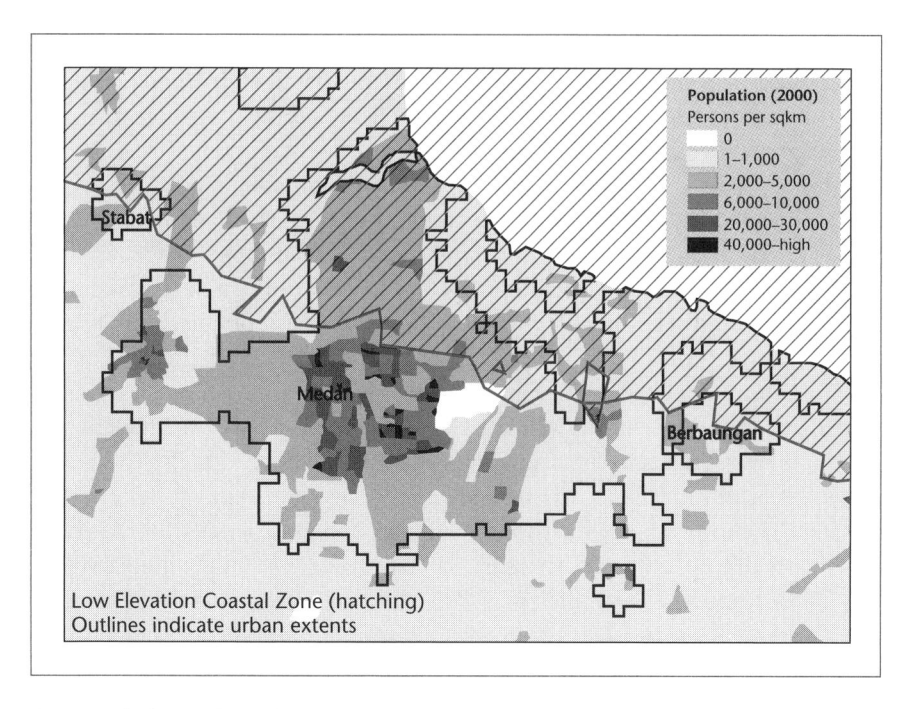

*Source:* Calculations by Deborah Balk (Baruch College, New York) based on the GRUMP database described in Balk (2009).

presents a map of Medan, Indonesia's third largest city located on the northern coast of Sumatra. The figure depicts the low-elevation coastal zone (in green) and underneath that layer, the city's administrative units, whose shades indicate the population of each such unit (darker shades represent larger populations). The outlined areas are taken from night-time lights satellite imagery; they suggest where population and economic activity is likely to be located within the urban agglomeration. This assemblage of data gives a reasonably detailed picture of urban exposure to risk. An Indonesian health planner, if provided with data such as these drawn from internationally accessible sources, could no doubt further refine and correct the maps on the basis of local understanding of flood histories and population location. Balk et al. (2009) explore such data in detail for cities in all developing countries.

## HEALTH AND THE URBAN POOR

Because the remainder of this volume examines urban health in some depth, the treatment here aims only to provide a measure of context, especially on the substantive issues and data limitations that are common to many health studies. We begin by noting a fundamental feature of urban populations that conditions health risks—their distinctive age and sex structure. We then proceed to give a brief account of the health differences associated with urban poverty, closing the section with a discussion of slum dwellers and the urban poor, two groups that are often assumed to be one and the same.

In many countries, the lower fertility that is characteristic of urban residents, coupled with the age pattern of migration, gives rise to a distinctive age profile in urban as against rural populations. Figure 3.5 illustrates the case of urban Ghana. The figure presents the urban age and sex distribution in relative terms, with (for men, and separately for women) the proportion of the urban population at a given age divided by the proportion of the rural population at that age. The age pattern depicted in the figure is commonly seen: when judged against the rural population, the urban areas of Ghana have relatively fewer children and relatively more residents in the prime reproductive ages (the early 20s to early 30s) as well as more residents in economically productive ages. The sex patterns seen here for Ghana vary a good deal across countries and time periods; for this particular case, the urban-rural differences in age structure are more pronounced for men than for women. In general, especially for diseases and risks that are strongly age- and sex-dependent, we would expect this distinctive urban population composition to be reflected in the urban burden of disease.

It is, unfortunately, uncommon for poor countries to be able to document the urban burden of disease by cause or condition, because very few of these countries have functioning and reliable vital registration systems. In the absence of such

FIGURE 3.5 Age and Sex Structure of Urban Ghana Relative to Rural Ghana

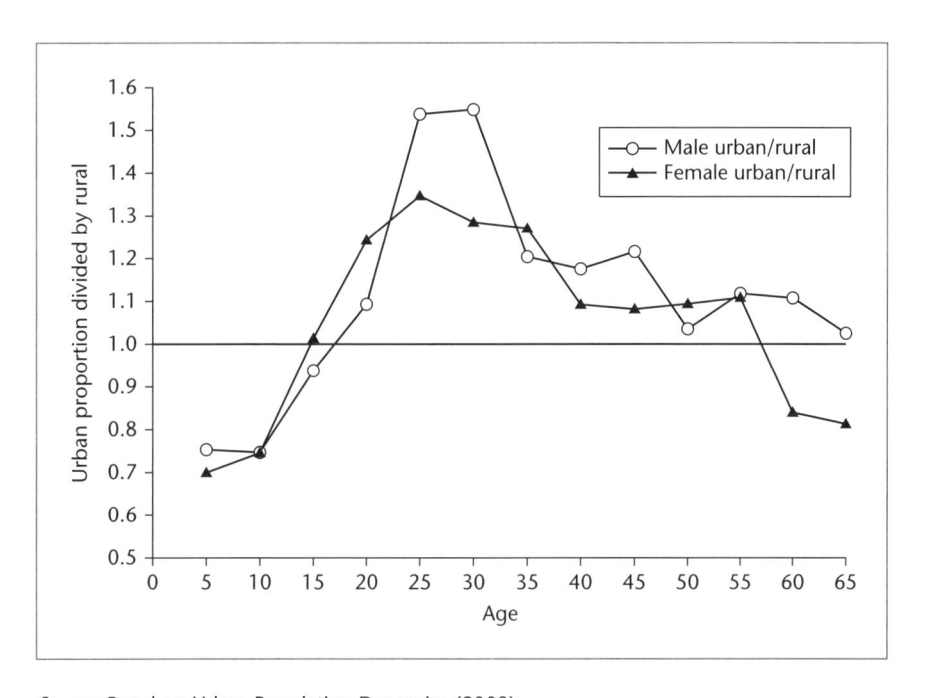

*Source:* Panel on Urban Population Dynamics (2003).

systems, health planners must draw insights mainly from sample surveys, the most prominent of which are the Demographic and Health Surveys (DHS) and the Multiple Indicator Cluster Surveys (MICS). It is becoming more common for these surveys to collect blood or tissue samples, but that effort is not undertaken in all surveys and, for reasons of cost, is usually restricted to subsamples of respondents. Therefore, the health conditions that can be studied are generally limited to those on which reliable information can be gathered in interviews. Skilled and sensitive interviewers can elicit reliable information from respondents on the survival of their infants and children and the age at death, but credible cause-of-death information cannot generally be obtained. Adult mortality is measured only indirectly, via questions about the survival of a respondent's siblings. Urban life expectancy cannot therefore be assessed through such surveys. Men are increasingly, but not always, interviewed in these survey programs.

In addition, as explained by the Panel on Urban Population Dynamics (2003), the major international survey programs focusing on health have not generally provided sufficient locational information in the samples released to the public domain

## 38 URBAN HEALTH

to identify small and medium-sized cities. The city-size dimension of health is consequently far more difficult to document than might have been supposed. Also, as mentioned earlier, the sample sizes of nationally representative surveys may allow a country's urban residents to be studied as a group, but are generally too small to provide reliable estimates of health in any given city. In short, there are major if understandable gaps in the health record that can be compiled through sample surveys.

### Relative Poverty

A further limitation, which comes to the fore in any effort to understand inequities in urban health by standard of living, is that the surveys in these international programs do not attempt to gather information on income or consumption expenditures. Measures of urban (and rural) living standards must therefore be based on proxy variables (Montgomery and Hewett 2005).

Figure 3.6 for India provides a sample of the health differentials that can be seen in many countries, using proxies for relative living standards. Here

**FIGURE 3.6 Any Prenatal Care: Urban and Rural India (1998–2000)**

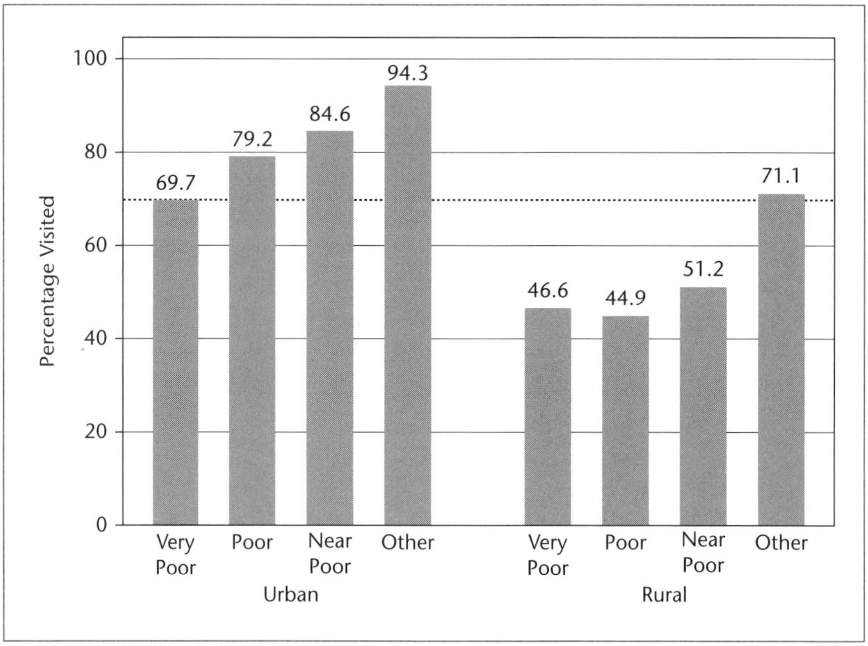

| Group | Urban | Rural |
|---|---|---|
| Very Poor | 69.7 | 46.6 |
| Poor | 79.2 | 44.9 |
| Near Poor | 84.6 | 51.2 |
| Other | 94.3 | 71.1 |

*Source:* 1998–2000 Demographic and Health Survey for India.

we consider a basic measure of reproductive health—whether a pregnant woman made at least one visit for prenatal care—as recorded in the 1998–2000 Demographic and Health Survey for India. The living standards measure is based on a ranking of urban households according to an index, which is summarized in relative terms. Rural households are ranked separately. As can be seen, the percentages of Indian women receiving prenatal care are notably higher for urban women than for rural, but within each sector, there are large differences evident by relative standards of living. Only 69.7 percent of very poor urban women in India receive any prenatal care—which is not much different from the percentage for rural women in the top half of the rural living standards distribution.

A similar picture is evident in the percentages of Indian children who are stunted, that is, shorter by two standard deviations or more from the height-for-age median of an international reference population. Figure 3.7 shows the large differences in stunting by standard of living for urban children, but

FIGURE 3.7 Child Malnutrition: Stunting in Urban and Rural India (1998–2000)

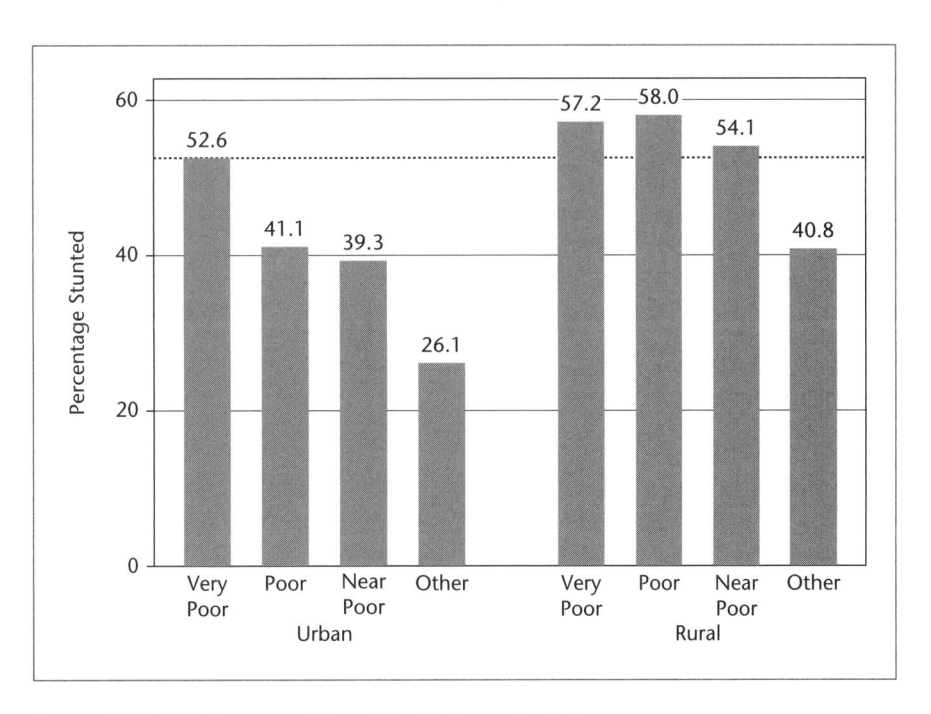

*Source:* 1998–2000 Demographic and Health Survey for India.

again, stunting among poor urban children is only slightly less common than it is among rural children.

Some of the differences in children's health are linked to provision of basic water and sanitation services. Table 3.1 documents the inequities by relative standards of living within urban populations as well as between urban and rural populations. The urban poor–urban nonpoor differences are very large indeed. Documentation such as this should put to rest the notion that urban dwellers are uniformly advantaged in terms of access to basic public services.

Finally, the differences in children's health and household access to services are also evident in measures of women's reproductive health. Table 3.2 summarizes modern contraceptive use, again distinguishing the urban poor from other urban

TABLE 3.1  Percentages of Poor Urban Households with Access to Services, Compared with Rural Households and the Urban Nonpoor

| DHS Countries in Region | | Piped Water on Premises | Water in Neighborhood | Flush Toilet | Pit Toilet |
|---|---|---|---|---|---|
| North Africa | Rural | 41.6 | 37.3 | 41.3 | 17.5 |
| | Urban poor | 67.3 | 27.8 | 83.7 | 8.5 |
| | Urban nonpoor | 90.8 | 7.8 | 96.3 | 2.6 |
| Sub-Saharan Africa | Rural | 7.8 | 55.7 | 1.1 | 47.6 |
| | Urban poor | 26.9 | 61.6 | 13.0 | 65.9 |
| | Urban nonpoor | 47.6 | 45.8 | 27.4 | 67.2 |
| Southeast Asia | Rural | 18.6 | 53.7 | 55.5 | 24.3 |
| | Urban poor | 34.0 | 53.7 | 61.8 | 22.9 |
| | Urban nonpoor | 55.8 | 40.1 | 89.0 | 9.4 |
| South, Central, West Asia | Rural | 28.1 | 53.6 | 4.3 | 55.4 |
| | Urban poor | 58.0 | 36.3 | 39.8 | 34.1 |
| | Urban nonpoor | 80.2 | 17.7 | 64.0 | 23.2 |
| Latin America | Rural | 31.4 | 36.4 | 12.6 | 44.0 |
| | Urban poor | 58.7 | 35.2 | 33.6 | 47.0 |
| | Urban nonpoor | 72.7 | 24.9 | 63.7 | 31.6 |
| Total | Rural | 18.5 | 50.7 | 7.5 | 46.6 |
| | Urban poor | 41.5 | 49.4 | 28.3 | 51.7 |
| | Urban nonpoor | 61.5 | 34.0 | 48.4 | 46.5 |

*Source:* Panel on Urban Population Dynamics (2003).

TABLE 3.2 Contraceptive Use by Women Aged 25–29 by Residence and, for Urban Residents, Poverty Status

| DHS Surveys in Region | All Rural | Urban Poor | Urban Nonpoor |
|---|---|---|---|
| North Africa | 0.26 | 0.37 | 0.48 |
| Sub-Saharan Africa | 0.08 | 0.13 | 0.22 |
| Southeast Asia | 0.44 | 0.40 | 0.47 |
| South, Central, West Asia | 0.33 | 0.35 | 0.44 |
| Latin America | 0.32 | 0.37 | 0.47 |
| Total | 0.22 | 0.26 | 0.35 |

Source: Panel on Urban Population Dynamics (2003).

dwellers. As is evident, levels of contraceptive use among the urban poor are midway between those of rural villagers and other urban residents, with trivial urban poor–rural gaps in use in South, Central, and West Asia, and also in Latin America. In Southeast Asia, rural women are slightly more likely to use contraception than poor urban women.

## Slum Dwellers and the Urban Poor

Although many focused and detailed studies of the health of slum dwellers have been undertaken, systematic studies and comparisons with other urbanites are still scarce. It is difficult to divide the overall health risks facing slum dwellers into those attributable to household poverty and the additional risks produced by the spatial concentration of poverty in slum neighborhoods. Although not definitive, Figure 3.8 is at least suggestive of the impact of concentrated poverty on child mortality in Nairobi, Kenya. In the slums of this city, child mortality rates are substantially above the rates seen elsewhere in the city; slum mortality rates are high enough even to exceed rural Kenyan mortality. The addition to risk that is apparent in the Nairobi slums may be due to multiple factors: the poor quality and quantity of water and sanitation in these communities; inadequate hygienic practices; poor ventilation and dependence on hazardous cooking fuels; the city's highly monetized health system, which for the poor delays or prevents access to Nairobi's modern health services; and the transmission of disease among densely settled slum dwellers.

But for health policies and programs to be properly focused, it is important to understand the circumstances of all urban poor, not only the sub-set of the poor

**FIGURE 3.8** Comparison of Child Mortality Rates (5q0) in the Nairobi Slums Sample with Rates for Nairobi, Other Cities, Rural Areas, and Kenya as a Whole

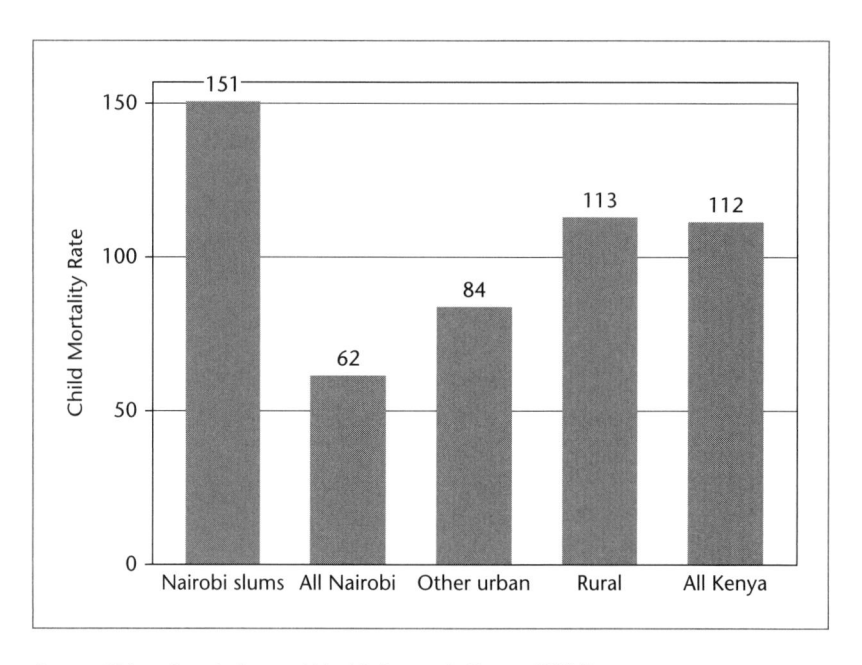

*Source:* African Population and Health Research Center (2002).

who live in slums. On the key question of what percentage of the urban poor are slum dwellers, there is surprisingly little that is known. One study of urban India, where the national authorities have taken care to distinguish slums from non-slums (and to further distinguish notified from non-notified slums) found that only one of every five poor urban households lives in a slum (Chandrasekhar and Montgomery 2009). This is doubtless an underestimate, as careful slum mapping efforts in India have generally uncovered many slum communities that were not included in the official records.[1] Even if the estimate is too low by half, however, an upward adjustment would not put slum dwellers in the majority of India's urban poor. Evidently, then, if urban health programs are to be correctly targeted, the poor living outside slums as such must be given due consideration. They may need to be approached through programs that operate in conjunction with municipal wards or other small-scale units of the municipal government, as in a recent innovative project carried out in urban Bangladesh where ward-level residents identified the poorest families in the area that were most in need of care (Pyle and Zannat 2007).

## SUMMARY

As we have argued, a substantial workload lies in store for the demographic and health research community if it is to assemble the data and methods needed for the upcoming urban era. At the aggregate level, the performance of UN forecasts of city and urban growth has been heavily criticized in recent years, and there is now general agreement on the need for a thorough critical review of forecast errors and the development of new methods (Panel on Urban Population Dynamics 2003; Bocquier 2005). Further effort will be needed to bring spatial specificity to the city population estimates in the form of geo-coded databases. Remote sensing methods will serve as a valuable supplementary tool, providing easily-updated information on spatial extents, if not on population as such.

Urban health information is currently being gathered on a systematic basis, mainly through the DHS and MICS international programs of sample surveys, which field nationally representative surveys. Sample surveys provide a less-than-ideal mechanism for documenting adult morbidities and mortality and for understanding asymptomatic health conditions. Even for infant, child, and reproductive health, these survey programs may need to be supplemented with more focused, possibly city-specific efforts such as have been carried out in urban Bangladesh (NIPORT and partners 2008). Among the many issues that merit further city-specific analysis, we would single out the urgent need to document where the urban poor live, and to consider intervention programs and methods that have the potential to reach the poor living outside as well as inside slums.

## REFERENCES

African Population and Health Research Center. 2002. *Population and health dynamics in Nairobi's informal settlements: Report of the Nairobi Cross-Sectional Slums Survey (NCSS) 2000*. Nairobi: African Population and Health Research Center.

Balk, D. 2009. More than a name: Why is global urban population mapping a GRUMPy proposition? In *Global mapping of human settlement: Experiences, data sets, and prospects*, ed. P. Gamba and M. Herold, 145–161. New York: Taylor and Francis.

Balk, D., T. Buettner, G. McGranahan, M. R. Montgomery, C. Small, D. Kim, V. Mara, M. Todd, S. Chandrasekhar, and S. Baptista. 2009. Mapping the risks of climate change in developing countries. Paper presented at World Bank Urban Research Symposium, June 28–30, in Marseille, France.

Bocquier, P. 2005. World urbanization prospects: An alternative to the UN model of projection compatible with mobility transition theory. *Demographic Research* 12(9):197–236.

Chandrasekhar, S., and M. R. Montgomery. 2009. Broadening poverty definitions in India: Basic needs in urban housing. Paper prepared for the International Institute for Environment and Development (IIED), February, in London.

Chen, N., P. Valente, and H. Zlotnik. 1998. What do we know about recent trends in urbanization? In *Migration, urbanization, and development: New directions and issues*, ed. R. E. Bilsborrow, 9–88. New York: United Nations Population Fund (UNFPA).

McGranahan, G., D. Balk, and B. Anderson. 2007. The rising tide: Assessing the risks of climate change to human settlements in low-elevation coastal zones. *Environment and Urbanization* 19(1):17–37.

Montgomery, M. R., and P. C. Hewett. 2005. Urban poverty and health in developing countries: Household and neighborhood effects. *Demography* 42(3):397–425.

NIPORT and partners. 2008, December. *2006 Bangladesh Urban Health Survey*. Dhaka, Bangladesh, and Chapel Hill, NC: National Institute of Population Research and Training (NIPORT), MEASURE Evaluation, International Centre for Diarrhoeal Disease Research, Bangladesh (ICDDR,B), and Associates for Community and Population Research (ACPR).

Panel on Urban Population Dynamics (M. R. Montgomery, R. Stren, B. Cohen, and H. E. Reed, eds.). 2003. *Cities transformed: Demographic change and its implications in the developing world*. Washington, DC: National Academies Press.

Pyle, D. F., and F. Zannat. 2007, October. *Municipal Health Partnership Program: Mid-term evaluation report*. Washington, DC: USAID–Municipality–Concern Worldwide, USAID/GH/HIPN.

Sivaramakrishnan, K., A. Kundu, and B. Singh. 2005. *Handbook of urbanization in India: An analysis of trends and processes*. New Delhi: Oxford University Press.

UN-HABITAT. 2006. *Meeting development goals in small urban centres*. London: UN-Habitat and Earthscan.

UNFPA (George Martine, lead author). 2007. *State of world population 2007: Unleashing the potential of urban growth*. New York: United Nations Population Fund.

United Nations. 2008. *World urbanization prospects: The 2007 revision*. New York: United Nations, Population Division, Department of Economic and Social Affairs.

World Bank. 2009. *World development report 2009: Reshaping economic geography*. Washington, DC: World Bank.

# CHAPTER FOUR

# MIGRATION, HEALTH SYSTEMS, AND URBANIZATION

NDIORO NDIAYE

MANUEL CARBHALLO

ROUGUI NDIAYE-COÏC

## LEARNING OBJECTIVES

- Understand the links among mobility of population, urbanization, and health system functioning in developing countries

- Understand how migration impacts disease patterns and access to health systems in urban settings

- See how migration trends affect economic and social development at the local and global levels

- Understand how to address factors in migration linked to "brain drain," poverty, and health system performance

- Show the need for new policies and new investments to address the effects of migration on health systems in Africa

It may at first seem unusual that a book devoted to urban health in the context of globalization should emphasize the role and importance of migration. The reason is that over the course of the last fifty years, but especially during the last decade, internal and cross-border migration has assumed an increasingly important position in defining the character of a nation's health as well as the urban profile of countries everywhere. In doing so, migration has necessarily, although somewhat late, caught the attention of national and international policy makers and is taxing the imagination of public health planners.

In 1993, Minister of Social Development of Senegal Dr. Ndioro Ndiaye shepherded a multidisciplinary study on what could be predicted about Senegalese women in 2015, which reported that, by 2025, at least 75 percent of the Senegalese population would be living in cities. The study pointed to the rapidly growing need for guidelines on planning for cities and suburban areas, taking into account the changing nature of social and economic indicators of Senegal and the impact that migration was already having on educational and health care systems.

At that time, the phenomenon of urbanization was still seen as a highly positive reflection of the labor demands generated by cities and the capacity of cities to absorb migrants economically and socially. This picture has since changed in many parts of the world, and questions are increasingly being raised as to the limits of cities' ability to take in new citizens.

In large part, the reason is that the growth in cities has occurred (and continues to take place) in regions of the world where economic development has been slow and where cities are no longer able to provide the basic amenities required for healthy life. Much of the growth in towns and cities has been in Africa and Asia, and the United Nations Department of Economic and Social Affairs estimates indicate that, by 2030, Africa will rank second to Asia in terms of total urban population.

## WHY MIGRATION IS SO IMPORTANT TODAY

The last fifty years have seen an unprecedented growth in the number of people moving within and between countries. Poverty and the need to seek new and better opportunities remain the main global drivers of migration, but changing patterns of climatic conditions are also forcing more and more people to leave regions that were previously capable of sustaining agriculture and life. This is likely to become even more evident in years to come and will constitute the foremost challenge facing national governments and the international community. In addition to these drivers of migration, conflicts and political instability continue to push people from their homes and communities, and prompt refugee and internally displaced movements of massive proportions.

In the contemporary world, factors facilitating migration have emerged. Improved road and air transport have made it increasingly possible for people to move farther and faster than ever before. A global media has helped to create a vision of the world in which people in poor countries and in deprived areas within wealthier countries are constantly being exposed to images of what life could be like if only they moved.

The number of international migrants has at least doubled over the last twenty-five years. The real figure may be considerably more, because relatively little is known about the number of people moving irregularly across borders or people moving within their own countries from rural to urban areas.

Migration is largely a market-driven process and responds to both push and pull factors. As such, it is a dynamic process that will become even more dominant in years to come. For if cities are perceived as hubs of opportunity, rural poverty grows, and climate change makes some parts of the world less attractive, and movement becomes more feasible, people will continue to move in ever-growing numbers. As they do, the need for new policies and practices in both sending and receiving communities and countries will increase.

The need for new policies and practices is also driven by the fact that the direction and very nature of migration is changing. Some regions and countries that were originally considered sending regions and countries, such as much of Western Europe, have suddenly become receiving countries that are seemingly ill-prepared for this role. Other sending countries in developing regions of the world have become transit countries where migrants spend long periods of time trying to earn money and pay for the next step in their journey.

## MIGRATION AND GLOBALIZATION

Globalization has had a far-reaching impact on the structure and nature of the world economy and the distribution of wealth and well-being. While it has done much to bring countries into a closer dependency relationship, globalization has also emphasized many of the gross social and health disparities that exist between countries. It has also become apparent that the costs and benefits of globalization have not been equally distributed, either between or within countries. Some of these disparities have been reflected in the ongoing need for people to move in search of economic and political security. They have also been reflected in the emerging health disparities between and within countries.

Migration, be it international or within national borders, has become a pivotal development theme. Not addressing it in a comprehensive way will be dangerous for all countries and for all people. The WHO Commission on Social Determinants of Health (2008) brought together leading practitioners and scientists and also policy makers, researchers, and civil society actors to consider the social factors (such as environment, housing, work, and wealth) that affect health and social development. Their findings focused on twelve thematic areas: early child development, creating healthy communities and living spaces, healthy employment, universal health care, comprehensive social protection, fair financing, market responsibility, gender equity, shared responsibility, political empowerment, good global governance, and capacity-building. The commission recognized that improving the health of the world's population is not simply a question of technical or scientific progress, or even a question of the availability of financial resources; it is an inclusive and participatory process of social change that calls for the empowerment of people, communities, and countries. Understanding the social determinants of health and coordinating and integrating actions to address them with national development strategies is an important good governance exercise, notably for developing countries. It will promote national development processes in poor countries by creating synergies between social and wealth production sectors to make the health system deliver quality services and address health inequities that undermine global agreements on universal human rights.

## Urbanization and Health

Because cities have become (as they always have been) the focus of industry and production and have drawn and depended on (as they always did) workers from rural areas, cities have grown rapidly everywhere. However, in developing countries, the pace of urbanization has not been consistent with the real demand for labor or the capability of absorbing newcomers. Therefore, cities have been unable to develop and maintain health and sanitation systems in a way that would have allowed them to keep up with the needs created by these new populations. Shantytowns and slums have come to characterize emerging cities and have become centers of health and socioeconomic crises. Poverty and inadequate water and sanitation systems in the context of massive rural-urban migration have opened the door to diseases that were previously considered essentially and only rural in nature. Despite many of the assumptions that cities are likely to be able to provide health and social services more rationally and cost-effectively than is the case when people are distributed over large rural areas, the reality is that this is so only if and when investments in health and social services are able to keep pace with demographic growth.

## Migration and Health

Despite the fact that migration is as old as history, it remains a complex and often difficult process that potentially brings with it an element of human wastage. Migration affects the health of people in many different ways. In some cases, the same factors that prompt people to move continue to play a role in defining the nature of their migration, their resettlement, and their health. People move with their health prints, their medical histories, and their cultural belief systems that, in turn, influence what they believe can be done to promote and protect health. The conditions they are exposed to along the route to their final places of settlement expose them to new diseases and/or reactivate old ones.

Educational history and economic background are critical factors in this, and gender is also a key variable in determining the type of health risks and insults migrants are exposed to. While some countries, such as Thailand, are seeking to integrate migrants (regular and irregular) and respond to their needs through local health systems, many others have not, and migrants often remain peripheral to whatever services are otherwise available.

## Good Practices

Most developing countries have yet to develop good practices to address the health issues of migrants within their borders. Thailand, as are all destination countries, is facing regular and irregular movement. Its program called Healthy Migrants for Healthy Thailand helps increase understanding and cooperation in providing health services to the non-Thai population through the cooperation of the International Organization for Migration's (IOM) Migration Health Dialogue with relevant government and nongovernmental organizations. The program provides both financial and technical support to the minister of public health (MOPH) in organizing biannual border health meetings and establishing provincial health-coordination committees in all of the five targeted provinces. Good practices have also been developed in other countries, and a recent EU presidency meeting has published a series on them (Castles and Delgado-Wise 2008).

# HEALTH IMPACTS OF MIGRATION ON RECEIVING COUNTRIES

The following sections discuss migration with respect to working conditions, living conditions, language and culture, communicable and noncommunicable diseases, and reproductive health in receiving countries.

## Role of Working Conditions

There are multiple reasons why migrants and newcomers of all kinds have typically been at risk for health insults and problems. The most obvious one is that newcomers tend to accept work in occupations or industries that nationals (or those who arrived earlier) will not. Some of these, such as mining, construction, heavy civil projects, and intensive agriculture, require activities that are high risk by the very nature of the work involved, the technologies involved, and the pesticides or other products to which workers are exposed. Today, these continue to account for high rates of industrial accidents and diseases among migrants.

## Role of Living Conditions

Even when migrants are not exposed to new risks as a result of the work they do, their living conditions often have adverse health effects. Poor economic conditions drive them into low-income, poor quality, and old housing where safety cannot be assured and where rental requirements cause them to accept highly overcrowded living conditions. In countries that continue to attract massive numbers of workers for mining and plantation industries, the tendency to put large numbers of men into small barrack-like constructions similarly continues to play an important role in heightening the risk of exposure to new diseases or the stimulation and spread of old ones, such as tuberculosis.

## Role of Language and Culture

Underlying many of these problems is also the fact that linguistic, cultural, and legal backgrounds of migrants often place them on the margins of their host societies, and they are unable to access or use health care systems and services effectively. Late presentation for diagnosis and care of serious health problems is common, as is poor compliance with the solutions proposed to them. Therefore, even when care is available, the inability to participate fully in the health care process makes disease outcomes among migrants worse than they are among nonmigrants.

## Migration and Communicable Diseases

Communicable diseases have long been the accepted (often exaggerated) threat associated with migration and migrants, and fear of them has led to a variety of screening and quarantine policies and practices whose effectiveness has been varied and rarely very good. Contemporary migration into Europe and North America is nevertheless fast changing patterns of HIV, STIs, tuberculosis, and hepatitis in these regions and is calling for new measures to prevent and respond to them. In some cities, urban malaria, urban schistosomiasis, and urban leishmaniasis, formerly thought to be only health problems of rural communities, have become threats to health and to the functioning of cities.

How best to do this while concurrently respecting the right of people to move will tax policy makers for years to come. But in the meantime, there should be concern about return migration to countries of origin being equally fraught with the possibility of importing diseases.

### Migration and Noncommunicable Diseases

There is growing evidence that migrants may also be more at risk than others for noncommunicable diseases, such as type-2 diabetes, hypertension, stroke, and cardiovascular events. These are beginning to be understood as the result (in part) of the stress that migrants are exposed to and, in many cases, the ways that they cope with this stress. Abuse of tobacco, alcohol, and other drugs is not uncommon in the panoply of coping mechanisms that migrants (as well as others) turn to. Inappropriate food consumption patterns also play into this and help create situations where migrants progress more quickly than other people to diseases of lifestyle.

### Migration and Reproductive Health

Within the spectrum of noncommunicable disease problems that migrants are confronted with, reproductive health and mental health are also very prominent. In general, migrants tend to have less access to reproductive care services or to understand the need for them. Throughout Europe and North America, there is evidence that female migrants are more likely than nonmigrant women to have unwanted pregnancies and to seek abortions to deal with them.

## IMPACT OF MIGRATION ON COUNTRIES OF ORIGIN

### Brain Drain

Migration does not always or only involve low-skilled and poorly educated people. The last twenty years have seen a massive recruitment of doctors, nurses, teachers, engineers, and other highly skilled graduates from developing countries. The IOM estimates the figure is over 100 million, and the number of doctors and nurses trained in Africa who were estimated to be working in OECD countries in 2006 was one in four and one in 20, respectively. At the outset of the 1990s, the

United States had received over half of the world's skilled migrants coming from developing countries (Carrington and Detragiache 1999) and now employs the greatest number of foreign-trained doctors and nurses, followed by the United Kingdom.

The brain drain continues to deplete developing countries of people in which they have invested massively through public educational systems in early and higher education. According to the World Health Organization, approximately 23 percent of physicians trained in ten sub-Saharan African countries are currently working in eight OECD countries, particularly in Anglophone countries (WHO Commission on Social Determinants of Health 2008). The brain drain has meant that some thirty-six countries in sub-Saharan Africa cannot meet their target of one doctor per 5,000 people; even in non-conflict-affected zones, such as Zambia and Ghana, there is only one doctor for more than 10,000 people. Outmigration has done much to diminish access to health care services in developing countries (Marchal and Kegels 2003), and low health-worker density and diminished access to services has contributed to stagnating, if not increasing, maternal and young child mortality.

## Resource Constraints

For developing countries, the challenge is a difficult one. Many of them do not have the resources needed to achieve stated goals for investment in their health care systems. This shortage of financial resources means that retention based on competitive financial remuneration is not likely to be the answer. Nor is it easy to persuade highly qualified staff to work in rural areas where whatever health care facilities do exist are poorly staffed and equipped and offer few, if any, possibilities of putting knowledge gained into practice. For health care staff that are expected to move there from urban university centers, the paucity of educational facilities and poor housing makes it unattractive from a family point of view.

One way to reverse this phenomenon is to mainstream migration priorities into the National Debt Reduction Strategy Paper, particularly the health sector.

# PERSPECTIVES AND SOLUTIONS

## Growing Awareness of the Problem

The twenty-first century has seen a growing sensitivity to some of these disparities, and countries and regional intergovernmental structures, such as the EU, are now looking for ways that the health and welfare of migrant workers can be improved. As far as the movement of highly qualified people is concerned, new initiatives are also under way. In some countries, ethically driven decisions have been taken to stop proactive recruitment of highly trained staff from developing countries and to accelerate professional training and education of nationals to achieve self-sufficiency in the face of changing local demands. For example, the United Kingdom's national need for nurses is now being met through the accelerated training of personnel in the United Kingdom itself and far less through nurses from abroad. In other parts of the world, recruiting countries are seeking ways that they can invest in professional training programs in sending countries, so that for all who are trained and attracted away, an equal number will be trained and encouraged (with incentives) to stay.

## Long-Term Solutions to the Brain Drain

The real solution will only come when the international community works together to develop intergovernmental plans that are evidence-based, ethically driven, and internationally sensitive. Predicting how many doctors, nurses, engineers, and others a country will need is not in itself difficult to do, and applies to both rich and poor countries alike. Understanding the ethical component of proactive recruitment is similarly not difficult in a world that has already agreed on its millennium development agenda. What is difficult and has eluded so many countries in the past has been the political will to see migration as part of a much larger and long-term development agenda that applies to sending and receiving countries alike; it is very likely to be fundamental to effective development policy for decades to come.

## Regional and International Responses

The migration of highly skilled personnel, especially but not only doctors and nurses, has not been totally ignored. A number of initiatives have been taken at a national and an international level. Some countries have already begun to address the issue. Countries such as Jamaica, Mauritius, and the Philippines all have increased their production by expanding class size or establishing medical and nursing schools that specifically prepare their students for migration to other countries. They have often become massive exporters of trained medical personnel as a matter of national economic policy, because health workers who emigrate remit significant income (for some countries up to 40 percent of annual revenues) to their families in their country of origin. However, maintaining a balance that assures an adequate health workforce for the exporting countries can be challenging.

## The Situation in Africa

Africa is now the only continent in the world that still faces all the classic obstacles to successful development: educational and health systems are deteriorating throughout much of the continent; armed conflicts and civil wars are common and repetitive; millions of people are being forced from their homes and communities; natural hazards, such as drought, are growing in intensity; and the pressure on cities is increasing as a result of uncontrolled rural migration. Meanwhile, the brain drain is depriving African countries of a very significant part of their skilled human resources.

As noted above, the effects of the brain drain on health care systems throughout Africa are becoming more evident and more far-reaching, but most African countries are failing to respond to the health needs of their populations. Some of this problem is related to general lack of resources that do not permit African heads of state to achieve their own goals for investing 15 percent of GDP in the health sector. Other parts of national infrastructures are also failing as a result of resource constraints and brain drain: the loss of engineers, teachers, and other highly trained key personnel is rendering development more difficult than it was twenty years ago. If Africa as a whole is to respond to the dilemma of interrupted development, it must pay special attention to the theme of migration and understand three aspects of the phenomenon within their country—international, subregional, and internal migration—to develop effective action plans. To address international migration, especially the migration of highly skilled workers, the international community must work with African countries to reach solutions that, while not forbidding free movement of talent, nonetheless place it into a larger policy context of mutually supportive development.

Much could be gained from larger and more focused international investments in strengthening vocational and higher education in Africa to increase and strengthen faculty and infrastructure. This would permit expanded enrollment of traditional health professionals and new programs for cadres of new health workers to meet specific community needs. Bilateral agreements between receiving/recruiting and sending/training countries, designed to create the economic and social environment might help to create quality practice environments, featuring continuing professional development opportunities that might persuade more people to stay. This could mean the introduction of salary or other financial incentives or of nonfinancial incentives, such as better physical working (health facilities) conditions, better and more up-to-date supplies and equipment, better housing for staff, educational allowances for their children, and more frequent professional in-service training. However, to attract providers to less desirable areas, rural or inner-city, remuneration and benefits should be structured accordingly.

While, to date, much of the competition has been focused on highly skilled migrants from developing countries, with time the need for less skilled personnel will grow as well. At that time, it will become more important than ever that developed countries enter into well-planned and evidence-based agreements with sending countries to properly compensate sending countries for the loss of personnel. Much will depend on to what extent creative investments in education and socioeconomic development can be made, and the extent to which migration is channeled into official patterns that allow migrants to be counted and supported from a health and welfare perspective.

Much of the discussion above has referred to international migration, but in reality, the same concerns (and in many cases even greater concerns) are emerging with respect to migrants arriving in cities from rural areas. Few, if any, countries have developed the types of health policies required to take account of the growing number of rural migrants arriving in cities that can no longer provide them with employment opportunities, safe housing, healthy environments, and access to quality health care. Urbanization for such countries has become a threat to human security and health; many of them are poor, all of them are confronted with unplanned and uncontrolled internal migration, and many of them are in ecological zones where the threat of rural diseases being imported into cities is high. The mix of these rural diseases, such as malaria, and the classic diseases of urban poverty, such as tuberculosis and hepatitis, threaten to produce new and difficult-to-manage challenges to public health in cities.

## MIGRANT HEALTH, HUMAN RIGHTS, AND ACCESS TO CARE

The end of the twentieth century saw health increasingly spoken about as a right. While the nuances of this continue to be discussed, there is no doubt that the right to health care has been largely accepted by the world. Achieving the right to health care still remains a distant objective for many countries, and much remains to be done if the Millennium Development Goals for health are to be achieved. However, for most of the developed countries that have become the receiving focus of migration, providing access to quality health care is less of a challenge. What has become a challenge is ensuring the right to quality health care for migrants. A host of factors has made the task difficult.

Migrant access to quality health care has become complex because of many reasons. Not least among these factors has been the emergence of different categories of migrant. In some instances, legal long-term migrants have been followed by irregular migrants, whose real number remains unknown and who remain relatively invisible to local and national health authorities. Poorly understood in terms of their health care needs, these migrants remain poorly served. In some instances, their legal access to routine health care is not clear; in others their capacity to access medical insurance (where it is required) remains equally ill-defined.

Everywhere, there is a growing recognition that irregular migrants typically only access emergency services, and even those only when it is late, in terms of the evolution of disease. Unless more is done to change this situation and regularize the access to health care for all migrants irrespective of their legal status, the potential danger of communitywide ill health undermining the economic productive capacity of these migrants will grow, and with it, so will the dangers to host societies.

## WHAT CAN BE DONE?

Migration has always been a positive force for development. It has underpinned much of the economic growth of countries everywhere. Nevertheless, uncontrolled and poorly managed migration today presents opportunities for disaster, especially because people are moving in unprecedented numbers. They are also moving faster and over greater distances than ever before. The health needs they carry with them are likely to become more complex and more demanding of attention than receiving cities and countries have been willing or capable of providing to date. If these implicit threats are to be reduced and migration is to be made the positive force that it can be, a number of steps are required.

The first of these is the development of international rules that will govern the rights of migrants and the obligations of both sending and receiving countries. The responsibility for global health is global, and migrant health is today one of the most global features of public health.

The second step is that much more research is needed to map and understand the health dynamics of migration. Unless more is done in this area, it will be impossible to predict and proactively respond to the changing patterns of global public health. Migration is a complex process and possibly becoming more complex. How migrants move, from where to where, under what circumstances, with what medical histories, and with what exposure along the way are features that must be better understood. Similarly, much more needs to be known about how migrants resettle, under what conditions, and with what risks to their health and access to health care.

The third step is that policy for recruitment of skilled personnel requires new and more cooperative agreements between sending and receiving countries participating as equals in defining conditions that ensure all are winners. Developing countries must not be allowed to invest in and then lose their scarce human resources. Equally, developed countries must not be faced with losing critical workers to advance their own development agendas. Concurrently, skilled workers must be allowed to benefit from the principle of free movement and the right to migrate. This will call for creative and "out-of-the-box" ideas and policies.

The special challenges of migration in the context of rapid urbanization calls for urgent policies from national governments, with the help of the international development community. The current pattern of urban growth—much of it related to migration—left unchecked is unlikely to be able to sustain healthy life; it could become more associated with social problems and political instability, and it will inevitably be associated with the emergence of new and difficult-to-manage health problems. Making rural areas attractive, developing new towns and cities with adequate health infrastructure, and expanding health and other services to rural areas may help stem the flow. However, cities historically have been a magnet for economic opportunity through formal and informal economies. Health care systems and professionals need appropriate support in order to address urban health as migration continues from rural to urban areas. Overall, more holistic national development policies that place health at the center of the equation are needed.

## SUMMARY

Urbanization has been a consequence of population mobility, and migration has implications for disease patterns and access to health care in cities. Migration also impacts economic and social development at the local and global levels. While much attention is paid to the migration of the poor from rural to urban settings (particularly in low- and middle-income countries), another aspect of migration that impacts the health of urban residents is the "brain drain"—the departure of professionals for perceived greater opportunity and higher standards of living in more developed settings. This form of migration compounds the overall health problems of populations in low- and middle-income countries—especially the poor—through less access to quality preventive and curative care. To address these needs, policy makers at the national and international levels will need to recognize the patterns of migration, invest in cities with adequate health care for all, and create policies and conditions that will entice health professionals to provide quality care in these underserved settings.

# REFERENCES

Carrington, W. J., and E. Detragiache. 1999. How extensive is the brain drain? *Finance and Development* 36(2):46–49.

Castles, S., and R. Delgado-Wise. 2008. *Migration and development: Perspectives from the south.* Geneva: International Organization for Migration.

Marchal, B., and G. Kegels. 2003. Health workforce imbalances in times of globalization: Brain drain or professional mobility? *International Journal of Health Planning and Management* 8 Suppl. 1:S89–S101.

WHO Commission on Social Determinants of Health. 2008. *Closing the gap in a generation: Health equity through action on the social determinants of health.* Geneva: World Health Organization.

# CHAPTER FIVE

# IMMIGRANT HEALTH IN AMSTERDAM, THE NETHERLANDS

### ARNOUD P. VERHOEFF
### ROEL A. COUTINHO

---

### LEARNING OBJECTIVES

- Discuss the dimensions of a multicultural urban population in determining local urban health policy
- Identify concerns and approaches to addressing health promotion of a multicultural urban population

## CHARACTERISTICS OF AMSTERDAM

The city of Amsterdam, capital of the Netherlands, is a medium-sized European city with around 750,000 inhabitants. Whether a city can be classified as an "urban area" depends not only on the absolute number of inhabitants but also on other characteristics. For example, the population density of Amsterdam is around 4,500 per square kilometer, with around 2,300 houses per square kilometer (Van Zee and others 2008). Another major characteristic of an urban population is diversity with respect to social economic status, cultural background, ethnicity, and household composition.

The Amsterdam population consists of people from more than 170 different countries around the world. Only half of the population is of Dutch descent, which will further decrease in the coming years. In 2030 about 40 percent of the population will be from nonindustrialized countries, mainly from Morocco, Turkey, Suriname, and the Dutch Antilles. People from Morocco and Turkey came to the Netherlands during the 1960s as labor migrants. Originally, this was seen as temporary migration. As time passed, it turned out to be a permanent stay for most, and family reunions increased the migration influx. At present, approximately 5 percent of the Amsterdam population has Turkish ancestry, and 8 percent has Moroccan ancestry. Suriname is a former colony of the Netherlands. After independence in the 1980s, almost half of the Surinamese population migrated to the Netherlands and especially to Amsterdam, where people of Surinamese descent now account for almost 10 percent of the population. The Dutch Antilles are still part of the Kingdom of the Netherlands: around 2 percent of the Amsterdam population comes from the Dutch Antilles. Recently, migration from West African countries—primarily Ghana and Nigeria—has become important. Presently, people coming from this region account for around 2 percent of the Amsterdam population (Van Zee and others, 2008). These data are based on the population register of the city, which does not include undocumented immigrants. No estimation of the size of this last group is available.

Around 20 percent of Amsterdam households have a family income below 105 percent of the legal social minimum wage, and almost three-quarters of them have lived below this minimum for over three years; this proportion is considerably higher than the country's total population. The proportion of single-person households and single-parent households are larger in Amsterdam—around 35 percent and 15 percent respectively (Van Zee and others 2008). Finally, the gay community is overrepresented in the Amsterdam population. Based on interviews of a random sample of the adult male population in the Amsterdam population register, about 10 percent of males 18–55 were homosexual or bisexual, which is 4–5 times higher than elsewhere in the country (Veugelers and others 1993). Drug users are also overrepresented: in 1997, the number of heroin users in Amsterdam was estimated—by capture/recapture—at 4,130 (Buster, Van Brussel, and Van den Brink 2001).

## Health Status of Amsterdam's Population

As indicated above, Amsterdam's population is characterized by great ethnic diversity. About 10,000 children are born annually; about 60 percent are of migrant descent. Perinatal infant mortality rate during 2002–2006 in Amsterdam was 11.8 per 1,000 live births, considerably higher than for the rest of the Netherlands (apart from the four largest cities)—9.3 per 1,000 live births (De Graaf and others 2008). Within the city, perinatal mortality is higher in deprived neighborhoods, with a relative risk of 1.36 for non-Western women and 1.52 for Western women. The higher perinatal mortality rate is primarily related to more premature deliveries and lower birth weights. Here we already see differences between different ethnic groups and socioeconomic status. For example, a lower birth weight is primarily found among Surinamese infants, and premature deliveries primarily among infants of Turkish and Surinamese descent. Infant mortality during the first year of life is higher in Amsterdam than in the Netherlands as a whole. Mortality is especially higher among infants of Turkish and Moroccan descent. These differences are probably related to differences in an increase of prenatal healthcare and differences in lifestyle factors during pregnancy (Alderliesten and others 2007; Van Eijsden 2008). Twenty percent of non-Western pregnant women did not receive prenatal health care within 18 weeks of conception compared to only 5 percent of pregnant women of Dutch descent. Among pregnant Turkish women, 30 percent were still smoking.

Lifestyle determinants are also related to ethnic background. (Uitenbroek and others 2006). Overall, around 30 percent of the adult population smokes; the highest prevalence is found among Turkish men (45 percent), the lowest among Moroccan women (2 percent). About half the population struggles with overweight, comparable with the national figure. Around 40 percent of the Moroccan and Turkish women are obese. The lower mean figure is probably related to the overrepresentation in the Amsterdam population of the 20–45 age group. The mean prevalence of diabetes is approximately 4 percent, with the highest prevalence for the Moroccan population (10 percent). The health status of the Surinamese population with respect to cardiovascular risk factors is between that of the Turkish and Moroccan populations on one hand and the Dutch population on the other hand (Dijkshoorn 2006). So far, no information is available about the prevalence of cardiovascular risk factors of the West African population in the city.

Previous research in the Netherlands indicated a higher prevalence of depression and anxiety disorders in the urban populations, with the highest prevalence in the city of Amsterdam. These studies included only the Dutch population. A recent study in Amsterdam also included the migrant population. In general, 7 percent of the population had depression or an anxiety disorder in the last month based on the Composite International Diagnostic Interview (CIDI). Among the Turkish population, this was 19 percent, and among the Moroccan population, 10 percent. Turkish women and Moroccan men seem the populations most at risk (De Wit and others 2008).

Because risk groups such as men having sex with men (MSM) and (young) migrants are overrepresented in Amsterdam, the incidence of sexually transmitted infections (STIs) and HIV/AIDS is also higher. About 40 percent of all HIV positives registered in the national HIV register are from Amsterdam; most new HIV diagnoses are among MSM and to a lesser extent among migrants from sub-Saharan Africa. Among heterosexually active men and women between 15–40 years, the prevalence of *Chlamydia trachomatis* (CT) was found to be close to 5 percent, over two times higher than in the non-urban Dutch population (Van den Hoek and others 1999). There were considerable differences by ethnic group. The highest CT prevalence was found among black Surinamese women (12.4 percent) and Antillean men and women (around 10 percent). Relatively low CT prevalences were found among Turkish women (2.5 percent) and Moroccan women (3.5 percent).

## PUBLIC HEALTH POLICY IN AMSTERDAM

The responsibility for public health in the Netherlands is partly at the national level and partly at the local level.

The national law on public health (*Wet Publieke Gezondheid*) regulates the control and prevention of infectious diseases and some other public health requirements at both the national and local level. For the control of infectious diseases, the local health service is responsible, with the exception of large outbreaks that involve other parts of the country and certain severe infectious diseases like hemorrhagic fevers. Interventions are carried out locally and directed to specific target groups, for example, migrants or MSM.

For other public health issues, like obesity tobacco and alcohol use, and depression and anxiety disorders, the responsibility is also at the local level. The national law prescribes that each municipality must regularly formulate its own public health policy, based on the local public health situation. Concurrently, the national government formulates priorities that should be taken into account in the local health policy plan. The latest national health policy plan for 2007–2010 sets the following priorities: prevention of overweight, diabetes, depressive disorders, tobacco use, and excessive alcohol use. Based on the health status of the Amsterdam population, at the local level the following priorities were added for 2008–2011: sexual health (prevention of STI and HIV infections, prevention of teenage pregnancies and abortions), psychosocial health (including depressive and anxiety disorders, behavioral problems among young people, social isolation among the elderly, and the prevention of suicides), and drug abuse (in addition to tobacco and alcohol, also cannabis and party drugs). In general, priority is given to the most vulnerable groups within the Amsterdam population, primarily the population with a low socioeconomic status. Depending on the public health problem, further specification is needed, for example, for the prevention of STI and HIV infections and overweight. For some issues targeting of different age

FIGURE 5.1   The Influence of General Socioeconomic, Cultural, and Environmental Conditions on Individual Health

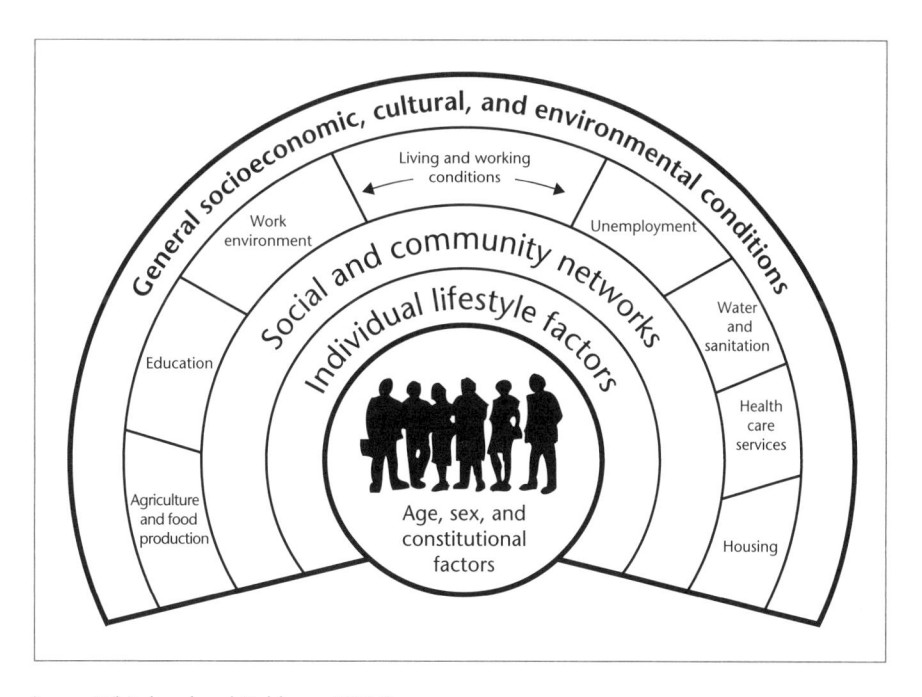

*Source:* Whitehead and Dahlgren (2006).

groups is needed, as in the case for sexual health and drug abuse (Verhoeff and Acda 2007).

Health promotion within the Netherlands (and Amsterdam) has long been dominated by the so-called classic form of health education solely directed to the individual. Now, a more integrated approach is used as it is well known that programs solely directed to health behavior of the individual are not capable of reducing health disparities within the (urban) population. It is well known that not only individual behavioral factors influence health, but also social factors on which an individual has little or no influence. This includes economic and cultural factors, quality of the physical environment, quality of housing, working conditions, and access to and quality of health care (see Figure 5.1; Whitehead and Dahlgren 2006). In view of this, Amsterdam's public health policy promotes a more integrated approach. This means strong cooperation among different fields of public policy within the city. It also strengthens the importance of cooperation with other parties outside the local municipality like health care providers, health care insurance companies, private companies, and community organizations.

## HEALTH PROMOTION IN THE MULTICULTURAL POPULATION OF AMSTERDAM

In general, health promotion interventions should take into account factors like setting and nature of the target population—among others—to be effective. Amsterdam's public health policy prioritizes a culturally competent approach to health in the city. Health and sickness are typically related to culture. Assuring the development and implementation of culturally sensitive interventions in Amsterdam is mainly achieved through community participation. HIV and STI prevention illustrates this through the effort of migrant health educators in different health care settings in the city.

### HIV and STI Prevention

As indicated in the previous sections, the incidence of HIV and STI infections is higher among certain migrants within the Amsterdam population, namely, Surinamese, Antilleans, and West Africans. It was apparent that the mainstream health promotion campaigns to promote sexual health and safe sex were not effective for these high-risk groups. Reasons included language difficulties—especially for the West African population—and cultural factors. Although the message was the same, the approach used in the mainstream campaigns did not take into account the specific settings relevant to reach these groups. Therefore, in 2005 the public health service developed a specific community-tailored approach to make the interventions more effective. Starting that year, community-based organizations, such as religious groups, welfare groups, and youth groups, were invited to develop their own prevention projects with support of the Amsterdam public health service. Members of community organizations were invited to be trained on sexual health issues and safe sex to ensure these community leaders had the essential knowledge regarding HIV and STI prevention. They were also given proposal writing support. Projects could receive a maximum of around $10,000 for implementation. The public health service aimed at capacity building as well, bringing together different community organizations with comparable proposals to promote cooperation. Since the start of this annual approach, around twenty-five different projects have been implemented. Activities range from group educational sessions, peer education, interactive radio programs, soap series on local radio and television stations, interactive theater productions, and comedy shows to large-scale public events. This mix of activities reaches a large proportion of the target population. The approach is continuously monitored to get insight about the projects' quality and the results of individual projects. Ongoing attention is needed to assure that the content of the messages of the projects remains in line with the scientific knowledge about HIV and STI prevention. At least twice a year, meetings are organized by the public health service for community leaders' supplementary training.

Whether this approach is successful in decreasing the incidence of new HIV and STI infections is not known. Ideally, a randomized controlled trial should be performed, but one using infection outcomes is not feasible. For some of the projects, tailored research is carried out using intermittent outcomes such as measuring knowledge about HIV and STI prevention and attitudes toward safe sex and voluntary testing. The results are positive for at least short-term effects such as increased knowledge and a more positive attitude among participants in these programs (results not published yet). Interestingly a similar approach has recently started in Suriname, supported by the Amsterdam public health service.

Apart from HIV and STI prevention, community-based health promotion is also used in Amsterdam for other main public health issues like obesity and the promotion of physical exercise and the consumption of healthy foods.

## Migrant Health Educators

The example described above illustrates the necessity for targeted interventions for different groups within the urban population, first recognized twenty-five years ago in Amsterdam. At that time, a small initiative started to educate a number of first-generation Turkish and Moroccan migrant women as "migrant health educators." They were trained primarily as peers to communicate with women of the same background about health issues and the organization of the Dutch health care system. Most first-generation migrants have little education; basic information about the biology of the body, health, sickness, and health care is a real need for this group. The experience of health and sickness is strongly related to the culture in which a person is raised and lives.

With the growing epidemic of HIV in the 1980s, not only women but also men with different cultural backgrounds were trained as health educators, at first only on the issue of safe sex and later more broadly to encompass other public health issues.

Concurrently, general practitioners working in deprived city neighborhoods experienced an increasing workload and dissatisfaction with the quality of care they provided, especially for patients of migrant descent. General practitioners face not only language barriers but also cultural differences. For example, Turkish and Moroccan patients have other expectations of primary health-care practitioners than what is usual in the Dutch health care system; in general, these patients expect a prescription or referral to a specialist, whereas the Dutch system is reluctant to prescribe medicines and relies more on the personal responsibility of the patient. To support general practitioners in deprived areas, migrant health educators were trained to work as intermediaries between general practitioners and migrant patients. They bridge the gap by clarifying the patient's demand for medical aid on one hand and the treatment proposed by the medical doctor on the other hand. The advantage of a migrant health educator instead of a translator as an intermediary is that the health educator also has basic medical knowledge and skills for culture-specific discussions. Evaluation of the impact of this intermediary function showed increased satisfaction of the quality of care experienced by both the general practitioners and the patients (Gerits and others 2001). Also, the health educators facilitate preventive activities for the patients within the practice of the general practitioner—mainly in the format of group sessions on major public health issues.

In view of the positive results among the general practitioners, migrant health educators are now also working as intermediaries in other health care facilities like mother-and-child centers (to promote a healthy lifestyle during pregnancy and to support young migrant women in the care of their babies) and mental health care (to educate migrants about psychosocial stress and depressive and anxiety disorders and to improve access to mental health care; Hesselink and others, in press).

## SUMMARY

In view of the large cultural diversity of the Amsterdam population and related health problems, interventions to promote public health have to take this diversity into account to be effective. The city of Amsterdam has chosen a community-based approach by developing interventions together with migrant community organizations and supporting migrant health educators to bridge the gap between the (mainly) Dutch health care professionals and migrant patients. This approach has proven to be successful in reaching the specific risk groups within the population and improving the (perceived) quality of health care. Whether this approach also leads to an improvement of the health status of the Amsterdam population as a whole needs further evaluation.

## REFERENCES

Alderliesten, M., T.G.M. Vrijkotte, M. F. van der Wal, and G. J. Bonsel. 2007. Late start of antenatal care among ethnic minorities in a large cohort of pregnant women. *British Journal Obstetrics and Gynecology* 114:1232–1239.

Buster, M.C.A., G.H.A. Van Brussel, and W. Van den Brink. 2001. Estimating the number of opiate users in Amsterdam by capture recapture: The importance of case definition. *European Journal of Epidemiology* 17:935–994.

De Graaf, J. P., A.C.J. Ravelli, H.I.J. Wildschut, S. Denkta, A.J.J. Voorham, G. J. Bonsel, E.A.P. Steegers. 2008. Perinatal outcomes in the four largest cities and in neighbourhoods in the Netherlands. *Ned Tijdschr Geneeskd* 152:2734–2740.

De Wit, M.A.S., W. C. Tuinebrijer, J. Dekker, A.T.F. Beekman, W.H.M. Gorissen, A. C. Schier, B.W.J. H. Penninx, I. H. Komproe, and A. P. Verhoeff. 2008. Depressive and anxiety disorder in different ethnic groups: A population based study among native Dutch, and Turkish, Moroccan, and Surinamese migrants in Amsterdam. *Social Psychiatry and Psychiatric Epidemiology* 43:905–912.

Dijkshoorn, H. 2006. *The health status of the Surinamese population in Amsterdam*. Amsterdam: Public Health Service.

Gerits, Y. C., D. G. Uitenbroek, H. Dijkshoorn, and A. P. Verhoeff. 2001. The communication between the general practitioner and Turkish and Moroccan patients closer examined. *Tijdschrift voor Gezondheidswetenschappen* 79:16–20

Hesselink, A., A. P. Verhoeff, and K. Stronks. In press. Ethnic health care advisors: A good strategy to improve the access to health care and social welfare services for ethnic minorities? *Ethnicity and Health*.

Uitenbroek, D. G., J. K. Ujcic-Voortman, A. P. Janssen, P. J. Tichelman, and A. P. Verhoeff. 2006. *The Amsterdam Health Monitor 2004*. Amsterdam: Public Health Service.

Van den Hoek, J.A.R., D.K.F. Mulder-Folkerts, R. A. Coutinho, N.H.T.M. Dukers, M. Buimer, and G.J.J. Van Doornum. 1999. Opportunistische screening op genitale infecties met Chlamydia trachomatis onder de seksueel actieve bevolking in Amsterdam; meer dan 90% deelname en bijna 5% prevalentie. *Ned Tijdschr Geneeskd* 143:668–672.

Van Eijsden, M. 2008. *Ethnicity, nutrition and pregnancy: Food for thought.* Amsterdam: University of Amsterdam.

Van Zee, W., E. De Boer, C. Hylkema, and J. Slot. 2008. *Amsterdam in figures 2008.* Amsterdam: Amsterdam Office of Statistics.

Verhoeff, A. P., and A. Acda. 2007. *All inhabitants of Amsterdam healthy: Framework policy document for Amsterdam's public health policy 2008–2011.* Amsterdam: Public Health Service.

Veugelers, P. J., G. Van Zessen, J.C.M. Hendriks, T.G.M. Sandfort, R. A. Coutinho, G.J.P. Van Griensven. 1993. Estimation of the magnitude of the HIV epidemic among homosexual men: Utilization of survey data in predictive models. *European Journal of Epidemiology* 9:436–441.

Whitehead, M., and G. Dahlgren. 2006. *Levelling up: A discussion paper on concepts and principles for tackling social inequities in health.* Liverpool: WHO Collaborating Centre for Policy Research on Social Determinants of Health, University of Liverpool.

## CHAPTER SIX

# GLOBAL CLIMATE CHANGE AND CITIES

### TORD KJELLSTROM
### PATRICIA MONGE

---

**LEARNING OBJECTIVES**

- Identify evidence for climate change at the global, regional, and local levels
- Define the "heat island effect" in urban areas
- List the components of damaging health exposures
- List the range of clinical health and work-related impacts for heat exposures
- Identify elements required for mitigation of global climate change
- Describe the role of the health sector and other sectors (such as urban planning, infrastructure development, workplace management) in prevention of adverse urban health effects related to climate change

**C****LIMATE** change presents a threat to the ecological systems that support life and health of humans as well as all other species on this planet (IPCC 2007). Human beings have evolved within temperature, humidity, wind movement, and solar radiation—environments that have not varied much during thousands of years. The human core body temperature needs to be kept close to 37°C, which requires adaptation to the different climate zones on Earth, but there is a limit to our ability to adapt to heat, and the ongoing global climate change may well bring many areas beyond this limit. People also depend on local food systems, water systems, and other natural ecological services, which are not easily able to adapt to a changing climate. The greatest global health challenges may come from lack of food and water, direct effects of heat, extreme weather, and wider spread of certain infectious and vector-borne diseases (Costello and others 2009).

Cities are human creations with a distinctive impact on the climate. They produce heat due to the density of populations and their daily activities. Cities retain heat from sun radiation in their concrete and asphalt surfaces—the "heat island effect" (Oke 1973). They are also differentially vulnerable to floods and sea level rise, due to their location at rivers or sea coasts. Each of these features can create health risks to city populations.

But cities can also provide cooled environments via good urban design and other features that protect human health from climate extremes. However, city people will still depend on the natural ecological services from their surroundings, and low-income people may not have the resources to create a healthy living environment as global heating continues due to climate change.

## GLOBAL AND REGIONAL CLIMATE CHANGE TRENDS

Global climate change leads to an increase of average global temperature, changes of rainfall patterns and to more and longer periods of extreme weather (mainly extremely hot or violent weather, but in some places also extremely cold weather). The temperature increase may be between 1.8 and 4.0°C (average of the estimated increase is 3.0°C) until 2100 (IPCC 2007), depending on which actions

---

We acknowledge inputs from research colleagues during the drafting of this text, particularly the heat exposure trend modeling carried out by Bruno Lemke, and financial support from the universities we represent. Some of the text builds on analysis carried out for the World Health Organization by Tord Kjellstrom.

are taken during future years to limit greenhouse gas emissions. Different places on Earth will experience different degrees of change, but all populated areas are expected to get hotter (IPCC 2007).

The expected sea level rise (IPCC 2007) will create particular problems. In low- and middle-income countries with long coasts (for example, Bangladesh, India, and China) it will not be possible to protect large parts of the currently inhabited areas. Millions of people in both rural and urban areas will be affected by flooding, lack of access to food and safe drinking water, and associated health risks.

Climate conditions that are most directly related to urban health are the local climate trends in the geographic area of the city's location, where people actually spend time. Table 6.1 summarizes the trends in temperature change for eleven cities around the world. The greatest increases are seen in Shanghai, Osaka, Bangkok, Athens, and Cairo. In many cities, a part of the temperature increase is caused by the urban "heat island effect" (Oke 1973; USEPA 2009). This creates higher heat exposure in densely populated modern urban settings where large areas are covered by concrete buildings or tar-sealed roads that absorb and store solar heat radiation. The time trends for other urban environmental hazards (Kjellstrom and others 2007) will also influence heat-related health risks. This is particularly important for urban air pollution but applies also to water access and water quality, food storage and transport, occurrence of disease-carrying vectors,

TABLE 6.1  Summary of Temperature Change in Selected Cities, 1980 to 2007 (Degrees Per Century)

| City | Maximum (°C) | Average (°C) | Minimum (°C) |
|---|---|---|---|
| Johannesburg | +2.97 | −1.27 | −3.86 |
| Atlanta | −0.89 | +1.85 | +3.77 |
| Managua | +0.27 | +1.29 | +3.51 |
| Cairo | +2.62 | +4.84 | +6.58 |
| Athens | +4.09 | +5.30 | +5.14 |
| Delhi | +2.08 | +0.53 | +0.18 |
| Chennai | +2.87 | +0.41 | −0.43 |
| Bangkok | +4.52 | +5.19 | +5.37 |
| Chiang Mai | −1.13 | +0.22 | +0.77 |
| Osaka | +4.76 | +5.25 | +5.96 |
| Shanghai | +7.06 | +7.77 | +11.79 |

*Source:* Kjellstrom (2009a).

and vulnerability through people living and working in places exposed to impacts of weather extremes.

Several billion people will be affected by the increasing heat exposure due to ongoing local climate change. Air conditioning is not an option for outdoor activities (work, travel, exercise, and other daily activities) and low-income groups cannot afford it or live in ramshackle buildings in slums without windows or walls. The energy consumption of air conditioning contributes to the greenhouse gases that cause global warming (IPCC 2007), and large numbers of air conditioning units in an urban area adds to the heat island effect (for example in Hong Kong; Giridharan, Lau, and Ganesan 2005). Alternative methods to create an acceptable indoor climate are therefore of great importance, including building design that creates natural ventilation, building materials that isolate against heating of the indoor air, and urban design that reduces direct heat exposure and the "heat island effect" (USEPA 2009).

The time trends of other climate variables (for example, rainfall, cloud cover, air humidity, and wind movement) are also of importance for changes of the local heat exposure. For example, in Delhi where the average temperature is increasing (Table 6.1), the air humidity is also increasing, adding to the heat exposure trend.

The average hourly temperatures are important for heat exposures, generally peaking in the afternoons. Figure 6.1 shows hourly temperatures in the coolest

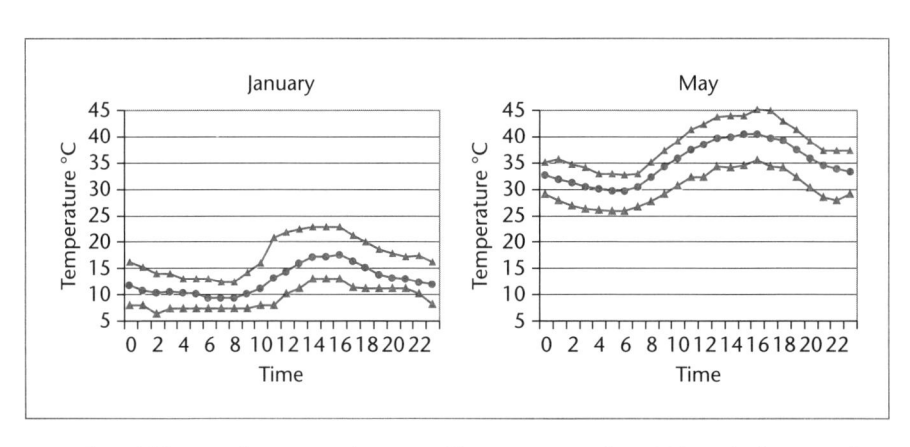

FIGURE 6.1 Hourly Air Temperatures, Delhi, for the Coldest and Hottest Months, 1999

*Note:* The middle curve is average; the top and bottom curves show 95th and 5th percentiles, between which lies 90 percent of daily observations.

*Data source:* NOAA hourly database.

(January) and hottest (May) months in Delhi. To accurately assess the potential health impact of increased direct heat exposure in different cities around the world, it is essential that seasonal and diurnal variations are estimated and described (Kjellstrom 2009a).

## DOCUMENTED AND POTENTIAL HEALTH THREATS OF CLIMATE CHANGE

The changes in the urban climate described in Figure 5.1 may have major health impacts via different environmental exposure pathways (Figure 5.2). Each pathway is important for health in cities, and actions to reduce exposures and effects can be taken at any stage in the pathways (Kjellstrom and others 2007).

The greatest changes in climate change-related health hazards are likely to take place in tropical low- and middle-income countries among poor people (Patz and others 2007; WHO 2008b). They do not have access to preventive measures, such as air conditioning (in homes, offices, cars, schools, and shops), strong housing design, or efficient escape mechanisms during floods. They also have less access to health services. Climate change mitigation and adaptation need to go hand-in-hand with the global efforts to achieve health equity (Friel and others 2008).

The local heat island effect (Oke 1973), due to poorly designed urbanization, contributes to the global health impacts of climate change (Figure 6.2). The population growth in urban settings has been particularly high in low- and middle-income countries. For example, in Asia between 1975 and 2000, urban population increased from 600 million to 1,400 million (WHO 2008a). This trend is expected to continue during the coming decades with a doubling of urban population by 2030.

The high population density in urban areas creates a high density of local air conditioners contributing to the heat island effect (Oke 1973) and a high density of motor vehicles contributing to health damaging air pollution. Densely populated urban neighborhoods with industrial areas and few trees have maximum temperatures during the day 1–3°C higher than parks or open landscape areas (Blazejyk and Kuhnert 2009). This aspect of urbanization and climate is amenable to preventive interventions via urban design, tree planting, and other shade creation.

In low- and middle-income countries, many of the people who migrate to urban areas end up in "slums," where the additional heat exposures due to climate change and the indirect risks (for example, extended lack of good quality drinking water) are much greater than in other parts of cities (WHO 2008a). The "slum" inhabitants may also use building materials (such as black corrugated steel panels

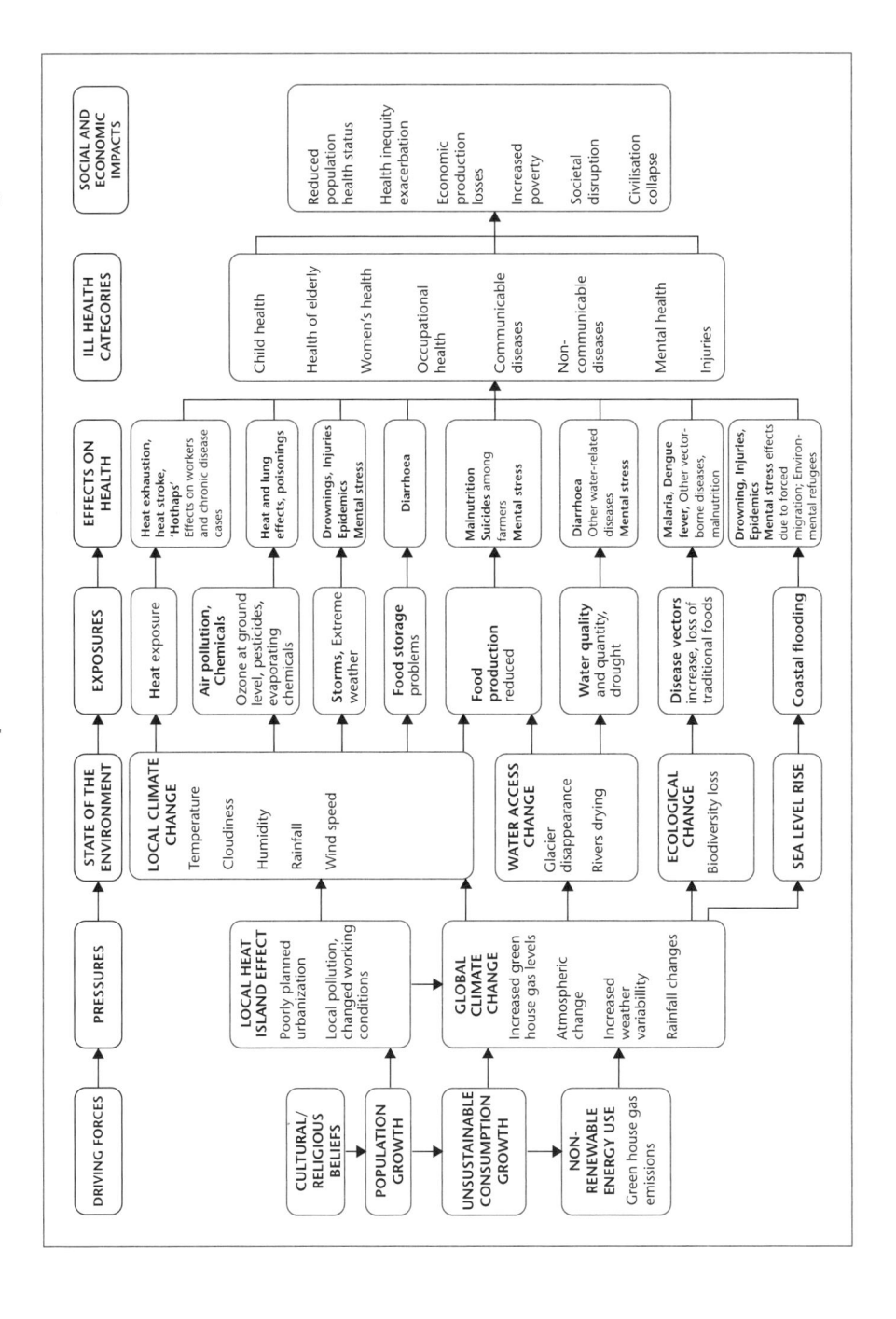

FIGURE 6.2 Health-Relevant Exposures and Effects of Global Climate Change

for roofs and walls) that attract heat from the sun and create intolerable "indoor" heat exposures.

Aging is another factor of importance because elderly people are vulnerable to climate-change health effects, and an increasing number of elderly with chronic diseases presents challenges for the health services (McMichael and others 2003).

## Impacts via Direct Heat Exposure

An increased mortality during heat waves has been reported from many cities around the world: United States (Luber and McGeehin 2008), Europe (Poumadere and others 2005), and developing countries (Hajat and others 2005). In France, 15,000 people died during the two-week heat wave in August 2003, and a similar number died in other countries of central and southern Europe. Extreme heat mortality is primarily a result of the cardiovascular system being "overloaded" due to the physiological reactions to heat exposure (Parsons 2003). In addition, acute hospital admissions and emergency ambulance transport for heart disease, asthma, and acute kidney diseases increases (Knowlton and others 2008; Hansen and others 2008; Kjellstrom, Butler, and others 2010). The most vulnerable people are children, the very elderly, and, for kidney diseases, middle-aged men.

Apart from temperature, other climate variables are important for the human health impacts: humidity, wind speed, and heat radiation (especially from the sun). Several heat stress indices incorporating these variables have been developed (Parsons 2003); the most widely used is the Wet Bulb Globe Temperature (WBGT), which is the basis for the widely used international standard for occupational heat exposure (ISO 1989). When WBGT exceeds 26°C, serious heat stress can occur among people working at high physical intensity, and WBGT above 32°C affects all working people (Kjellstrom, Holmer, and Lemke 2009). To avoid heat stroke, working people need to reduce physical activity (Parsons 2003), which reduces work output and daily productivity.

WBGT is ideally measured with special equipment, but measurements from weather stations can be used to calculate the WBGT for each hour, using an elaborate computer program (Liljegren and others 2008). Using the calculated WBGT heat stress values, one can estimate the need for rest periods to avoid core body temperature exceeding 38°C (ISO 1989). Work capacity is the remaining percentage of each hour that is left for actual work (Kjellstrom, Holmer, and Lemke 2009). In Delhi in May (Figure 6.3) between 09.00 and 17.00, WBGT exceeds 26°C and work capacity goes below 25 percent. This fits with work practices in India, where, for instance, during the hottest season, outdoor construction

**FIGURE 6.3  Calculated Hourly WBGT Outdoors in the Sun and Resulting Hourly "Work Capacity" for Workers in Heavy Labor Jobs (500 watts), Delhi, 1999**

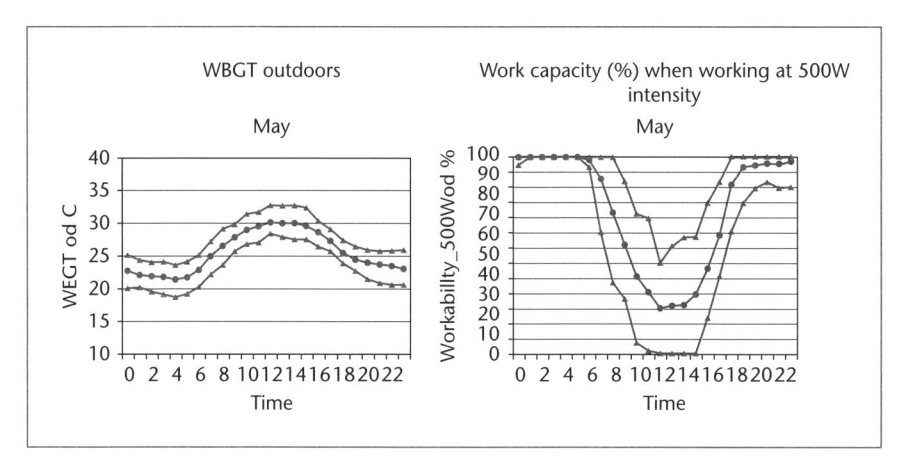

*Note:* The middle curve is the average; the top and bottom curves show 95th and 5th percentiles, between which lies 90 percent of daily observations.

These calculations have been updated and changed from similar figures in a previous report; Kjellstrom, 2009a.

workers take a five-hour "lunch break" and, in a car factory, two people have to be employed to cope with one person's job (Kjellstrom 2009b).

Heat exposure creates a need for additional liquid intake due to sweating (up to 10 liters per day; Parsons 2003). If sufficient water is not consumed, dehydration occurs with potential damage to the kidneys (Schrier and others 1967). Military personnel deployed in hot, arid climates have increased occurrence of kidney stones (Cramer and Forrest 2006). Kidney stone incidence is also highest in hot parts of the United States (Brikowski, Lotan, and Pearle 2008), such as during severe heat waves in Chicago (Semenza and others 1997). In Adelaide, Australia (Hansen and others 2008), there was increased emergency hospital admissions for acute renal failure and co-morbidity of renal disease.

An issue of importance is to what extent men and women are affected differently by the climate change health hazards (Jämting 2008; United Nations Gender and Climate Change [GENCC] 2008). In developing countries, women are more exposed to "double job schedules," since they work 8–10 hours in their usual jobs and are also in charge of household activities, most of them exposed to extra sources of heat (for example, cooking, ironing) and/or physical activities (cleaning, washing, carrying water and supplies). There are indications that biological differences make women less tolerant to heat stress than men (Duncan 2007). Women sweat less and have a higher metabolic rate and thicker subcutaneous fat that prevents them from cooling themselves as efficiently as men. During the heat wave in France in 2003 (15,000 deaths), female mortality was 15 to 20 percent higher than male mortality in the older age groups (Poumadere and others 2005). Among younger adults, men had higher mortality than women, which may be associated with occupational heat exposures, but no analysis of this has been carried out. Moreover, women generally endure more mental stress than men as the primary caregivers during and after extreme events, when health effects on children and elderly family members create stress.

If heat exposure is high enough to force a person to slow down daily physical activities, the time women in poor communities of tropical countries spend on collecting water, food, or firewood gets longer, and the time available for other important activities in the household gets shorter (Kes and Swaminathan 2006). This is likely to be a particular issue in rural areas, but in urban slums and other poor urban areas, extreme heat will affect daily life in a similar way.

For Delhi, we made a tentative estimate of the impact of current and future heat exposure on the work capacity in outdoor work (Figure 6.4). The current

FIGURE 6.4 Impact of Climate Change on the Annual Number of "Fully Workable Days" (out of 365 days) in Delhi at Two Levels of Work Intensity (200 and 500 watts)

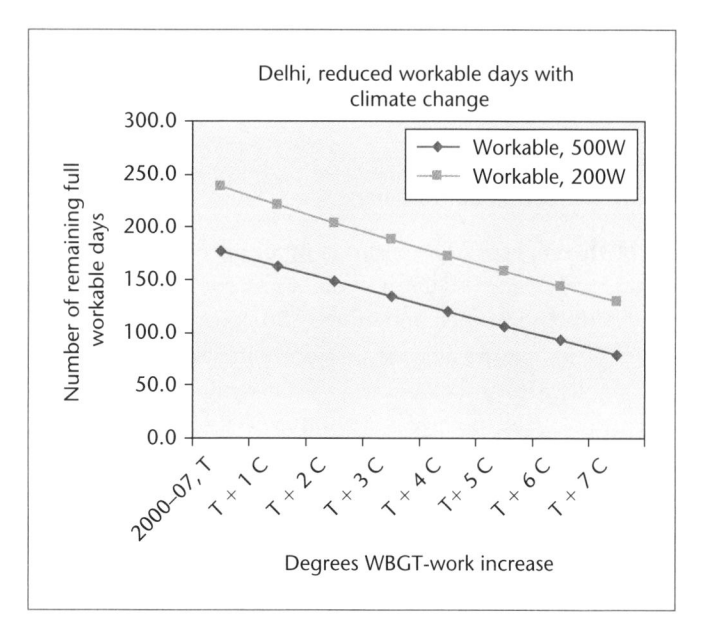

Note: WBGT-work is the heat stress level during daylight hours.

daily WBGT distribution was estimated tentatively with a formula published by the Australian Bureau of Meteorology (ABM 2009). Daily work capacity was estimated from the recommended rest periods by ISO (1989). The projected WBGT heat stress values are likely to increase at a rate slower than the climate-change-related temperature increase. Using this approach, the annual equivalent number of "workable days" might be substantially reduced with climate change (Figure 5.4).

Currently, heavy labor outdoors (500 watts) is restricted by heat to approximately 175 days per year (out of 365 days; Figure 5.4). As heat increases by 3°C, the fully workable day equivalent is reduced to 130 days, a loss of 45 working days per year or approximately 25 percent of current outdoor work productivity. These estimates are tentative, but a downward trend of outdoor workers' productivity in cities is certain unless working conditions are drastically changed.

Central America is another tropical area where urban health has been considered in relation to climate conditions as a part of the SALTRA (Salud y Trabajo en América Central) program in occupational health and safety (http://www.Saltra.info). The lowlands of Central America are generally hot, humid, and often plagued by disease, and the most important cities are located in the lowlands, with a few exceptions. A variety of job activities are developed in urban areas with high heat exposure: construction, transport, services (sales, sanitation, recreation, tourism, communication), manufacturing without air conditioning, and some professional activities (education, social work). Agriculture for the local urban market is often practiced close to the cities. People working in agriculture are particularly exposed to high heat stress due to their exposure to sunlight (Table 5.2), but this also applies to construction workers and some others. Many sun-exposed workers reside and work in urban areas.

## Impacts via Increased Air Pollution

One of the effects of increasing temperatures in cities is an increasing level of ground level ozone (Figure 6.2) due to motor vehicle emission interactions with solar UV radiation (Bell and others 2007); ozone formation is faster and greater when air temperature increases. Ozone increases incidence and mortality of heart and lung diseases and causes respiratory symptoms (WHO 2006).

Particulate air pollution is another well-known and widespread health hazard (for example, Brunekreef and Holgate 2002; Brunekreef and Forsberg 2005; WHO 2006). A significant proportion of the finest particles are secondary organic particles, condensed from gaseous $SO_2$ and $NO_2$ pollution, which are expected to increase over coming decades (WHO 2006). Studies where both heat and particulate air pollution were included in time series daily mortality analysis have

TABLE 6.2  Proportion of Male and Female Workers Regularly
Exposed to Sunlight During Work, Costa Rica

| ICEA II[a] | Job Activity | Men[b] | Women[b] |
|---|---|---|---|
| 113 | Agriculture | 0.85 | 0.3 |
| 120 | Forestry | 0.75 | 0.75 |
| 130 | Fishing | 0.85 | 0.3 |
| 500 | Construction | 0.60 | 0.3 |
| 711 | Land transportation | 0.13 | 0.13 |
| 719 | Services related with transportation | 0.50 | 0.5 |
| 941 | Recreational and cultural services | 0.40 | 0.4 |

[a] International Classification of Economic Activities, United Nations.
[b] Proportion of workers with exposure, among the total population of workers for the specific job activity.

*Source:* Chaves and others (2004).

shown a significant combined effect (for example, Hales and others 2000). Thus, an increased health impact of air pollution in cities is a likely outcome of climate change (Bernard and others 2001).

A particular type of air pollution that is associated with climate is pollen from selected plants, which causes allergies (Beggs 2004). Approximately 15–20 percent of young adults in Sweden are allergic to pollen (SOU 2007), and pollen allergies represent 40 percent of all allergies in Sweden. Reports from Europe and North America indicate that the start of the pollen season is moving to earlier dates, most likely due to climate change (IPCC 2007).

## Impacts via Increased Chemical Exposures

When the climate gets warmer, certain environmental toxic chemicals will evaporate more easily and cause higher exposure via air in workplaces and in the general environment (Figure 6.2). Absorption through skin may also increase (Johanson and Boman 1991). This climate change health risk is likely to be of importance both in rural and urban environments. In particular, the poor working conditions in urban slums may interact with climate change to create additional health risks (WHO 2008a). There will also be changes in the long-distance transport of environmental chemicals, such as the "persistent organic pollutants" (POPs; Grandjean, Bjerregaard, and Weihe 2009). Extreme weather and floods can also cause chemical contamination from industries, damaged sewage systems, or hazardous waste dumps, all having importance in densely populated urban areas.

### Impacts via Extreme Weather

Climate change is likely to create more extreme weather incidents (IPCC 2007), which will cause droughts, floods, and landslides that block roads and damage houses; windy typhoons or hurricanes damage electricity supply, water supply, buildings, and so on (Figure 6.2). A variety of health impacts and threats can be predicted in cities: drowning, injuries, food shortages, contamination of or lack of drinking water, vector-borne diseases, lack of health services, and so on (McMichael and others 2003). The most vulnerable will be poor people and people with pre-existing chronic diseases or disabilities. The effects of flooding in New Orleans on elderly rest home patients and other poor people, who suffered lack of transport for evacuation, showed what might happen in affected urban areas (Sharkey 2007).

Other groups that are particularly affected by extreme weather events are emergency workers, firefighters, and police involved in efforts to reduce the health impacts on a local population. In addition to burns, injuries, and heat stress, these occupations are affected by mental stress symptoms, depression, and post-traumatic stress disorder (for example, Hurricane Katrina in New Orleans; Tak and others 2007; West and others 2008; NIOSH 2007).

### Impacts via Malnutrition

Malnutrition was estimated to be the greatest contributor to climate-change-related mortality 1990–2000 (McMichael and others 2004). This is primarily due to droughts and other climate calamities affecting subsistence farmers in rural areas of low-income countries (Figure 6.2). It will also indirectly affect access to food in urban areas. The estimated impact of climate change on agricultural production by 2080 shows reductions in all highly populated tropical and subtropical areas (Cline 2007). Lack of local food production will lead to rising prices, and poor people are most likely to be affected, an important aspect of the health equity threats that climate change will bring (Friel and others 2008).

Malnutrition is a major cause of ill health in young children, being linked to specific nutritional deficiency diseases and common diseases, such as diarrhea and acute respiratory infections. Pregnant women with low nutrition status give birth to low-birth-weight children, a major health hazard for children. Fetal, antenatal, and childhood undernutrition or malnutrition affects health status in later life (Gluckman and Hanson 2006) and contributes to cardiovascular disease, obesity, diabetes and other metabolic disorders in later life (Barker 1999).

## Impacts on Infectious and Vector-borne Diseases

Assessments of specific medical conditions related to climate change have focussed on infectious and vector-borne diseases in developing countries (McMichael and others 2003), and their causal pathways clearly involve climate factors (Gage and others 2008; Figure 6.2). Climatic conditions such as temperature, precipitation, sunshine, and wind can affect and accelerate their dispersion and their increase. Infectious diseases and toxin food poisoning can be caused by contamination and too-high storage temperatures (Hall, D'Souza, and Kirk 2002), for example, *Staphylococcus aureus*, *Clostridium perfringens*, and *Salmonella*.

Several vector-borne diseases have been reviewed by Gage and others (2008) and categorized by vector type and pathogen (Table 6.3). Malaria and dengue fever are of particular concern at the global level, but as Table 6.3 indicates, a number of locally important diseases may also be influenced by climate change.

TABLE 6.3  Climate-related Vector-borne Diseases by Vector and Pathogen Types

| Vectors or Pathogens | Parasites | Arbo-viruses | Bacteria and Rickettsia |
|---|---|---|---|
| Mosquitoes | Malaria | Dengue fever | |
| | | Yellow fever | |
| | | Chikungunya fever | |
| | | West Nile virus | |
| | | Rift Valley fever | |
| | | Ross River virus | |
| Ticks | | Tick-borne encephalitis (TBE) | Lyme borreliosis |
| | | | Tularemia |
| | | | Human granulocytic anaplasmosis |
| | | | Human monocytic ehrlichiosis |
| Other | | | Plague |
| Sand flies | Leishamniasis | | |
| Triatomine bugs | Chagas disease | | |
| Black flies | Onchocerciasis | | |

*Source:* Gage and others (2008).

### Impact on Chronic Diseases

A disease that strongly interacts with heat exposure is multiple sclerosis (MS; Selhorst and Saul 1995). Direct heat exposure can also interact with other chronic diseases by worsening the clinical state of prevalent cases (Kjellstrom, Butler, and others 2010).

Obesity has been shown as a risk factor for heat disorders, even among young, relatively fit military personnel (Chung and Pin 1996). It should also be noted that heat reduces a person's ability and inclination to carry out physical activity, impacting on exercise activities and active transport, which are important for obesity prevention, particularly in modern cities with sedentary lifestyles.

### Other Effects and Concerns

Figure 6.2 includes some other effects such as mental stress associated with extreme weather, lack of food, and forced migration (Berry and others 2008; Berry, Bowen, and Kjellstrom 2009). Adaptation to climate change may cause mental stress in urban areas through major changes in people's "normal" lives.

## CITY POLICIES AND ACTIONS TO REDUCE THE HEALTH IMPACTS OF CLIMATE CHANGE

There are many ways that cities can protect and improve urban health through policies and actions related to climate impacts on health. Table 6.4 shows a number of examples, but the list could be made much longer if specific detailed actions that have been implemented in individual cities were reviewed.

Many of the studies of heat-related mortality have been carried out at city level, but few attempts have been made to estimate the future urban health impact as climate change progresses. One analysis for Australian cities (McMichael and others 2002) calculated that hundreds of additional heat-related deaths would occur, but this, of course, depends on the extent to which preventive interventions are implemented. After the extreme heat-wave mortality in France in 2003, the local health authorities implemented improved climate control in old age homes and other places, and the heat mortality risk was significantly reduced in subsequent heat waves (Fouillet and others 2006).

Studies in Shanghai, Delhi, and a number of cities in high income countries have shown that daily mortality is associated with increasing temperature, not only during heat waves, but also as a basic phenomenon (McMichael and others 2003). The examples given in Figure 6.1 and Table 6.1 indicate the increasing exposures and potential effects of climate change in cities.

TABLE 6.4   Examples of City Policies and Actions that Can Reduce Climate Change Impacts

| Climate Issue | Policies and Actions | Type |
|---|---|---|
| Local green house gas emissions | Encourage active transport (walking, bicycling) and use of energy efficient public transport (reduce unnecessary private motor vehicle use) | M |
| | Discourage unnecessary air transport to and from the city, for instance, by establishing convenient and cost-effective broadband access and videoconferencing facilities | M |
| | Design new buildings for improved heat insulation, natural ventilation and cooling (reduce unnecessary air conditioner use) | M |
| | Encourage growing of food in local urban spare land or on rooftops (reduce unnecessary long-distance transport of certain food items) | M |
| Urban heat island effect | Plant trees for shade along urban buildings and walkways | PA |
| | Provide light color on roofs and walls | PA |
| | Limit tar seal areas by proactive urban planning, including underground vehicle parking and transport | PA |
| | Provide fountains, ponds, parks, and other water features (evaporating water reduces local heat) | PA |
| Climate in living spaces | [Same as actions above] | PA |
| | Improve insulation against cold and heat in buildings to reduce heating and cooling needs | M+PA |
| | Shade overhangs on sidewalks, bicycle ways, and walkways (common practice in Australia) | PA |
| | Double wall and roof panels to provide natural insulation from heated building materials (common practice in Australia) | PA |
| | Adjustable outside window blinds to reduce direct sunlight on windows, or outside window shutters totally closed during hot days (common practice in South Europe) | PA |
| | Natural cooling ventilation in building design | PA |
| | Reduce excessive crowding | PA |
| Climate in working spaces | [Same as above for industrial and office buildings, to the extent possible] | PA |
| | Shield outdoor workers from direct sunlight via light roofs on wheels | PA |
| | Shield indoor workers from direct heat radiation sources | PA |
| | Provide fans or air conditioning in general work space when possible | PA |
| | Provide air conditioned small rooms or vehicle cabs within larger hot area when workers are relatively stationary | PA |

*(Continued)*

**84  URBAN HEALTH**

TABLE 6.4 (Continued)

| Climate Issue | Policies and Actions | Type |
|---|---|---|
| Climate in public spaces and commercial areas | *[Same as above for shops, schools, health services, sports facilities, and other community buildings]* | PA |
| | Provide swimming pools for cooling down and exercise purposes | PA |
| Vulnerability to weather extremes | Avoid buildings next to rivers or streams that may flood and next to seacoasts potentially affected by sea level rise or storm surges | PA |
| | Encourage design of buildings that can sustain strong storm winds and major rainfall | PA |
| | Develop warning systems, evacuation plans, and emergency preparedness (health services and access to water, food, energy, information, and transport) | PA |
| Vulnerability to diseases: vector-borne, communicable and chronic | Improve general population health status that reduces vulnerability (less occurrence of diseases that can be prevented with good primary health care) | PA |
| | Develop health and vector monitoring systems that provide early warning of increasing risks | PA |
| | Develop health services for early treatment of any climate-related diseases that may occur | PA |

*Note:* M = mitigation, PA = preventive intervention and adaptation.

Most of the policies and actions in Table 6.4 would be the responsibility of community sectors other than the health sector. This highlights the need for a broad awareness among professionals and in the community about health threats caused by climate exposures. Such threats occur already now, and they will increase in the future.

Table 6.4 starts with environmental issues concerning climate change, which need to be addressed via mitigation that reduces greenhouse gas emissions (see also Figure 6.2). For the health sector, maybe the most important issues are those concerning the population's vulnerability to climate-related exposures. It is important to note that improvement of the general population's health status in poor communities (where infectious diseases, vector-borne diseases, and a low level of nutrition are common) will provide significant protection against the health threats of climate change. In the assessment of the impact on mortality due to global climate change from 1990 to 2000 (McMichael and others 2004), it was found that more than 90 percent of the assessed deaths occurred in low- and middle-income countries with a generally poor level of population health.

The risks of climate-change-related malnutrition, infectious diseases, vector-borne diseases, and health impacts of extreme weather events are likely to be much lower in communities with a good population health status. Most of the preventive interventions listed in Table 6.4 can be considered as "adaptations" to climate change, but they are in fact of value for health protection already in the current climate situation.

## SUMMARY

Climate change is already occurring, and the climate in cities is more affected than in rural areas because of the "urban heat island effect." The additional climate change during this century will create great challenges for health in cities. A changing climate can cause a variety of direct and indirect health effects. Many of them depend on the extent of climate change in the local area, whereas others are more influenced by regional or even global climate change. The health sector in cities has a crucial role in raising awareness about hazards related to climate variables and in providing expertise concerning preventive interventions. It is also clear that a poor general population status in poor communities creates particular vulnerability to climate variables and climate change. Therefore, policies and actions by the health sector to improve population health are important for climate change vulnerability reduction. Most of the other policies and actions for mitigation and preventive interventions are outside the main responsibilities of the health sector, but encouragement toward action by other sectors is an important role of the health sector.

## REFERENCES

Australian Bureau of Meteorology (ABM). 2009. The WBGT heat stress index. http://www.bom.gov.au/info/thermal_stress/.

Barker, D.J.P. 1999. Fetal nutrition and cardiovascular disease in later life. *British Medical Bulletin* 53: 96–108.

Beggs, P. J. 2004. Impacts of climate change on aeroallergens: past and future. *Clinical & Experimental Allergy* 34:1507–1513.

Bell, M. L., R. Goldberg, C. Hogrefe, P. L. Kinney, K. Knowlton, B. Lynn, J. Rosenthal, C. Rosenzweig, and J. A. Patz. 2007. Climate change, ambient ozone, and health in 50 U.S. cities. *Climate Change* 82:61–76.

Bernard, S. M., J. M. Samet, A. Grambsch, K. L. Ebi, and I. Romieu. 2001. The potential impacts of climate variability and change on air pollution-related health effects in the United States. *Environmental Health Perspectives* 109, Suppl. 2:199–209.

Berry, H. L., B. J. Kelly, I. C. Hanigan, J. H. Coates, A. J. McMichael, J. A. Welsh, and T. Kjellstrom. 2008. *Rural mental health impacts of climate change*. Commissioned report for the *Garnaut Climate Change Review*. Canberra: The Australian National University.

Berry, H. L., K. Bowen, and T. Kjellstrom. 2009 (in press). Climate change and mental health: a causal pathways framework. *International Journal of Public Health*.

Blazejzyk, K., and A. Kuhnert. 2009. Bio-thermal conditions in Warsaw. http://nargeo.geo.uni.lodz.pl/~icuc5/text/P_1_8.pdf.

Brikowski, T. H., Y. Lotan, and M. S. Pearle. 2008. Climate-related increase in the prevalence of urolithiasis in the United States. *Proceedings of the National Academy of Sciences* 105(28):9841–9846.

Brunekreef, B., and B. Forsberg. 2005. Epidemiological evidence of effects of coarse particles on health. *European Respiratory Journal* 26:309–318.

Brunekreef, B., and S. T. Holgate. 2002. Air pollution and health. *The Lancet* 360:1233–1242.

Chaves, J., and others. 2004. Occupational exposure matrix for carcinogens and pesticides in Costa Rica (Matriz de exposiciones ocupacionales a agentes carcinogénicos y plaguicidas en Costa Rica). Serie Informes Técnicos IRET No 2. Heredia, Costa Rica: Universidad Nacional, Instituto Regional de Estudios en Sustancias Tóxicas.

Chung, N. K., and C. H. Pin. 1996. Obesity and the occurrence of heat disorders *Military Medicine* 161:739–742.

Cline, W. R. 2007. *Global warming and agriculture: Impact estimates by country*. Washington, DC: Center for Global Development, Peterson Institute for International Economics,

Costello, A., M. Abbas, A. Allen, S. Ball, S. Bell, R. Bellamy, S. Freil, and others (Lancet-University College London Institute for Global Health Commission). 2009. Managing the health effects of climate change. *The Lancet* 373:1693–1733.

Cramer, J. S., and K. Forrest. 2006. Renal lithiasis: addressing the risks of austere desert deployments. *Aviation, Space and Environmental Medicine* 77:649–653.

Duncan, K. 2007. Global climate change and women's health. *Women & Environments International Magazine* 74/75:10–11.

Fouillet, A., G. Rey, F. Laurent, G. Pavillon, S. Bellec, C. Ghihenneuc-Jouyaux, J. Clavel, E. Jougla, and D. Hémon. 2006. Excess mortality related to the August 2003 heat wave in France. *International Archive Occupational Environmental Health* 80:16–24.

Friel, S., M. Marmot, A. J. McMichael, T. Kjellstrom, and D. Vagero. 2008. Global health equity and climate stabilization: A common agenda. *The Lancet* 372:1677–1683.

Gage, K. L., T.R. Burkot, R. J. Eisen, and E. B. Hayes. 2008. Climate change and vector-borne diseases. *American Journal of Preventive Medicine* 35:436–450.

Giridharan, S., S. S. Y. Lau, and S. Ganesan. 2005. Nocturnal heat island effect in urban residential developments in Hong Kong. *Energy & Buildings* 37:964–971.

Gluckman P. D., and M. A. Hanson. 2006. Adult disease: echoes of the past. *European Journal of Endocrinology* 155:S47–S50.

Grandjean P., P. Bjerregaard, and P. Weihe. 2009. Climate change implications for contaminant exposures in the Arctic. In IOP Conference series: Earth and Environmental Science 6. http://www.iop.org/EJ/article/1755-1315/6/14/142004/ees9_6_142004.pdf?request-id=92671412-dbb1-4768-815d-8ba2b0f2e4b9.

Hajat, S., and others. 2005. Mortality displacement of heat-related deaths: A comparison of Delhi, São Paulo and London. *Epidemiology* 16:313.

Hales, S., C. Salmond, I. C. Town, T. Kjellstrom, and A. Woodward. 2000. Daily mortality in relation to weather and air pollution in Christchurch, New Zealand. *Australian and New Zealand Journal of Public Health* 24:89–91.

Hall, G. V., R. M. D'Souza, and M. D. Kirk. 2002. Food-borne disease in the new millennium: Out of the frying pan and into the fire? *Medical Journal of Australia* 177:614–618.

Hansen A. L., P. Bi, P. Ryan, M. Nitschke, D. Pisaniello, and G. Tucker. 2008. The effect of heat waves on hospital admissions for renal disease in a temperature city of Australia. *International Journal of Epidemiology* 37:1359–1365.

Inter-governmental Panel on Climate Change (IPCC). 2007. *Fourth assessment report*. Cambridge: Cambridge University Press. Also available online at http://www.ipcc.ch.

International Standards Organization (ISO). 1989. Hot environments—Estimation of the heat stress on working man, based on the WBGT-index (wet bulb globe temperature). ISO Standard 7243. Geneva: ISO.

Jämting H. 2008. Gender and climate change. Report for Society, Nature and Change course. Uppsala: Swedish University of Agriculture Science.

Johanson, G., and A. Boman. 1991. Percutaneous absorption of 2-butoxyethanol vapour in human subjects. *British Journal of Industrial Medicine* 48:788–792.

Kes, A., and H. Swaminathan. 2006. Gender and time poverty in Sub-Saharan Africa. In *Gender, time use and poverty in Sub-Saharan Africa*. World Bank working paper no. 73, ed. C. M. Blackden and Q. Wodon, 13–38. Washington, DC: World Bank.

Kjellstrom, T. 2009a. Climate change exposures, chronic diseases and mental health in urban populations—A threat to health security, particularly for the poor and disadvantaged. Technical report to the WHO Kobe Centre. Kobe: World Health Organization.

Kjellstrom, T. 2009b. Climate change, direct heat exposure, health and well-being in low and middle income countries. *Global Health Action* 2:1–4. Also available online at http://www.globalhealthaction.net/index.php/gha/article/view/1958/2183.

Kjellstrom, T., S. Friel, J. Dixon, C. Corvalan, E. Rehfuess, D. Campbell-Lendrum, F. Gore, and J. Bartram. 2007. Urban environmental health hazards and health equity. *Journal of Urban Health* 84:i86–i97.

Kjellstrom, T., A. J. Butler, R. M. Lucas, and R. Bonita. 2010. Public health impact of global heating due to climate change: Potential effects on chronic non-communicable diseases. *International Journal of Public Health* 55(2):97–103.

Kjellstrom, T., I. Holmer, and B. Lemke. 2009. Workplace heat stress and health—An increasing challenge for low and middle income countries during climate change. *Global Health Action*. http://www.globalhealthaction.net/index.php/gha/issue/view/282.

Kovats, R. S., and S. Hajat. 2008. Heat stress and public health: A critical review. *Annual Review of Public Health* 29:9.1–9.15.

Knowlton, K., M. Rotkin-Ellman, G. King, and others. 2008. The 2006 California heat wave: Impacts of hospitalizations and emergency department visits. *Environmental Health Perspectives* 117:61–67.

Liljegren, J. C., R. A. Carhart, P. Lawday, S. Tschopp, and R. Sharp. 2008. Modeling the wet bulb globe temperature using standard meteorological measurements. *Journal of Occupational and Environmental Hygiene* 5(10):645–655.

Luber, G., and M. McGeehin. 2008. Climate change and extreme heat events. *American Journal of Preventive Medicine* 35:429–435.

McMichael, A. J., R. Woodruff, P. Whetton, K. Hennessy, N. Nicholls, S. Hales, A. Woodward, and T. Kjellstrom. 2002. Human health and climate change in Oceania: A risk assessment. Canberra: Commonwealth of Australia, Department of Health and Ageing.

McMichael, A. J., D. Campbell-Lendrum, S. Kovats, S. Edwards, P. Wilkinson, T. Wilson, R. Nicholls, S. Hales, F. Tanser, D. Le Sueur, M. Schlesinger, and N. Andronova. 2004. Global climate change. In *Comparative quantification of health risks*, Vol. 2, ed. Ezzati and others, 1543–1650. Geneva: World Health Organization.

McMichael, A. J., D. Campbell-Lendrum, K. Ebi, A. Githeko, J. Scheraga, and A. Woodward. 2003. *Climate change and human health: risks and responses*. Geneva: World Health Organization.

National Institute of Occupational Safety and Health (NIOSH). 2007. *Hurricane Katrina response*. NIOSH health hazard evaluation report, HETA no. 2005-0369-3043. Atlanta: NIOSH.

Oke, T. R. 1973. City size and the urban heat island. *Atmospheric Environment* 7:769–779.

Parsons, K. 2003. Human thermal environment. In: Parsons, K., ed. *The effects of hot, moderate and cold temperatures on human health, comfort and performance*. 2nd ed. New York: CRC Press.

Patz, J. A., H. K. Gibbs, J. A. Foley, J. V. Rogers, and K. R. Smith. 2007. Climate change and global health: Quantifying a growing ethical crisis. *EcoHealth* 4:397–405.

Poumadere, M., C. Mays, S. Le Mer, and R. Blong. 2005. The 2003 heat wave in France: Dangerous climate change here and now. *Risk Analysis* 25:1483–1494.

Schrier, R.W., H. S. Henderson, C. C. Tisher, and R. L. Tannen. 1967. Nephropathy associated with heat stress and exercise. *Annals of Internal Medicine* 67:356–376.

Selhorst, J. B., and R. F. Saul. 1995. Uhthoff and his symptom. *Journal of Neuroophthalmolology* 15:63–69.

Semenza, J. C., J. E. McCullough, D. Flanders, M. A. McGeehin, and J. R. Lumpkin. 1997. Excess hospital admissions during the July 1995 heat wave in Chicago. *American Journal of Preventive Medicine* 16:269–277.

Sharkey, P. 2007. Survival and death in New Orleans: An empirical look at the human impact of Katrina. *Journal of Black Studies* 37:482–501.

SOU. 2007. Climate and vulnerability investigation (Klimat-och sårbarhetsutredningen). Report no. 60. Stockholm: SOU.

Tak, S., R. Driscoll, B. Bernard, and C. West. 2007. Depressive symptoms among firefighters and related factors after the response to Hurricane Katrina. *Journal of Urban Health* 84:153–161.

United Nations Gender and Climate Change [GENCC]. 2008. Written submission by Centre for Organisation Research and Education. http://www.un.org/esa/socdev/unpfii/documents/E_C19_2008_CRP_5.pdf.

U.S. Environmental Protection Agency (USEPA). 2009 (last updated July 9). Heat island effect. http://www.epa.gov/heatisld/about/index.htm.

West, C., B. Bernard, C. Mueller, M. Kitt, R. Driscoll, and S. Tak. 2008. Mental health outcomes in police personnel after Hurricane Katrina. *Journal of Occupational Environmental Medicine* 50:689–695.

World Health Organization (WHO). 2006. *WHO air quality guidelines for particulate matter, ozone, nitrogen dioxide and sulphur dioxide*, global update 2005. Summary of risk assessment. Geneva: World Health Organization.

World Health Organization (WHO; chair and lead writer T. Kjellstrom). 2008a. *Our cities, our health, our future: Acting on social determinants for health equity in urban settings*. Kobe, Japan: World Health Organization, Centre for Health Development.

World Health Organization (WHO). 2008b. *Protecting health from climate change: World Health Day 2008*. Geneva: World Health Organization.

# CHAPTER SEVEN

# AGE-FRIENDLY NEW YORK CITY

**RUTH FINKELSTEIN**

**JULIE NETHERLAND**

## LEARNING OBJECTIVES

- Discuss the age-friendly cities paradigm for planning for the needs of older urban residents

- Identify how a specific urban environment, New York City, impedes and facilitates active aging

- Describe a model for engaging public and private stakeholders in planning to address urban health challenges

**THIS** chapter will introduce readers to the Age-friendly New York City project, a private-public partnership to address the growing numbers of older urban residents in New York City. After providing some general demographic and descriptive information about New York City and its older adult population, this chapter explains how New York used a new paradigm for planning to engage local government and the private sector in a comprehensive assessment of the needs of older New Yorkers. It concludes with a description of the findings from that assessment and plans for moving toward the implementation of concrete steps to insure that older residents can participate fully in the life of the city.

## OVERVIEW OF THE CITY

New York City is home to more than 8.2 million people (NYC DOHMH 2008). With 321.8 square miles of land and a city budget of more than $53 billion, New York is a large and complex urban environment and one the most ethnically and racially diverse cities in the United States. New Yorkers come from all corners of the globe; more than 174 languages are spoken in New York City. According to figures from the 2000 census, 44 percent (2.9 million) of the adult population is foreign-born; 46 percent of the population speaks a language other than English at home (NYC Department of City Planning 2004). Of those who are foreign born, 53 percent are from Latin America, 19 percent are from Europe, 24 percent are from Asia, and 3 percent are from Africa (NYC DOHMH 2008). In 2000, 35 percent of New Yorkers were white, 25 percent were Black, 27 percent were Hispanic, 10 percent were Asian, and 4 percent were another race or multiple races (NYC DOHMH 2004).

Compared to the United States average, New Yorkers are more likely to live below the poverty line (21 percent versus 12 percent; NYC DOHMH 2004). New York is also a city with tremendous economic disparities—the wealthiest 20 percent of residents enjoy about 50 percent of the city's income, while the poorest 50 percent of the population earn less than 20 percent of the city's income (NYC DOHMH 2004).

On average, New Yorkers enjoy good health. The average life expectancy for someone born in 2006 is 75.9 years for men and 81.7 years for women (NYC DOHMH 2008). The death rate of 6.5 per 1,000 has been steadily declining for the past several decades (NYC DOHMH 2008). By far, the single largest cause of death is heart disease (40 percent), followed by lung cancer (5 percent), cerebrovascular disease (3 percent), and AIDS (2 percent; NY State Department of Health 2008).

Unfortunately, the disparities in health status based on race and income are stark. For example, the life expectancy of those living in New York City's poorest neighborhoods is eight years less than those living in its wealthiest ones (NYC DOHMH 2004). Black males, on average, live six years less than their white male peers, and there is a difference of three years in the life expectancy of Black and white females (NYC DOHMH 2004). In fact, Black men living in Harlem are less likely to reach the age of 65 than men in Bangladesh (Marmot 2001). Those living in New York City's low-income neighborhoods do more poorly on a host of health indicators, including hospitalizations for asthma, diabetes, and drug use. Besides having high rates of morbidity and mortality, Blacks and Hispanics, who are disproportionately poor, have more trouble accessing health care (NYC DOHMH 2004) and are much more likely to live in poor housing conditions (NYC DOHMH 2004). New York has always been a city of neighborhoods, and health disparities are concentrated in particular communities (NYC DOHMH 2004).

## GOVERNANCE AND RANGE OF PUBLIC HEALTH INTERVENTIONS

New York City has a mayoral-council system and a city charter that gives the executive branch significant control over a number of functions, including public health. The commissioner of health is appointed by the mayor and sets priorities for the Department of Health and Mental Hygiene (DOHMH). DOHMH is advised by an eleven-member board of health comprising experts from a broad range of health disciplines who are appointed by the mayor with the consent of the city council to oversee the city's health code. Although DOHMH has established three district health offices in neighborhoods with the greatest health disparities, most functions remained centralized. The city council passes bills and regulations related to the health of city, and local community boards make decisions about zoning that affect the built environment. However, in New York City, the executive branch plays a particularly prominent role in public health because of the governance structure of the city and the funding available to it. New York City also has a well-developed health care infrastructure, including a system of public hospitals and clinics and some of the world's leading academic medical centers.

NYC DOHMH has been seen as a leader in public health innovation. In 2004, under the leadership of Thomas Frieden, MD, the commissioner of DOHMH at the time, the department launched a major campaign called Take Care New York that provided an evidence-based framework for its comprehensive health promotion agenda. For each of ten priority areas, DOHMH set goals for improvement and suggested steps individuals, health providers, businesses, and community- and faith-based organizations could take to improve the health of New Yorkers. In the first four years of the program, progress was made on nine of the ten goals: smoking rates decreased from 21.6 percent to 16.9 percent; colonoscopy screening increased 48 percent; and infant mortality fell by 10 percent (NYC DOHMH 2009). In addition to education and direct service programs, DOHMH's success also may be due to the fact that many of its strategies include structural interventions as well as regulatory and policy changes, such as prohibiting smoking in public places, taxing tobacco products, banning the use of trans fats by restaurants, and requiring chain restaurants to post calorie counts.

## URBAN INTERVENTION

Despite New York City's relatively good health and innovative prevention policies, the city is facing an enormous challenge borne out of its shifting demographics. In New York City—as in other urban centers—globalization, urbanization, and aging have converged to place unprecedented demands on city infrastructure and planning.

### Overview of Older New Yorkers

The number of people over the age of 65 in New York City is projected to rise 44.2 percent, from 938,000 in 2000 to 1.35 million in 2030 (NYC Department of City Planning 2006). The city's total population is projected to increase by almost one million over the next twenty years—an increase due in part to increased immigration and longevity (NYC Department of City Planning 2006). New Yorkers are living longer than the average American: by 2030, one in every five New Yorkers will be over age 60. Currently, one million older adults call New York City home; this number is expected to increase to 1.35 million by 2030 (NYC Department of City Planning 2006). Also by 2030, there will be more older people than school-age children in the city (NYC Department of City Planning 2006). The diversity of New York's older population is also expected to grow as the current African American, Hispanic, and Asian populations (in the aggregate representing over 50 percent of the total population) age and immigrants of all ages continue to move into city.

New York City has a number of features that make it an extremely attractive place for older adults, including good public transportation, cultural richness, excellent medical centers, proximity of stores, and a wide array of social services. However, New York also poses a number of unique challenges. The high cost of living burdens many, particularly the large numbers of older poor living in the city.

Almost one-third of older New Yorkers live in poverty, according to the New York City Center for Economic Opportunity (Finkelstein and others 2008). There are also gaps in the accessibility and coverage of public transportation, and appropriate and affordable housing for older New Yorkers is already in short supply.

The diversity of New York City, a tremendous source of the city's strength, also creates difficulties in ensuring culturally appropriate services. Like older people everywhere, older New Yorkers face significant health and mental health challenges (AARP 2002; NYC Department for the Aging 2007). Disability rates among older New Yorkers are higher than comparable rates nationally. In 2005, 42 percent of the total elderly population aged 65 and over in the civilian non-institutionalized population reported some form of disability (Walker and Mayer 2007). Older New Yorkers, particularly the disabled, face a number of barriers to their full participation in city life. Leaving the workforce, the relocation of family members, ageism, and the difficulty in navigating inaccessible housing, sidewalks, and businesses all contribute to isolation. Ensuring that older New Yorkers are able to stay connected, active, healthy, and participate fully in the life of the city is the primary goal of the Age-friendly New York City project.

## A New Planning Paradigm

New York, like other major cities, is at the nexus of two global trends—population aging and urbanization. As of 2007, over half the world's population lived in cities, and by 2030, that proportion will rise to about three out of every five people in the world. At the same time, improvements in public health have led to more and more people living longer lives. As a result, the proportion of people aged 60 and over will likely double from 11 percent of the world's population in 2006 to 22 percent by 2050 (WHO 2007).

These trends require new approaches to planning. Traditionally in the United States, urban planning efforts have addressed the challenges of aging by implementing a set of "aging services" targeted to the old and infirm—an approach that fails to maximize either the potential of older adults or the strengths of the urban environment. The idea of an age-friendly city came out of the World Health Organization's (WHO) Ageing and Life Course program and shifts this paradigm by asking planners, policy makers, researchers, and residents to view all aspects of urban life through the lens of aging and to imagine a city that fosters active aging. Active aging is the process of optimizing opportunities for health, participation, and security to enhance quality of life as people age. The ability of individuals to remain active and engaged depends in part on their level of functionality and their health, but external social, environmental, and economic factors also influence whether older people are able to remain independent.

Using the active aging framework, WHO established a network of thirty-five cities around the globe to conduct research on what older people themselves identify as the factors that foster or impede an age-friendly city. The resulting *Global Age-Friendly Cities: A Guide* offers age-friendly indicators for eight domains: access to outdoor spaces and buildings, transportation, housing, respect and social inclusion, social participation, communication and information, civic participation and employment, and community support and health services (WHO 2007).

## Engaging Political Leadership

The New York City Age-friendly Cities (AFC NYC) project took the Global Age-friendly Cities project as its starting place and adapted it to meet the unique political and social environment of New York City. It is rich in research and policy institutes, but too often the recommendations of these institutions are never implemented because the city's political and community leaders have not been engaged in the process from the beginning. To avoid producing another report that would sit on the shelves of policy makers, the first step we took was to meet with political leaders. We approached the New York City Departments of Aging and Health, the leadership of the city council, and the mayor's office because we knew that to shift the planning paradigm for older residents, we needed to engage most, if not all, city agencies.

Getting the buy-in of these government leaders required both educating them about the new approach and assuring them that the project would be a true partnership between the public and private sectors. Political leaders were already grappling with how to meet the demands of the city's growing population of older adults, and they recognized that older adults are among their most politically active and engaged constituents. City officials, on the other hand, understood that older residents are high users of city services. The age-friendly cities approach appeals to political leaders because it addresses a real need among a key constituent group in a way that optimizes the strengths of the city. Moreover, this paradigm generates recommendations for change that can be built into future planning and resource allocation decisions. This may be no or low cost and/or can be implemented by government as well as businesses, cultural institutions, religious groups, and nongovernmental agencies. In fact, creating an age-friendly city requires the involvement of all sectors.

## Assessment of City Agencies

Once committed to the project, government leaders were instrumental in engaging city agencies. Using the WHO *Global Age-friendly Cities: A Guide* as a basis, the mayor's office asked city agencies to assess how "age-friendly" each agency was and what could be done to improve the way they addressed the needs of older residents. Seeing their services through the lens of aging marked a breakthrough for agencies that would normally not see themselves as focused on addressing aging issues. For example, under the leadership of the deputy of Health and Human Services, the departments of Homeless Services, Health and Mental Hygiene, Parks and Recreation, and Transportation; the Human Resources Administration/Department of Social Services (which provides temporary help to individuals and families with social service and economic needs); the Administration for Children's Services; the Department for the Aging; the Health and Hospitals Corporation; the departments of Corrections, Probation, and Juvenile Justice; and the Office of Health Insurance Access all participated in assessments of their agency's age-friendliness. As a result, each agency generated a list of activities and policy changes that it could implement to make New York City more age-friendly. Other agencies, such as the Department of Cultural Affairs, have not conducted formal assessments but have worked with the project to identify programs and services that already do or could be adapted to better serve older New Yorkers.

## Assessment of Community Needs

While city agencies were assessing themselves under the direction of the mayor's office, the New York Academy of Medicine (NYAM) worked closely with the city council to conduct a community assessment to collect the opinions and views of aging experts and older New Yorkers. An important tool in this process was the use of Geographic Information System (GIS) mapping. GIS mapping has gained in popularity in recent years and is a particularly effective tool for engaging policy makers and elected officials, because they can see for themselves how their own constituencies are affected by the issue at hand to guide local planning. The AFC NYC report included nine maps, which visually displayed the distribution of key variables planners need to consider in meeting the needs of older New Yorkers. For example, the maps displayed the distribution of people older than 65 across the five boroughs as well as the proportion of disabled older people, older people living in poverty, neighborhoods with high percentages of buildings without elevator access, distance to bus stops, sidewalk cleanliness, and the walkability of different neighborhoods. This visual display revealed nuances difficult to pick up in tabular data. For instance, a map of older New Yorkers whose rent is unaffordable illustrated that older New Yorkers are struggling to meet their basic housing needs in every neighborhood, even in the most affluent areas (see maps at http://www.agefriendlynyc.org/maps.html). The report included a transparent overlay that allows policy makers to see the data outlined by their city council or community board districts and to compare their jurisdictions to others. These data help to set priorities regarding what problems should be addressed in specific communities.

New York City is a diverse and complex city, and we used a number of direct assessment activities and methods:

- Expert roundtables to discuss current practices and innovative ideas in the areas of business, housing development, civic engagement, transportation and outdoor spaces, tenants' rights, social services, and health
- Fourteen community forums to gather the experiences, ideas, and opinions of older adults and service providers
- A widely disseminated request for information soliciting policy and programmatic ideas
- Focus groups and interviews with underrepresented older New Yorkers (e.g., low-income, formerly homeless, and immigrant)

In all, we consulted with more than 1,500 older adults and dozens of policy makers, service providers, and researchers. Each community forum was cosponsored by one or more city council members, and the staff from the city council were active partners throughout the assessment. Data from these activities were analyzed and published in the fall of 2008 in *Toward an Age-Friendly New York City: A Findings Report* (Finkelstein and others 2008). To supplement these qualitative findings and to build an evidence base for moving forward, NYAM also conducted a comprehensive literature review and identified best practices and existing programs. This work, along with the GIS maps created for the report, will provide guidance and a research base for local intervention efforts.

## MAJOR FINDINGS OF *TOWARD AN AGE-FRIENDLY NEW YORK CITY*

### Social Inclusion and Participation

Many of the older adults loved aging in New York City and felt that their neighborhoods were centrally important to their lives. Proximity to stores and services and a sense of connection and familiarity were important. For example, several long-time residents of public housing discussed the benefits of knowing their neighbors and living in close proximity for decades. Despite living in a relatively high-crime neighborhood, they described feeling safe and connected to their environment, because, as one woman told us, "I know most faces." Despite the protective features of many neighborhoods, the relocation of family, urban development, and ageism made some older residents feel excluded and/or isolated. A woman from the East Harlem forum noted, "Once children get married, they leave the community because they want a better life, and there's nothing for them here."

Older New Yorkers were well aware of the perils of becoming isolated and saw social and civic engagement as essential to health and well-being. Many of the older people we spoke with are very active, currently occupying many critical roles that form the backbone of civil society and community service in the city. They serve on community and nonprofit boards, lead advocacy efforts, play important roles as family caregivers, and work in paid or volunteer positions. "Older people carry the community around here," one woman said. Older New Yorkers are enthusiastic users of all the city has to offer and want to stay active and involved. However, affordability, physical accessibility, transportation limitations, and linguistic barriers stand in the way of ongoing participation for many.

## Employment

Researchers estimate that 41.2 percent of persons 55 and older and 9.6 percent of those 75 and older in New York City will be in the workforce in 2014 (U.S. Department of Labor 2005). Many older adults we spoke with want or need to participate in the workforce. As one focus group participant explained, "I waited five years longer than I wanted to retire because I needed the income." Job flexibility, phased retirement, and changing health insurance and pension policies were just a few of the needed improvements identified.

## Physical Environment and Accessibility

The ability of older New Yorkers to stay involved in the workforce and social and civic activities is directly related to how safe and accessible the city is. While actual crime rates are very low in New York City, some older New Yorkers, especially those who are frail, expressed feelings of anxiety about their safety and cited a number of modest improvements that would tremendously improve their ability to stay active, including places to rest on sidewalks, more public restrooms, clean and debris-free sidewalks, and more bus shelters. People from many neighborhoods discussed poorly lit and maintained sidewalks and crowded sidewalks that discourage them from going outside. These obstacles make it especially difficult for older people with low vision, poor balance, or who use wheelchairs or walkers. Many of the housing policies that make New York City affordable for older people also force some people to remain in housing that is no longer appropriate for them, like "walk-ups," and accessible and affordable housing are concerns for many older people. Similarly, people saw New York City's public transportation system as an enormous benefit, and they made recommendations for solutions to problems of affordability and accessibility.

### Health and Human Services

Informal caregivers provide the bulk of care and support for older New Yorkers, often with little support or recognition. Older New Yorkers want to age in place, but the existing formal service paradigm, focused on acute- and long-term care, is complex and fragmented; caregivers and older adults alike have difficulty navigating the existing services system. As one older person put it: "Agencies that are supposed to address the problems of the elderly should have some sort of [mechanism] to better coordinate programs for the elderly. We don't know where to go sometimes." As elsewhere in the country, affordability and training for the health and social services workforce are major concerns. One participant begged, "Please get people skills training for employees in the social services. The younger employees tend to think anyone with gray hair is either deaf or mentally incompetent."

### Information and Communication

The city's centralized information line, 311 (a 24-hour service that provides information on all city services in several languages), was reported to be helpful for those who knew about and had tried using it. However, many older adults, particularly those whose first language was not English, were unaware of the service.

Older New Yorkers consistently indicated that information is fragmented and inaccessible, impeding their ability to access opportunities, services, and benefits. While some older adults saw opportunity in the move to web-based information sources, many were challenged by new technologies. Older New Yorkers expressed a strong preference that information should be available through a variety of media, in multiple languages, and accessible to the visually or hearing impaired. They also indicated a pattern of getting information from local newspapers and other community sources. One older woman who speaks only Chinese said, "I'm blind because I cannot read documents written in English. I'm deaf because people speak to me in English and I don't understand. And I'm mute because I cannot communicate with anyone who does not know my language."

## MOVING TOWARD IMPLEMENTATION

The *Findings Report* was released at a press conference at City Hall with all the major stakeholders and many of the research participants in attendance, and it has been widely disseminated and well received. Based on this report, NYAM convened work groups from nongovernmental sectors, including leaders from civil society, health and social services, business, academia, and research. Each sector was asked to make specific commitments for how it can contribute to making New York City more age-friendly. Concurrently, both the city council and city agencies developed recommendations and commitments. The New York City government action plan for an Age-friendly New York City was released at a mayoral press conference where the co-chairs of a public-private partnership, an Age-friendly New York City Commission, were introduced and the commission's role in overseeing the implementation of the government and private-sector commitments was announced. The commission will include high-level representatives who have an understanding of the structures, systems, and programs that affect the lives of the elderly and who can provide leverage for meaningful action. The commission will convene work groups to synthesize evidence, design policies and programs, engage additional partners, build private-public partnerships, conduct additional research if needed, develop indicators of success, and report progress to the public.

At the same time that progress is being made on citywide recommendations and policy initiatives, the Age-friendly New York City Commission will work with communities to help them develop plans to transform their neighborhoods to be more age-friendly. For some, this will mean local changes in the built environment, a re-visioning of neighborhood services, or community outreach and education campaigns. Community boards, local planning groups, business improvement districts, and borough-level decision makers have indicated an interest in learning how to incorporate the perspectives and needs of older people in their planning and decision making, and these interests will be actively pursued by the staff of the commission and its members.

## LESSONS LEARNED

Every city is unique, but Age-friendly New York City has led to a number of conclusions about what might work in other urban areas. The AFC NYC project captured the imagination of many, in part, because "age-friendliness" is a simple, intuitive concept. The "age-friendly" frame is one that generates wide support and little opposition. Similarly, the concept of healthy aging that frames the age-friendly cities movement offers a new paradigm for thinking about the best ways to meet the demographic challenge of an aging population. The commitment to having voices of older people themselves lead the assessment and problem-solving process reinforces the important role older people will and must play in the change process. This not only makes good planning sense; it also engages participants and is persuasive to policy makers. Rather than having the policy process dominated by concerns over services for the most frail and disabled, the healthy aging approach challenges policy makers to think about the whole urban environment through the lens of older people and to consider what can be done to optimize the health and independence of all people as they age.

The AFC NYC project also has wide appeal because, rather than focusing solely on the city's deficits, it builds upon the city's existing strengths. We worked with older New Yorkers to identify what they love about the city and how it already works to keep them actively aging. This focus generates hope and optimism that the barriers are not insurmountable and that New York City can make modest changes and incorporate age-friendliness into future infrastructure design.

Getting government buy-in early gave the initiative both stature and momentum and helped ensure that the assessment would lead to concrete policy change. Working with government partners requires an investment of time and a willingness to compromise—both well worth the effort.

## SUMMARY

This case study presented a project used in New York City to address rapid growth in the population of older residents. Rather than using a traditional planning model that focuses on designing aging-specific services to meet the health and social service needs of older adults, the Age-friendly New York City initiative adopted a healthy-aging perspective. Viewing all of city life through the lens of aging, the project conducted assessment of the needs of older residents that started with their opinions and built on these to look at all facets of city life—from outdoor spaces to social inclusion. The inclusive assessment process involved more than 1,500 older New Yorkers, service providers, and community leaders and asked them to identify what made the New York City a good or a difficult place to grow old. GIS mapping was used to identify specific areas of need and to present data in a visually compelling way that resonated with policy makers and planners. By engaging public officials (both elected and appointed) from the earliest stages of the project, the initiative was able to build a public-private partnership that brought together leaders from government, business, academia, social services, health care, and civil society. This new paradigm of planning takes advantage of the strengths of the urban environment and engages multiple sectors in addressing the needs of older urban residents.

# REFERENCES

AARP. 2002. *Beyond 50: A report to the nation on trends in Health Security*. Washington, DC: AARP Public Policy Institute.

Finkelstein, R., A. Garcia, J. Netherland, and J. Walker. 2008. *Toward an age-friendly New York City: A findings report*. New York: The New York Academy of Medicine.

Marmot, M. 2001. Inequalities in health. *New England Journal of Medicine* 345(2):135–136.

New York City Department for the Aging. 2007. *Annual plan summary 2009–2010*. New York: New York City Department for the Aging. Also available at http://www.nyc.gov/aging.

New York City Department of City Planning. 2004. *The newest New Yorkers: Immigrant New York in the new millennium*. New York: Population Division.

New York City Department of City Planning. 2006. *New York City population projections by age/sex and borough, 2000–2030*. New York: Population Division.

New York City Department of Health and Mental Hygiene (DOHMH). 2004. *Health disparities in New York City*. New York: Bureau of Epidemiology.

New York City Department of Health and Mental Hygiene (DOHMH). 2008. *Summary of vital statistics 2007 City of New York*. New York: Bureau of Vital Statistics.

New York City Department of Health and Mental Hygiene (DOHMH). 2009. *Take care New York: Fourth year progress report*. New York: Bureau of Chronic Disease Prevention.

New York State Department of Health. (2008). County Health Indicator profile. Available from: www.health.ny.us/statistics/chip/newyorkcity.htm.

U.S. Department of Labor. December 2005. *Civilian labor force participation rates by sex, age, race and Hispanic origin, 1984, 1994, 2004, and projected 2014*. Washington, DC: Bureau of Labor Statistics.

Walker, J., and M. Mayer. (2007). *Under the radar: Poverty among older adults in New York City*. New York: New York Citizens' Committee.

World Health Organization (WHO). 2007. *Global age-friendly cities: A guide*. Geneva: Ageing and the Life Course Program, World Health Organization.

# CHAPTER EIGHT

# GLOBAL INFECTIOUS DISEASES AND URBANIZATION

## THOMAS C. QUINN
## JOHN G. BARTLETT

### LEARNING OBJECTIVES

- Identify the association between urbanization and infectious diseases
- Identify eight factors inherent in urban centers that contribute to spread of infectious diseases
- Discuss case examples of six infectious diseases that have affected cities
- Discuss recommendations for prevention and control of infectious diseases in cities

## GLOBALIZATION AND INFECTIOUS DISEASES

In this era of globalization, with increasing mobility of humans, animals, food, and feed products and with the associated growth in the population and increasing trends in urbanization, the threat of infectious diseases continues to be a major challenge to the health of the human population. While new global markets have created economic opportunities, the benefits in financial growth have not been distributed equally, and the associated health risks among the poor have risen dramatically and foster the spread of infectious diseases, particularly in our cities. Although the burden is greatest for the developing world, infectious diseases, which thrive on poverty, population crowding, and mobility, remain a growing threat to all nations.

## URBANIZATION AND THE GROWTH OF INFECTIOUS DISEASES

This trend of the interconnectedness between urbanization and the spread of infectious diseases is not new. Historically, in the eighteenth and nineteenth centuries, industrialization and the growth of cities in our developed nations led rapidly to the spread of sexually transmitted infections, cholera outbreaks, and many other infectious causes of diarrhea, leading to increased mortality and shortened life expectancy (Coetzee and Schneider 1996; Olshansky and others 1997). During the twentieth century, despite renewed optimism from breakthroughs in vaccine development and improved sanitation, we witnessed the resurgence of influenza pandemics, the new appearance and rapid expansion of HIV/AIDS as a deadly global pandemic, increases in multiple-drug-resistant tuberculosis (TB) and the rise and fall of new diseases like severe acute respiratory virus (SARS), scenarios where urbanization played a key role in the expansion of these infectious diseases.

The current era of globalization is now viewed as an intensification of trends that have occurred throughout history. Never before have so many people moved so quickly throughout the world, whether by choice or force. Never before has the population density been higher, with more people living in urban areas. Never before have food, animals, commodities, and capital been transported so freely and quickly across political boundaries. And never before have pathogens had such ample opportunity to hitch global rides on airplanes, people, and products.

Infectious diseases today are responsible for 26 percent of all reported causes of mortality worldwide. However, the burden is far greater for the developing world. In Africa infectious diseases are responsible for over 60 percent of all reported cases of mortality (WHO 1999, 2007). From the perspective of urbanization, the developing world has recorded the greatest rate of growth of mega-cities, rapidly expanding from less than two to greater than ten megacities in less than twenty-five years (Smolinski, Hamburg, and Lederberg 2003). Every year, new infectious diseases are being recognized and pose daily threats to the public health of societies. Because of rapid mobility of populations worldwide, a new emerging infectious disease in one area of the world can be a threat the next day in another area of the world. The worldwide resurgence of dengue fever, the introduction of West Nile virus to New York City in 1999, the rapid spread of human immunodeficiency virus (HIV) infection, and the global spread of multidrug-resistant tuberculosis (TB) are but a few examples of the profound effects of globalizing forces on the emergence, distribution, and spread of infectious diseases. No nation or city is immune to the growing global threat that can be posed by an isolated outbreak of infectious diseases in a seemingly remote part of the world. Today, whether carried by an unknowing traveler or an opportunistic vector, human pathogens can rapidly arrive anywhere in the world at any time.

# EMERGING INFECTIOUS DISEASES

Emerging infectious diseases cause a significant burden on global economies and public health. Their emergence is driven largely by socioeconomic, environmental, and ecological factors (Binder and others 1999; Lederberg, Shope, and Oakes 1992; Morens, Folkers, and Fauci 2004). Between 1940 and 2004, 335 emerging infectious disease events were reported and demonstrated nonrandom global patterns (Jones and others 2008). Emerging infectious disease events have arisen significantly over time even after controlling for reporting bias, with their peak incidence concomitant with the HIV pandemic at the end of the twentieth century. Over 60 percent of emerging infectious diseases are dominated by zoonoses, the majority (71.8 percent) originating in wildlife, such as SARS, and are increasing significantly over time, particularly as large populations of people within cities encroach into our more rural and forested woodlands. Half of these emerging infectious disease events were caused by bacteria or rickettsiae, reflecting a large number of drug-resistant microbes in the reports. The origins of these diseases are in fact significantly correlated with socioeconomic, environmental, and ecological factors and provide a basis for identifying regions where emerging infectious diseases are most likely to originate (hot spots; Morse 1995; Smolinksi, Hamburg, and Lederberg 2003). They also reveal a substantial risk of wildlife zoonotic and vector-borne emerging infectious diseases, originating at lower latitudes where the reporting effort is low (Daszak, Cunningham, and Hyatt 2000). Global resources to counter disease emergence are poorly allocated, with the majority of scientific and surveillance effort focused on countries where the next important emerging infectious diseases are least likely to originate. These findings support calls for international investment and the capacity to detect, identify, and monitor infectious diseases targeted at regions of the world where the need is greatest.

# FACTORS AFFECTING MICROBIAL SPREAD

## International Travel

International travel is one of the fastest-growing industries worldwide. Yearly international tourist arrivals are expected to pass the one-billion mark by 2010. Every region of the world is experiencing this increase. An estimated 700 million tourists cross international borders each year. About 60 million people from other countries travel annually to the United States; around the same number of U.S. citizens travel internationally and then return. In a one-year period, the three New York City airports experience nearly five million international arrivals. The most rapid increase in international air travel has been in Africa and the Middle East, places where many new infectious diseases are emerging (Wilson 1995). Not only do international travelers themselves pose the risk of spreading an infectious disease, but the airplanes on which they travel and the cargo that accompanies them also serve as potential sources of vector introduction.

Like air travel, cruise ship travel has increased dramatically, with nearly seven million people in North America traveling by this mode annually. And although cruise ships are increasing in size and becoming more complex in design, they are still fairly densely populated. The average duration of stay on one of these ships is about two average incubation periods, which range from three to ten days for microorganisms responsible for many emerging infectious diseases. These "floating cities," where people gather from all over the world for short periods of time, represent a unique environment for disease dissemination, amplification, and dispersal. Large aggregates of tourist populations not only serve as potential source for the rapid spread of disease but also are very difficult to monitor. While travelers on board a cruise ship are at risk of contracting infectious diseases, the people they come into contact with when they leave the ship are also at risk. A 1999 outbreak of influenza A virus (Sydney) in Alaska, which affected about 30,000 people, was preceded by the introduction of an influenza A virus strain via a cruise ship the previous year.

## Urbanization

Urbanization, particularly in poor countries, is expected to become a key demographic feature of the world over the next fifteen years as more than 90 percent of the population growth in poor countries will be in cities and will serve as a key determinant in health (Dye 2008; Dobson and Carper 1996). The world's urban population increased from 1.7 billion (39 percent) in 1980 to 2.7 billion (46 percent) in 1997 and is expected to reach 5 billion (60 percent) by 2030. Over the next twenty-five years, urban populations in Africa are expected to more than double (Leon 2008). Those in Asia will almost double, and those in Latin America and the Caribbean are expected to increase by almost 50 percent. The density of humans will increase disproportionately because the higher proportion of those people will live in cities, compared to today.

The mass relocation of rural population to urban areas is one of the defining demographic trends of the latter half of the twentieth century. The world's cities are currently growing at four times the rate of their rural counterparts, and at least 40 percent of their expansion is the result of migration rather than natural increase. Each day, approximately 160,000 people move from the countryside to metropolitan areas, and almost 50 percent of the world's population now lives in urban centers. Rural-to-urban migration in cities without adequate infrastructure has serious health consequences, not the least being the spread of infectious diseases (Ackerman 1997; Gushulak and MacPherson 2004). Impoverished rural migrants typically live in unusually crowded living conditions as a result of housing costs and relatively large family sizes, which further contribute to the spread of communicable diseases. Infants in poor and more crowded portions of cities are at least four times more likely to die from diseases such as tuberculosis and typhoid than infants in more affluent neighborhoods. Moreover, many young women who migrate to cities in search of economic opportunity are able to gain economic security only through commercial sex, and men often travel far from home to seek work in cities where their reliance on the commercial sex trade increases the risk of HIV and other sexually transmitted diseases (Pick and Cooper 1997). Migrants who contract HIV in urban areas generally return to their villages to be cared for by their families, often perpetuating transmission. Other health concerns associated with increased urbanization include lack of access to clean water and sanitation, absence of adequate shelter, and health hazards posed by open sewers and people living in close association with animals (Sutherst 2004).

## URBAN FACTORS AND THE SPREAD OF INFECTIOUS DISEASES

### Population Size and Density

About two-thirds of all fatal infectious diseases are spread person-to-person; greater population density increases transmission by bringing people into closer contact with each other. Size matters, as there is often a minimum number of susceptible people required to sustain and propagate future generations of epidemics, as in the case of measles.

## Health Systems

The stress on already weak health systems in many poor countries is increasing, and this is particularly severe in urban centers. This includes weak public health systems for surveillance, detection, and control. Diversity of populations within cities also places a burden on the health systems in developed and developing countries due to cultural differences and effective outreach for disease control. For example, the area with the lowest rate of influenza immunization in New York City is Flatbush, which has a significant minority immigrant population—despite extensive efforts of the health department and the local medical community, the influenza immunization rate has not budged in years. New approaches, including community partner and engagement models, need to be considered so that health systems can be responsive to endemic levels and, importantly, epidemics and pandemics.

## Urban Infrastructure

Water and sanitation systems are weak or lacking in many urban areas of less economically developed countries, increasing susceptibility to contaminated water-borne diseases. This is particularly true for cities in developing countries, such as the recent outbreak of cholera in Lusaka, Zambia, but also applicable to developed countries, as evidenced by an outbreak of cryptosporidiosis in Milwaukee, Wisconsin, due to contaminated water purification plants within the city.

## Slums

The huge peri-urban slums that tend to develop around many major cities in developing countries are typically poor areas that lack infrastructure and resources. This, combined with warm water and low latitudes of most of these regions, make these slums ideal sites for the spread of infectious diseases. For example, squatters often settle in marginal lands that are undesired by cities because their geography is prone to flooding, mud slides, pooling of water from poor ground drainage, and consequently are often not serviced by the city—all that can contribute not only to disasters but also to transmission of water-borne infectious diseases (David and others 2007).

## Hubs of Domestic and International Travel

Because urban centers service international travelers, an infectious traveler could potentially and unknowingly set off a worldwide epidemic. More than 5,000 urban center airports worldwide have regularly scheduled international flights. The International Air Transport Association projection for 2011 is 2.75 billion passengers; 900 million will be international. Cruise ships ("floating cities") carry millions of people per day (up to 5,000 per ship per day) and are essentially closed urban systems for transmitting diseases like norovirus-induced diarrheal epidemics. Transportation of infected people or cargo (36 million tons of cargo in 2011) containing infectious vectors can lead to spontaneous epidemics within a city. The classic examples of SARS and West Nile virus will be described later. Other examples of travel include transport of cargo within country, as in the spread of HIV by truck drivers in Africa and India.

## Animal Importation

Animal importations are another potential source to introduce infectious diseases known as zoonoses. Every year, cities across the world receive millions of animal importations from countries where a variety of diseases are endemic. In a single year, there were more than 2.8 million international animal importations into New York City, most of which were amphibians (61 percent) and birds (36 percent). In 1996, the port of Miami received more than 30 million animal imports; most (96 percent) were fish and aquatic invertebrates. These figures represent only legally imported animals, and there is also a large trade in illegally imported animals. The emergence of monkey pox in Midwestern cities, such as Milwaukee, is a classic example of the importation of animals harboring potentially severe and deadly human pathogens.

Another related issue is the expanding margins of cities near or adjacent to woodlands, with implications for emerging and reemerging infections. Lyme disease is a classic example of the spread of a zoonosis exacerbated by the increasing interface of urban growth near rural woodlands where deer and ticks, the vector of Lyme disease, reside (Bradley and Altizer 2006).

## Cities as Heat Islands

Another variable for the spread of infectious diseases is the effect of global temperature change on infectious microbes and on global movement—related to rural droughts that drive some of the rural-urban migration (noted previously). Cities are known to have higher temperatures due to the built environment, including the sacrifice of green space for pavement, and have consequences related to temperature. As many large urban centers are located on coasts and waterways, they are prone to weather-related events that can create considerable damage to people, property, and infrastructure—creating a basis for transmission of infectious disease. Other factors in cities that contribute disproportionately to climate change include industrialization; burning fossil fuels for heat and transportation; and deforestation, most common near our urban centers, contributing to increasing levels of greenhouse gases and eliminating carbon sinks (Patz and others 2005). Many aspects of vector behavior, including the range of habitability, are at least partially driven by temperature. The consequences of higher temperatures have led to increased malaria, dengue, and other vector-borne diseases in temperate areas (Hay and others 2002; Rogers and Randolph 2000). Interestingly, although most diseases are associated more with areas of concentrated disadvantage, the epidemiology of dengue is more "democratic," posing a broader health challenge in cities.

## Food Availability and Transport

With urbanization, there is a greater need for the transportation of food. The globalized food supply raises questions about food safety and opens the door for potential spread of infectious diseases, either from infectious microbial contamination or via intentional contamination (bioterrorism). Several hundred known food-borne microbial agents, including bacteria, viruses, and parasites, pose potential dangers on a daily basis throughout the world. No one country or community has the capability to test for all potential hazardous agents in its imported food products, which make local control very important. Recent outbreaks have demonstrated the impact of imported produce in the occurrence of food-borne disease. In 1998, for example, an outbreak of multiple drug-resistant shigelloses infection occurred among patrons of restaurants in Minnesota. The culprit was imported parsley. Guatemalan raspberries were a classic example of a cash crop that resulted in an outbreak of cyclosporiasis throughout the urban centers of the United States and Canada. Local conditions also set the stage for a pathogen to enter the food supply. These outbreaks are similar to epidemics caused by bacterial pathogens, including enteric organisms such as *Campylobacter, Shigella, Salmonella*, cholera, shiga-toxin-producing *E. coli*, and *E. coli* O157:H7 in raw ground beef.

# SELECTED INFECTIOUS DISEASES

To illustrate the interaction between urbanization and the previously described factors for emergence of pathogenic microbes, selected epidemics of infectious diseases that have reemerged or newly emerged are described in the following paragraphs.

## Dengue

The worldwide resurgence of dengue illustrates the impact urban growth can have on the emergence of infectious diseases. Sustained transmission of dengue virus requires a population of between 150,000 and one million people. A growing number of tropical and subtropical urbanized areas are becoming large enough to favor the ongoing transmission of one or more of four dengue serotypes. These areas are typically littered with many discarded, nonbiodegradable items that provide ideal vector breeding sites for the vector *Aedes egyptii*. This vector, which carries both dengue and yellow fever viruses, lives almost exclusively in cohabitation with humans. Urbanization, combined with the subtropical and tropical temperatures that favor viral mobility, create a perfect setting for the emergence of dengue (Sutherst 2004). Dengue has reemerged with a vengeance in most of the Americas, where the number of cases rose from only a few to nearly one million by the turn of the century. Its reemergence coincides with the environmental presence of glass, plastic, and tires. Another vector, *Aedes albopictus*, has also adapted rapidly to breeding within these conditions and subsequently to transmitting all four dengue serotypes; all cause illness and have caused pandemics in the past. One of the more severe forms of the disease, dengue hemorrhagic fever or dengue shock syndrome, has a 10 percent mortality rate.

The history of dengue in the Americas demonstrates how a false sense of security can breed reemergence. Although a number of countries participated in eradication efforts of the vector and achieved local success by 1970, not all countries participated so the mosquito was not eradicated from the region. Over the past thirty years, with the increasing intensity of globalizing forces, such as trade and travel, *Aedes egyptii* has re-infested nearly every country in the Americas, except for Canada.

## Malaria

The resurgence of malaria is a dramatic example of the effects of globalization on disease trends. Twenty years ago, more than 80 percent of the world's population lived in malaria-free or controlled areas. Today, malaria is the most prevalent vector-borne disease, with more than 40 percent of the world's population living in endemic areas. Driving this resurgence in malaria is a variety of factors including global warming, increased air travel and human movement, crowded refugee camps, poor sanitation, and rapid growth of populations within urban centers (Hay and others 2002). Urbanization, though, may also have a modest or offsetting effect on decreasing malaria incidence within a country. In general, urban populations are subject to reduced levels of malarial transmission due to better access to health systems, including preventive and curative antimalarial measures, and the modified urban physical environment reduces the level of *Anopheles* breeding and, therefore, malaria transmission. However, in slums and other underdeveloped settlements, poor water supplies, poor drainage, and small-scale agriculture can create suitable breeding sites for the *Anopheles* vectors and so increase the risk of malaria (Utzinger and Keiser 2006). With increased rural-urban migration, malaria-infected migrants to these poor areas may spark a new round of malaria transmission that could be sustained in the absence of malaria control programs.

## HIV/AIDS

Perhaps one of the most striking examples of the convergence of globalization that involved mobility of the human population, urbanization, and the interface of humans with animals is the emergence of the AIDS pandemic. AIDS now ranks as one of the most important infectious diseases affecting humans for the last thirty years. Since its initial clinical descriptions, AIDS has resulted in the death of more than 40 million people worldwide. HIV-1, the primary cause of AIDS, has infected more than 80 million people during that time, and currently 33 million people are living with HIV infection (UNAIDS 2008).

Perhaps one of the most important variables in dissemination of HIV-1 was the massive migration and urbanization that occurred in Africa during this time (Mayer, Pizer, and Venkatesh 2008; Quinn 1994). Following independence in the 1960s, many African countries experienced dramatic demographic changes that may underlie the movement of HIV-1 from potentially remote areas to more populous areas. One of the most important types of migration during this period represented rural-urban movement, which was significant in the long-term spatial redistribution of populations (Quinn 1994). The number of cities with more than 500,000 inhabitants rapidly increased from three in 1960 to over one hundred by 2010 in sub-Saharan Africa. Though the total urban population in sub-Saharan Africa increased substantially, the average growth rates did not. By 2000, the proportion of people living in urban centers exceeded one-third of the national population in all regions except Eastern Africa. As a consequence of urbanization, the crude population density increased in every country with available data, averaging greater than 100 percent increase.

Unlike much of the industrialized world, where urbanization followed industrialization, urbanization and industrialization have largely taken place independently in sub-Saharan Africa. As a result, employment was frequently unavailable within these centers, social disruption became common, and many individuals reverted to commercial sex for means of survival. During this period, health officials noted marked increases in sexually transmitted diseases (STDs) within the urban centers. In one study in the Democratic Republic of the Congo (formerly Zaire), HIV-1 prevalence remained stable in a remote rural region between 1976 and 1985. In contrast, the capital city, Kinshasa, noted a massive increase in HIV-1 infection that was ten times higher than that documented in the rural region. This trend was duplicated in all the capital cities of African nations.

Once these viruses had reached the urban international centers within Africa, it was only a matter of time before further dissemination to other countries. International migration across national borders played a role in the movement of populations and HIV infection from one country to another. Early dissemination of HIV-1 outside of Africa is more difficult to trace, although there were reports of increasing numbers of HIV-1 cases in Port-au-Prince, Haiti, and in New York City, San Francisco, and Los Angeles. With international travel increasing over the same period, dissemination of these early HIV-1-infected cases soon were being reported in nearly every major city across the world (Quinn 1996).

Factors that contributed to HIV transmission in Southeast Asia included the commercial sex industry, international tourism, and injecting drug use (IDU). The majority of commercial sex workers were young women from poor rural areas who had migrated to urban centers as a means of addressing their economic situation. The circulatory nature of rural-urban migration and the substantial patronage of the sex industry by international tourists fueled HIV transmission throughout Thailand and neighboring countries. Similar factors were involved in the spread of HIV among IDUs.

Within the last decade, HIV/AIDS has also increased dramatically in Eastern Europe, primarily in urban centers where, once again, commercial sex work and injecting drug use are often intermixed and serve as primary routes of transmission. The number of cases is expected to rise in areas where poverty, poor health systems, poor access to health care services, and gender inequality are prevalent; where resources for health care and prevention are limited; and where a high degree of stigma and denial is associated with HIV infection.

# SARS

SARS (severe acute respiratory syndrome) is an acute viral respiratory infection caused by a coronavirus designated SARS-CoV. The story of its global transmission is tied to cities. The disease was first reported in Asia in February 2003, initially as an "atypical," sometimes fatal pneumonia in the province of Guangdong, in Southern China. The presumed initial source was transmission of the virus in the "wet market" by civets, a catlike mammal; however, human-human transmission by respiratory droplets was subsequently considered the major mechanism of transmission.

An unusual epidemiologic event was global dissemination when a physician from Guangdong, China, visited Hong Kong and stayed in room 911 of the Metropole Hotel. The physician had a respiratory illness that proved fatal due to SARS, and hotel occupants on the same floor subsequently became index cases for epidemics in Singapore, Toronto, Hong Kong, and Hanoi. When the SARS epidemic was all over, there were a total of 8,422 patients, and 916 (11 percent) died as a result of this infection.

This was almost exclusively an urban disease that was transmitted primarily within hospitals and households; in the early phases of the epidemic there was great confusion about cause, treatment, and prevention. Particularly important in defining the putative agent was Klaus Stohr at the World Health Organization (WHO), who convened a teleconference involving eleven highly accomplished virologists and virology laboratories throughout the world. They agreed to collaborate in defining the cause, and the group from Princess Margaret Hospital in Hong Kong was successful within days. Coronaviruses infect a variety of animals and cause a broad range of infections, but their menu of diseases in humans was limited to the common cold. So the SARS and coronavirus represents a newly recognized pathogen, and like so many new infections to humans, represents a zoonotic disease, but with the civet as the natural host.

Attempts to control the infection included airport screening, quarantines, hand hygiene, and masks. Health care workers were particularly vulnerable and accounted for about 10 percent of the cases. Although airport screening was aggressive, the retrospective analysis suggested little benefit despite the enormous impact on global travel and tourism to the metropolitan areas that were heavily impacted. In fact, most of the transmissions took place in the home and in the hospital. Reducing person-person spread and eliminating the source in the wet market best achieved ultimate control of the epidemic. It is now thought that the SARS-coronavirus continues to be present in civets and possibly other animal reservoirs in Asia, but the only human cases reported since WHO declared elimination of this disease in January 2004 have been in lab workers.

There are many learning points as a result of this epidemic: The concept of the "superspreader" was attributed to the patient who spent a single night in room

911 in Hong Kong and became the source of a global epidemic. There was a substantial delay in initial recognition in Southern China as the result of denial. This epidemic was yet another zoonosis, which seem to be the major source of new microbial pathogens in the modern era of urban sprawl. The cost to economies in East and Southeast Asia is estimated at about $60 billion. Caring for these patients represented a substantial risk to health care workers; Princess Margaret Hospital in Hong Kong had the largest number of patients—593 and 62 health care workers who became infected, presumably from occupational risk.

## Pandemic Influenza

Influenza is a continuous threat and particularly important in urban areas due to crowding, rapid contagion, extraordinary stress on existing resources, and high rates of morbidity and mortality. There have been thirty pandemics of influenza in the past four hundred years, three in the past century, and none for the past forty years, which accounts for expectations of a hit in the near future (IOM 2005; King and others 2006).

The highly pathogenic avian influenza is now endemic in much of Asia and has properties that resemble those of the 1918–1919 influenza pandemic, which was the greatest natural disaster in recorded medical history, with over 50 million deaths. The concern for this strain is marked by its extraordinary rate of mortality, approximately 62 percent compared to 2.4 percent for the 1918–1919 pandemic. Nonetheless, the number of cases showed a substantial decrease in 2008, largely attributed to control of the disease in poultry through vaccination and culling. However, there continues to be concern for this H5N1 strain and other novel influenza strains that have been transmitted to humans, including H7 and H9.

The more recent outbreak of swine, or H1N1, influenza in Mexico City with its subsequent global spread again illustrates the potential for rapid spread in urban areas. Although we are able to anticipate this type of epidemic, we are often unable to predict when, where, or what strain. For planning purposes, the World Health Organization classifies influenza into six stages that dictate policy recommendations and are generally accepted for what must be a global strategy, since all pandemics are global. The recent H1N1 epidemic was classified by WHO as a full worldwide pandemic with millions of cases, which is still ongoing.

## Antibiotic-Resistant Bacteria

Urban areas are facing increasing problems with resistant bacteria that appear to reflect the combination of use and abuse of antimicrobial agents in clinical practice, the inevitable development of resistance mutations during bacterial evolution, and the paucity of new antibiotics to deal with them. The result is a substantial challenge that is becoming increasingly more frequent in cities worldwide (Boucher and others 2009). Examples include methicillin-resistant *S. aureus* (MRSA), Gram-negative bacilli, and *Clostridium difficile*, which have shown permeability back and forth into the community.

# RECOMMENDATIONS

## Prevention of Emerging and Resurgent Infectious Diseases

Infectious diseases account for one-quarter of all human mortality and a similar fraction of morbidity. Infectious diseases of crops and livestock cost the global economy uncounted billions of dollars each year. Sudden epidemics of infectious diseases can deliver humanitarian and economic shocks on a scale difficult to absorb. The United Nations Millennium Development Goals have explicit targets for reducing the burden of human diseases (United Nations 2007). Prevention of infectious diseases requires using proven tools and developing and evaluating new ones. Vaccines provide excellent examples of proven, cost-effective disease prevention. Other proven prevention tools include screening and treatment of blood and blood products to prevent hepatitis and HIV transmission, and administering intrapartum antibiotics to women at high risk for transmitting group B streptococcus and HIV to their newborns.

Rapid detection of emerging and reemerging infectious diseases is essential to minimize illness, disability, death, and economic losses. Public health surveillance, ongoing systematic collection, analysis, interpretation, and dissemination of health data are the cornerstone of problem detection and response. The usefulness of augmenting routine surveillance with new technologies, such as molecular tools and rapid communication methods, has been demonstrated many times. For example, the national molecular subtyping network for food-borne disease surveillance, also known as PulseNet, has contributed to the identification of several multistate outbreaks with relatively few affected people in any given place. When intensive laboratory study of an illness with characteristics that suggest an infectious origin failed to identify a causative agent, creative approaches, such as searching for host mRNA response profiles that are age- and class-specific, may help solve the puzzle.

For some disease problems, such as antimicrobial resistance, effective approaches to prevention and control have been difficult to develop and implement. Overuse and misuse of antimicrobial agents are major contributors to antimicrobial resistance. Reducing inappropriate prescribing of antimicrobial agents requires intensive, sustained efforts; approaches that have been used with varying success include physician and patient education, peer review with feedback, computer-assisted decision support, and administrative intervention.

Most of the factors that contribute to disease emergence will continue, if not intensify, in the twenty-first century (Knobler, Mahmoud, and Lemon 2006; Weiss and McMichael 2004). These include social factors (lack of adequate health care and increase in international travel), demographic factors (aging of the population in developing countries, urbanization and population growth), and environmental factors (global climate change, lack of adequate sanitation and land use practices that result in human contact with previously remote habitats, and microbial evolution). The public health community must develop long-term strategies to respond to these challenges.

## Future Investments in Prevention

New understandings of human genetics may lead to immunizations, treatments, and other interventions tailored to an individual's genetic profile. New technologies, such as biosensors and high-density DNA microarrays, are likely to have profound effects on clinical medicine and public health practice. With increasing international travel and global commerce, prevention and control of emerging infectious diseases must involve global efforts, including insuring adequate supplies of safe food and drinking water, providing immunizations, improving personal hygiene, and reducing inappropriate antimicrobial use. The recent threat from H5N1 and H1N1 influenza in the last several years illustrates the importance of international communication and cooperation and the need for a global perspective.

The public health community also needs to work more actively with other sectors, such as agriculture, economic development, urban planning, and health care, with important roles and interest in reducing infectious diseases (Salama and others 2004). In recent years, the decision to slaughter cows that were potentially infected with bovine spongiform encephalitis and threatening the lives of people in London and elsewhere; the decision to slaughter poultry to stop H5N1 influenza infection in Hong Kong; and proposals to modify regulations governing the use of antimicrobial agents in food production are examples of multisector responses to infectious disease threats. Even greater collaboration will be necessary to deal with poverty, a particularly recalcitrant contributor to and consequence of infectious diseases. We must make a long-term commitment now to ensure the capacity to address current infectious disease problems as well as those that will occur in the future.

Although laboratory testing has been the basis for identifying many new diseases, clinicians are often the first to recognize new disease problems. Networks of medical specialists in emergency medicine, infectious diseases, and travel medicine have been formed recently to enhance collaboration about emerging infectious diseases. Physicians in these networks systematically collect data about difficult infectious disease problems and use the Internet and other means to rapidly circulate queries about diagnosis and management of uncommon or poorly understood infectious diseases. These capacities have been useful during influenza pandemics, SARS, and other infectious disease events.

Systems for detecting infectious disease problems must also be linked to systems for controlling them. In addition to ensuring adequate capacity for routine public health control functions, we must ensure surge capacity, ways of rapidly increasing laboratory, epidemiologic, and other staff and facilities to test specimens, conduct epidemiologic investigations, and otherwise respond to difficult and complex public health problems. This is particularly true for urban health departments.

The very interdependency and interconnectedness that creates such opportunities for the global spread of pathogens also offer mechanisms for innovative, multinational efforts to address the threat. A growing network of such efforts combined with global proliferation of technology and information continues to strengthen the global public health capacity to prevent and control the spread of emerging and reemerging infectious diseases (Wolfe, Dunavan, and Diamond 2007). Networks of surveillance systems distributed worldwide are constantly monitoring the emergence of new pathogens, and the importation of animals carrying potential human pathogens is strictly regulated and enforced. Although there may be lapses in these regulatory efforts to control infectious diseases, by and large they have limited the magnitude by which these diseases have infected individuals. The growth of antibiotics specific to unique pathogens has also reduced mortality: for example, the development of antiretroviral drugs, which are now distributed globally to limit the spread of HIV infection. So although the emergence of human pathogens is a continuous threat, society has responded in a variety of ways to limit their overall morbidity and mortality. This is a constant battle that will need to be fought on a daily basis, and nowhere more is that critically important than in our cities today.

## SUMMARY

With their population size and density, their proximity and association, urban areas are settings where infectious disease transmission can begin and become sustained. As the world is becoming increasing urbanized, cities are becoming more interconnected, meaning that transmission can quickly become global.

Infectious diseases such as pandemic influenza and SARS cross borders rapidly, primarily through travel hubs affecting urban residents. Other infectious diseases represent changing ecology of cities and climate change, such as peri-urban malaria and dengue. Others represent overtreatment with antibiotics in people and food. HIV infection has been associated with cities where size, density, and culture are a platform for transmission within and between cities.

Most of the factors that contribute to disease emergence will continue, if not intensify, in the twenty-first century. These include social factors (lack of adequate health care and increase in international travel), demographic factors (aging of the population in developing countries, urbanization, and population growth), and environmental factors (global climate change, lack of adequate sanitation, land-use practices that result in human contact with previously remote habitats, and microbial evolution). The public health community must develop long-term strategies to respond to these fundamental challenges.

The very interdependency and interconnectedness that create such opportunities for the global spread of pathogens also offer mechanisms for innovative, multinational efforts to address the threat. A growing network of such efforts, combined with global proliferation of technology and information, continues to strengthen the global public health capacity to prevent and control the spread of emerging and reemerging infectious diseases.

## REFERENCES

Ackerman, L. K. 1997. Health problems of refugees. *Journal of the American Board of Family Practice* 10:337–348.

Bartlett, J. D., and L. Borio. 2008. Healthcare epidemiology: The current status of planning for pandemic influenza and implications for health care planning in the United States. *Clinical Infectious Diseases* 46:919–925.

Binder, S., A. M. Levitt, J. D. Sacks, and J. M. Hughes. 1999. Emerging infectious diseases: public health issues for the 21st century. *Science* 284:1311–1313.

Bloom, B.R. 2002. Tuberculosis—the global view. *New England Journal of Medicine*, 346:1434–1435.

Boucher, H. W., and others. 2009. Bad bugs, no drugs: No ESKAPE! An update from the Infectious Disease Society of America. *Clinical Infectious Diseases*, 48:1–12.

Bradley, C. A., and S. Altizer. 2006. Urbanization and the ecology of wildlife diseases. *Trends in Ecology and Evolution* 22: 95–102.

Campbell, T., and A. Campbell. 2007. Emerging disease burdens and the poor in cities of the developing world. *Journal of Urban Health: Bulletin of the New York Academy of Medicine* 84(1):i54-i64.

Coetzee, D., and H. Schneider. 1996. Urbanisation and the epidemic of sexually transmitted diseases in South Africa. *Urban Health News*, 31:36–41.

Daszak, P., A. A. Cunningham, and A. D. Hyatt. 2000. Emerging infectious diseases of wildlife: Threats to biodiversity and human health. *Science*, 287:443–449.

David, A. M., and others. 2007. The prevention and control of HIV/AIDS, TB and vector-borne disease in informal settlements: Challenges, opportunities and insights. *Journal of Urban Health: Bulletin of the New York Academy of Medicine* 84(1):i65-i74.

Dobson, A. P., and E. R. Carper. 1996. Infectious diseases and human population history. *Bioscience* 46:115–126.

Dye, C. 2008. Health and urban living. *Science* 319:766–769.

Gushulak, B. W., and D. W. MacPherson. 2004. Globalization of infectious diseases: The impact of migration. *Clinical Infectious Diseases* 38:1742–1748.

Hahn, B. H., G. M. Shaw, K. M. DeCock, and P. M. Sharp. 2000. AIDS as a zoonosis: Scientific and public health implications. *Science* 287:607–614.

Hay S. I., and others. 2002. Climate change and the resurgence of malaria in the East African Highlands. *Nature* 415:905–909.

Institute of Medicine (IOM). 2005. *The threat of pandemic influenza: Are we ready?* Washington, DC: The National Academies Press.

Jones, K. E., N. G. Patel, M. A. Levy, A. Sotreygard, D. Balk, J. G. Gittleman, and P. Daszak. 2008. Global trends in emerging infectious diseases. *Nature* 451:990–994.

King, D. A., and others. 2006. Infectious diseases: Preparing for the future. *Science* 313:1392–1393.

Knobler, S., A. Mahmoud, and S. Lemon, eds. 2006. *The impact of globalization on infectious disease emergence and control.* Washington, DC: Institute of Medicine, National Academies Press.

Lederberg, J., R. E. Shope, and S.C.J. Oakes. 1992. *Emerging infectious diseases: Microbial threats to health in the United States.* Washington, DC: Institute of Medicine, National Academies Press.

Leon, D. A. 2008. Cities, urbanization and health. International *Journal of Epidemiology* 37:4–8.

Mayer, K., H. F. Pizer, K. K. Venkatesh. 2008. The social ecology of HIV/AIDS. *Medical Clinics of North America* 92:1363–1375.

Morens, D. M., G. K. Folkers, A. S. Fauci. 2004. The challenge of emerging and re-emerging infectious diseases. *Nature* 430:242–249.

Morse, S. S. 1995. Factors in the emergence of infectious diseases. *Emerging Infectious Diseases* 1:7–15.

Olshansky, S. J., B. Carnes, R. G. Rogers, and L. Smith. 1997. Infectious diseases: New and ancient threats to world health. *Population Bulletin* 52:1–52.

Patz, J. A., D. Campbell-Lendrum, T. Holloway, and J. A. Foley. 2005. Impact of regional climate change on human health. *Nature* 438:310–317.

Pick, W., and D. Cooper. 1997. Urbanisation and women's health in South Africa. *African Journal of Reproductive Health* 1:45–55.

Quinn, T. C. 1994. Population migration and the spread of types 1 and 2 human immunodeficiency viruses. *Proceedings of the National Academy of Sciences* 9:2407–2414.

Quinn, T. C. 1996. Global burden of the HIV pandemic. *Lancet* 348:99–106.
Rogers D. J., and S. E. Randolph. 2000. The global spread of malaria in a future, warmer world. *Science* 289:1763–1766.
Salama, P., P. Spiegel, L. Talley, and R. Waldman. 2004. Lessons learned from complex emergencies over past decade. *Lancet* 364:1801–1813.
Smolinksi, M. S., M. A. Hamburg, and J. Lederberg. 2003. *Microbial threats to health: Emergence, detection, and response*. Washington, DC: National Academies Press.
Sutherst, R. W. 2004. Global change and human vulnerability to vector-borne disease. *Clinical Microbiology Review* 17(1):140–151.
UNAIDS. 2008. *Report on the global HIV/AIDS epidemic*. Geneva, Switzerland: World Health Organization.
United Nations. 2007. *The millennium development goals report 2007*. New York: United Nations.
Utzinger, J., and J. Keiser. 2006. Urbanization and tropical health—Then and now. *Annals of Tropical Medicine & Parasitology* 100:517–533.
Weiss, R. A., and A. J. McMichael. 2004. Social and environmental risk factors in the emergence of infectious diseases. *Nature Medicine* 10:S70-S76.
Wilson, M. E. 1995. Travel and the emergence of infectious diseases. *Emerging Infectious Diseases* 1:39–46.
Wolfe, M. D., C. P. Dunavan, and J. Diamond. 2007. Origins of major human infectious diseases. *Nature* 447:279–283.
World Health Organization. 2005. *Addressing poverty in TB control: Options for national TB control programmes*. Geneva, Switzerland: World Health Organization, 10–20.
World Health Organization. 1999. Infectious diseases are the biggest killer of the young. In *Removing obstacles to healthy development*. Geneva, Switzerland: WHO.

# CHAPTER NINE

# CONFRONTING THE NEW EPIDEMICS IN OUR CITIES

STEPHEN LEEDER

ANGELA BEATON

CATHIE HULL

RUTH COLAGIURI

MICHAEL WARD

## LEARNING OBJECTIVES

- Explain the shift in the past fifty years in the global burden of disease from acute and infectious diseases to chronic and noncommunicable diseases
- Explain why the chronic disease is not evenly spread but increases with poverty and low levels of economic development
- Explain why the chronic diseases are made worse by aspects of urban living, often the same aspects that attract people to cities from rural areas
- Contribute ideas about possible long-term solutions to reduce chronic disease through the design of the environment and cities and the way life and commerce are regulated, to enable and support individuals in making choices that enhance their health

IN the long fresco of human history, the formation, defense, and maintenance of cities hold a position of honor among the themes of artistic representation. From ancient times, when a walled city set on a hill was a powerful expression of civil strength and military might, to today's brilliant cities of east and west, north and south, the city has been a magnet attracting those seeking a fuller, freer, safer, and progressive life. The proximity of services, the ease of exchanging goods, the competitive aggregation of skills and talents, the bustle, the sleeplessness, the anonymity, and the sheer force of life in cities has meant that, of all the ways we have explored to live, the city has increasingly become most people's choice of habitat. The current and recent movement of people to cities is the world's largest migration in all human history.

# THE RISE OF THE CITY

Cities—for good or bad—are taking over the world. Now, over half the 6.7 billion people that live on Earth do so in an urban setting. This setting need not be, and frequently is not, a large city. Nor are all cities places of great prosperity. An idealized view of the city can be easily disputed when one observes the complexity and contradictions of urban living. Around cities there exist penumbras of shantytowns, or poorer residential areas, the repository or dormitory communities of people who find menial employment in cities. Many towns and cities remain without adequate sanitary infrastructure and fresh water; basic amenities, such as transport and electricity, are missing from towns and cities in less economically advanced societies.

Cities have been growing fast in recent years. On the one hand we recognize the immense changes, most advantageous, that have attended the past two or three decades of economic growth and globalization. So much more of the world now participates in prosperity than it did at the beginning of this era that those interested in public health must turn their concern to what health gains they wish to see secured in an age of prosperity. Conversely, the forces of modernity that drive the construction of our towns and cities come at a cost and can damage our health.

# THE RISK OF CHRONIC DISEASE

Once that cost was expressed in highly visible disasters: rapidly spreading fires and explosive infectious disease epidemics, such as cholera and plague. Increasingly, it is now measured in lives lost or disabled through heart disease, stroke, diabetes, cancer, chronic alcohol abuse, and mental disorders. These chronic (meaning "taking a long time") diseases require years to develop; are closely aligned with the way we live, whether by free choice or constrained by circumstance; and often cause the sufferer distress for decades.

The frequency of chronic diseases is commonly underrecognized or underestimated. Chronic diseases are due to causal factors that are rooted in the social soil of our cities. We live with them for a long time without getting better. And they interfere with our quality of life, our capacity for work and earning income, our comfort, our relationships with family and friends, and our capacity for happiness.

## MYTHS ABOUT CHRONIC DISEASE

In 1542, when the Polish polymath Nicolaus Copernicus finally published his scientific theory that Earth was not a stationary planet around which the rest of the universe rotated, his ideas faced what might be politely termed a credibility gap. Fortunately for him, Copernicus died the next year; denigration of his ideas took decades to get started. So do the ideas suffer of those who mention that cities and urbanization—*despite* the manifold and precious achievements—set the stage for the slow emergence of noncommunicable chronic illness. It is worth exploring the objections to the notion that these diseases merit our collective attention and investment just as much as HIV, malaria, and tuberculosis do.

First, there are those who argue that chronic diseases are self-inflicted and do not deserve the attention given to the environmental determinants of infectious disease. People choose to smoke, choose to eat poor quality takeaway meals, and choose to be physically inactive. It is their problem: let them deal with it. We have seen this attitude before in relation to HIV, but it is durable and, like racism, ineradicable. We have to circumvent it.

Second, it is said that these diseases affect only older people who are of less economic value and who will, within a few years, die of *something*, so why worry what it is? Yes, chronic diseases do increase markedly with increasing age—no dispute. It is also true that chronic diseases do not kill many children, but it is untrue that they disable and kill only old people. In developing societies, and in many communities of Eastern Europe and Asia, they are killing the breadwinners in families and starting a poverty spiral for those they leave behind.

Third, there are those who mistakenly believe, despite strong evidence to the contrary, that chronic conditions are problems only of the prosperous and affluent and that they should pay the price of their indulgence and pay for their own suffering. Chronic diseases may start out that way, but in rapid order, the rich get smart, reorder their lifestyles, and chronic diseases fall principally on those who have few choices, are less affluent, or are poor.

When we look more carefully at these disorders, the argument for self-infliction becomes weak. Why are these disorders showing a predilection for less-affluent sectors of society? This is not because these people choose to eat damaging and fattening food, but rather because it is an economic necessity. The pressures of markets that thrive on providing fast, cheap, salty, and fattening foods are very powerful, and people respond to those pressures. Similarly, a city where development has proceeded without safe roads and sidewalks is a place where people will gain less physical activity. They will do more in a town or city that recognizes the value of walking or cycling and builds or modifies its roads and paths to that end. A town or other urban development that provides space for people to meet and feel safe is one where human assembly is likely to occur and where the social engagement may lead to a sense and reality of support, neighborliness, and community spirit. These factors contribute to the mental health of a community.

## THE CHANGING GLOBAL DEMOGRAPHY

It is worth pondering what is happening to the world's population. With increasing general prosperity, it has continued to grow, but not at the pace predicted. Indeed, it has slowed down somewhat, in large part in those countries where child survival has improved and parents spontaneously cut back on family size. The same factors that have decreased the scourge of infectious disease have helped us all to live longer and better lives. Most people in most countries of the world are living longer than ever before. More people than ever are living longer with developing forms of illness and disability that will take a varying and unpredictable course; many will cause their death. Some of them are not even able to be seen or felt, yet inevitably get worse, leading to constraints on well-being and the limitation of life.

There are demographic subtleties that deserve our attention as well. Many nations are currently experiencing a dependency holiday: they have fewer children to demand their support and not nearly as many older people as they will have around in a few years who might similarly expect state and community support (particularly in low- and middle-income countries; see Table 9.1). This window of opportunity for high productivity and organizing to prepare for a larger number of older people, including in our cities, will not remain open for long. If we wish to see lower levels of chronic illness among those who will be the old people of our communities in ten or fifteen years, we do not have long to act—we are racing against time (Leeder and others 2004).

TABLE 9.1  Percentage of Population in Low-, Middle-, and High-income Countries in 2005 (Estimated) and 2030 (Projected)

|  | Percentage of Population (15–64 years) | Percentage of Population (65+ years) |
|---|---|---|
| *Low-income countries* | | |
| 2005 | 56.6 | 3.6 |
| 2030 | 36.0 | 5.0 |
| *Middle-income countries* | | |
| 2005 | 66.0 | 6.7 |
| 2030 | 37.9 | 11.8 |
| *High-income countries* | | |
| 2005 | 67.3 | 14.6 |
| 2030 | 62.7 | 21.0 |

*Source:* World Bank, HNP statistics (http://go.worldbank.org/KZHE1CQFA0).

## THE MAGNITUDE AND SCOPE OF CHRONIC DISEASE

The stealth with which chronic diseases have replaced the dramatic infectious disease killers of earlier centuries has taken us by surprise. We have only recently taken them seriously. Developing countries must tackle the added challenge of a dual burden of disease: simultaneously dealing with "old" health problems, such as infectious and parasitic diseases with their declining mortality rates, and "new" health problems, such as noncommunicable chronic diseases affecting an aging population. This epidemiologic transition creates a complex situation in a developing country whose health infrastructure is often inadequate to deal with current needs and not agile enough to respond to emerging challenges through the development of preventive and other cost-effective interventions. Mexico is an example of a country currently undergoing an epidemiological transition (Rivera and others 2002), where standardized mortality rates attributed to diabetes, hypertension, and heart disease have increased dramatically, parallel to the prevalence of obesity.

No international aid agencies that profess an interest in health have yet committed funds in any meaningful way to the mitigation of chronic disease. Instead, an agenda for aid is established that concentrates on HIV, malaria, maternal survival, and immunization. This makes good sense—half good sense, in fact—but it is rather like taking an interest in the athletic development of one's left arm and leg and paying no interest to the limbs on the right.

Nothing, or next to nothing, is done about the chronic conditions that account for half the deaths in the world, even though one-third of those deaths due to heart disease and its relatives occur among people aged less than 65 who would otherwise contribute positively to family well-being and national productivity. In 2004, coronary heart disease, stroke, and other cerebrovascular diseases were the leading causes of death worldwide and in high- and middle-income countries and the second leading cause of death in low-income countries (WHO reference fact sheets).

Calculations of the burden imposed on the world by chronic disease indicate how big a problem these conditions are as a cause both of death and of disability and suffering. Combining death and suffering into a single indicator and expressing the impact in terms of years of quality life lost, the Global Burden of Disease (GBD) study reinforces that chronic diseases are the biggest challenge we face. The GBD study, conducted first in 1996 and then modified and developed on several occasions since, has revealed the long shadow cast by chronic disease. It stretches from the economically advanced nations, where heart disease deaths peaked in the mid 1960s and have now halved, to the economically developing nations. Today, death from chronic disease is as common in these developing nations as it is in economically advanced nations. It is no longer a set of disorders that are much more common in industrially advanced countries. On a case-to-population ratio, it is an even, toxic cloud that covers the whole Earth. It affects everyone, everywhere, men and women, and also young men and young women, especially in the case of diabetes. Ironically and somewhat paradoxically, it is best under control these days where city living is at its most affluent.

It is essential that policy makers appreciate the magnitude and scope of this escalating situation. As noted in Table 9.2, Mathers and Loncar (2006) estimate that by 2030 the two leading causes of death worldwide (and in high- and middle-income per capita countries) will be ischemic heart disease and cerebrovascular disease. In low-income per capita countries, the leading cause of death also will be ischemic heart disease, but HIV/AIDS will supplant cerebrovascular disease as the second leading cause of death. These trends not only highlight the epidemiologic transition associated with urban and economic development, but the strategic planning challenges that must be addressed to drive health policy development and priority-setting in developing countries.

## The Causes Behind the Causes

Individual factors that lead to chronic disease—tobacco, lack of physical activity, and excessive dietary intake of hydrogenated fats, alcohol, sugar, and salt—express

TABLE 9.2  Three Leading Causes of Death, by Income Group, 2030

| Income Group | Rank | Disease | Percent of Total Deaths |
|---|---|---|---|
| World | 1 | Ischemic heart disease | 13.4 |
|  | 2 | Cerebrovascular disease | 10.6 |
|  | 3 | HIV/AIDS | 8.9 |
| High-income | 1 | Ischemic heart disease | 15.8 |
|  | 2 | Cerebrovascular disease | 9.0 |
|  | 3 | Trachea, bronchus, lung cancers | 5.1 |
| Middle-income | 1 | Cerebrovascular disease | 14.4 |
|  | 2 | Ischemic heart disease | 12.7 |
|  | 3 | COPD | 12.0 |
| Low-income | 1 | Ischemic heart disease | 13.4 |
|  | 2 | HIV/AIDS | 13.2 |
|  | 3 | Cerebrovascular disease | 8.2 |

*Source:* Adapted from Mathers and Loncar (2006).

TABLE 9.3  "Causes Behind the Causes" of Chronic Disease

| Variables (Causes) | Examples |
|---|---|
| Social determinants | Lack of availability of social networks and support |
| Macrosocial determinants | Limited access to even poor quality foods  Poor physical infrastructure that inhibits exercise |
| Health services | Inequitable distribution and variable quality of health services |
| Environmental concerns | Air and noise pollution |

themselves in obesity, elevated blood pressure, high cholesterol and other lipid disturbances in the blood, diabetes, heart disease, stroke, and cancer.

Behind these individual factors and what they cause, elements can be found in the environment that "cause the causes" to a large or small extent (see Table 9.3). The international effects of globalization can affect health positively and negatively, especially of those in poorer countries. The opening up of world markets, instant international communications among countries, and sharing of labor, goods, and markets across national boundaries tends to favor the rich nations. This often increases the overall income of developing countries, while doing so with a differential that gives advantages to the better-off in developing countries; through loss of markets, protection, and reduced prices for their produce, this widens the gap in income for rural dwellers, which then limits availability of education and access to better nutrition.

City dwellers are worse off as globalization accentuates inequalities, and governments give priority to making cities attractive to foreign investment and industry or tourism, rather than investing in benefits to citizens. In India, Hyderabad is nicknamed "Cyberabad" because of its successful efforts to attract the information technology industry. Globalization of tobacco markets and of targeted advertising to the developing world with the decline in markets in the developed world add a growing burden of future illness, especially in urban areas where the products are freely available. People head to cities to benefit from jobs that globalization offers and add to the impetus for urban population growth. In their turn, these factors contribute to worsening health. Similarly, in the urban slums of Faridabad in India, the high prevalence of risk factors for chronic noncommunicable diseases across all age groups indicates the likelihood of a high future burden of disease (Anand and others 2007).

Signs of the new diseases do not show immediately, except perhaps in the stress experienced by people removed from their land, their villages, their extended families, and the ways of life that they knew. The risk factors and diseases lurk silently, such as asymptomatic high blood pressure or depression; or they develop slowly, such as obesity; or they are visible, in the case of a stroke.

These environmental forces are often the ones that do us so many favors as well—the operation of markets that underpin the growth of prosperity, which in itself can be associated with immense improvements in health. The falling rates of infant deaths that have accompanied economic reform and growth in countries such as India are witness to the amazing benefits that have come to so many people from increasing affluence.

As with concerns about human-induced climate change that have reached a serious pitch recently, we are growing in our awareness of the side effects of economic growth. Towns and cities are highly energy-dependent and their cars, factories, homes, and centers of culture, commerce, entertainment, sports, and learning all demand energy, whose release from fossil hydrocarbons adds to the global burden of greenhouse gases. So, too, urban pleasures of easy transport, reduced physical labor to procure food, the social pressures of eating (what we eat, how much we eat, and whom we eat with) and drinking, and the constant pressure of advertising that links consumption to satisfaction come at a price—part is chronic illness. Day by day, city dwellers walk less, their muscles change, their weight goes up, their metabolism alters and after a few decades, chronic disease is upon them. Illness leads to further losses: employment, opportunities for pleasure and interests, and a buoyant mood. With these losses, in poorer communities, there is also loss of work and livelihood; inability to maintain payment for housing; a shift into slum or shanty living conditions; worsening access to food, education, and transport; and further ill health.

The global financial crisis (GFC) has alerted all of us to the fragility of our social arrangements and has reminded us of the uncertainties we face, or often do not face. As economist Amartya Sen reminds us, when contemplating new approaches to problems, we spend far too little time, generally, thinking about the unintended side effects that may flow from our new proposal. To this consideration—in light of the GFC and what we are slowly learning about climate change—we should be adding a period for the intelligent contemplation of the sustainability of new efforts.

Generally speaking, what is good for the climate is good for chronic disease. Several writers have seen obesity as a metaphor for global warming. The same excessive use of energy that leads to one leads to the other, albeit with radically different outcomes. But to take Sen's point, when urban in-fill and replacement is under consideration, or a new town or city is being designed, there is value in asking questions about the extent to which it will make it easier to live a life that takes joy in physical activity (weather permitting), favors the use of the bicycle over other fuel-burning forms of transport, favors mass transit over the thrombotic overuse of cars, and enables access to markets where healthy food is easy to obtain.

Nor is urban design the only field that we should consider. What of the urban neighborhood itself? Some studies suggest that there has been an increase in the contribution of neighborhood socioeconomic factors to the socioeconomic gradient in heart disease (Chaix, Rosvall, and Merlo 2007). Even in a place where so many people live so close together, it is easy to drift into patterns of living that widen the spread of socioeconomic advantage. Surprisingly little progress has occurred in many countries in bringing the extremes of this spectrum together, and in many cities the gap has widened: the economically advantaged have become even more so, and while many have moved from poverty into less straitened circumstances, a good proportion of those who were poor remain so and, relatively speaking, worse off. It is among them that chronic disease does its worst. If poverty increases as the acid of the GFC trickles down through the layers of society, corroding structures and functions we once thought to be solid steel, then we will see more chronic disease, not less, in our towns and cities. The search for cheaper goods, a fragmenting labor market, and falling income all push the poor towards behaviors and patterns of consumption that will add to the burden of chronic disease. What then can and must be done?

## TAKING ACTION ON CHRONIC DISEASES

First, every opportunity should be taken for prophetic warnings about the coming tsunami of chronic disease. This is no joke, any more than climate change is. The conceptual foundations of aid agencies that are not yet funding the battle against chronic noncommunicable diseases need to be severely shaken. The evidence is sound and the case for action must be made wherever informed and articulate advocates can make it. This includes in national governments (well beyond the confines of departments and ministries of health and including treasuries) and international agencies. The World Health Organization should be energized to give chronic disease the emphasis it deserves. Their leadership through the treaty that binds countries to control tobacco—the Framework Convention for Tobacco Control—is a good beginning.

Second, a vast armamentarium of cheap, generic drugs to treat such conditions as high blood pressure and raised cholesterol, alone or combined in a "polypill," should be seen as weapons in the war against conditions such as heart disease and stroke. No person with diabetes should be without such treatment—anywhere, at any time.

Third, and considering the role of the city, we can no longer leave health aside when designing or redesigning our cities from the beginning, as they undergo change, or after disasters. We cannot confine our planning for health to concerns for clean water and waste disposal facilities, important as they are. It is time to design for the future demographic makeup of our cities, so that those with chronic disease and less mobility are not excluded from participating in the activities that cities offer. Green and environmentally thoughtful spaces for gathering, walkways that are safe and pleasant, access for older people to retail outlets for healthy food, and transport systems that encourage walking and bicycling but also enable older or disabled people to move around easily are all part of the design brief of a modern city.

The proximate risk factors for chronic disease—which is the metabolic equivalent of global warming—are expressed as individual behaviors (what we eat, smoke, and do for exercise), but they owe much to environmental circumstances.

The centrality of design to all forms of habitat, cities, urban transport systems, and the commercial and industrial worlds is well recognized in the sustainability movement. This movement seeks to mitigate global warming, reduce the use of fossil fuels, insulate buildings, and encourage walking as pollution-free way of getting about. Evidence suggests that urban areas in Northern Ireland remain less healthy than the more rural areas, and the association with respiratory disease and lung cancer suggests that air pollution may be a factor (O'Reilly and others 2007). Sustainability is aimed at maintaining quality of

> ### What Are Cities Doing to Counter Chronic Disease Risk?
>
> - The introduction of menu labeling laws is a potentially important legal tool to address the obesity epidemic in the United States. More cities and states are considering this move, having learned from New York City's efforts in this area (Rutkow and others 2008).
> - From 1995 to 1999, the World Health Organization (WHO) supported Healthy City projects in Cox's Bazar (Bangladesh), Dar es Salaam (Tanzania), Fayoum (Egypt), Managua (Nicaragua), and Quetta (Pakistan) to focus on improving the health and environmental conditions where poor people live. The main activities chosen by these community-based projects were awareness-raising and environmental improvements, particularly solid waste disposal (Harpham, Burton, and Blue 2001).
> - A number of effective innovative built environment and policy interventions have been implemented across the United States (Rutt, Dannenberg, and Kochtitzky 2008), recognizing the role of urban planning to create environments for health promotion, improving access to and consumption of healthy foods, protecting people against industrial pollution, and encouraging healthy corporate practices (Freudenberg and Galea 2008). In Philadelphia, Un Corazón Saludable: A Healthy Heart was developed in conjunction with a community-based organization to engage urban Latinas in physical activity and increase awareness of cardiac risk factors, highlighting the importance of addressing real-life barriers experienced by populations in low-income urban environments (Harralson and others 2007).
> - Concerted local action in New York City, with the implementation of a five-component tobacco control strategy, resulted in a sharp reduction in smoking prevalence (as measured from 2002 to 2003). Further progress will most likely require national action (Freiden and others 2005).

life across generations. It assumes, but less often examines, a role for health. This theme was pursued at the Sydney Summit (2008) of the Oxford Health Alliance (http://www.oxha.org), a network of concerned health advocates drawn from industry, academia, government, and the health professions. The conclusions of the summit were enshrined in a resolution (http://www.oxha.org/meetings/08-summit/sydney-resolution) calling for broad coalitions of support to combat the principal chronic diseases. The alliance is also active jointly through a program of "Grand Challenges" in chronic disease research and demonstration projects supported by the Ovations (United HealthCare Group) chronic disease initiative.

Promoting an understanding of health among those committed to sustainability is an important step. Arguing that efforts to prevent and limit chronic disease pay off for all societies through enhanced productivity and quality of life, and that putting money into health (including health-enhancing design) and, therefore, into prevention of chronic disease is an efficient investment for every government.

## SUMMARY

In the past fifty years, there has been a shift in the global burden of disease from acute and infectious diseases to chronic and noncommunicable diseases. These diseases are not evenly spread; they increase with poverty and low levels of economic development. These trends are compounded by aspects of urban living, often the same aspects that attract people to cities from rural areas. Now is the time to act and consider possible long-term solutions to reduce chronic disease. This may be achieved through the design of city environments and the way life and commerce are regulated to enable and support individuals in making choices that enhance their health.

## REFERENCES

Anand, K., and others. 2007. Are the urban poor vulnerable to non-communicable diseases? A survey of risk factors for non-communicable diseases in urban slums of Faridabad. *National Medical Journal of India* 20(3):115–20.

Chaix, B., M. Rosvall, and J. Merlo. 2007. Recent increase of neighborhood socioeconomic effects on ischemic heart disease mortality: a multilevel survival analysis of two large Swedish cohorts. *American Journal of Epidemiology* 165(1):22–26.

Freudenberg, N., and S. Galea. 2008. Cities of consumption: the impact of corporate practices on the health of urban populations. *Journal of Urban Health* 85(4):462–471.

Frieden, T. R., and others. 2005. Adult tobacco use levels after intensive tobacco control measures: New York City, 2002–2003. *American Journal of Public Health* 95(6):1016–1023.

Frieden, T. R., M. T. Bassett, L. E. Thorpe, and T. A. Farley. 2008. Public health in New York City, 2002–2007: Confronting epidemics of the modern era. *International Journal of Epidemiology* 37(5):966–977

Harpham, T., S. Burton, and I. Blue. 2001. Healthy city projects in developing countries: The first evaluation. *Health Promotion International* 16(2):111–125.

Harralson, T. L., and others. 2007. Un Corazón Saludable: Factors influencing outcomes of an exercise program designed to impact cardiac and metabolic risks among urban Latinas. *Journal of Community Health* 32(6):401–412.

Larson, K., and others. 2006. Public health detailing: A strategy to improve the delivery of clinical preventive services in New York City. *Public Health Reports* 121(3):228–234.

Leeder, S., S. Raymond, H. Greenberg, H. Liu, and K. Esson, eds. 2004. *A race against time: The challenge of cardiovascular disease in developing countries.* The Earth Institute at Columbia University. http://www.earth.columbia.edu/news/2004/images/raceagainsttime_FINAL_051104.pdf.

Lim, S., and others. 2007. Prevention of cardiovascular disease in high-risk individuals in low-income and middle-income countries: Health effects and costs. *Lancet* 370:2054–2062.

Mathers, C. D., and D. Loncar. 2006. Projections of global mortality and burden of disease from 2002 to 2030. *PLoS Medicine* 3(11):e442.

Ntandou, G., H. Delisle, V. Agueh, and B. Fayomi. 2009. Abdominal obesity explains the positive rural-urban gradient in the prevalence of the metabolic syndrome in Benin, West Africa. *Nutrition Research* 29(3):180–189.

O'Reilly, G., D. O'Reilly, M. Rosato, and S. Connolly. 2007. Urban and rural variations in morbidity and mortality in Northern Ireland. *BMC Public Health* 7:123.

Rivera, J. A., and others. 2002. Epidemiological and nutritional transition in Mexico: Rapid increase of non-communicable chronic diseases and obesity. *Public Health Nutrition* 5(1A):113–122.

Rutkow, L., J. S. Vernick, J. G. Hodge Jr., and S. P. Teret. 2008. Preemption and the obesity epidemic: State and local menu labeling laws and the nutrition labeling and education act. *Journal of Law and Medical Ethics* 36(4):772–789, 611.

Rutt, C., A. L. Dannenberg, and C. Kochtitzky. 2008. Using policy and built environment interventions to improve public health. *Journal of Public Health Management Practices* 14(3):221–223.

World Bank. 2009, August. Population projection tables by country and group. Health, nutrition and population (HNP) statistics. http://go.worldbank.org/KZHE1CQFA0.

# CHAPTER TEN

# CHRONIC DISEASE CARE IN NAIROBI'S URBAN INFORMAL SETTLEMENTS

## CATHERINE KYOBUTUNGI

## ALEX EZEH

### LEARNING OBJECTIVES

- Describe the chronic disease situation among residents of poor slum settlements in Nairobi City, with a focus on cardiovascular disease conditions
- Describe how the existing health care system is unresponsive to the needs of the urban poor affected by such chronic diseases
- Learn about a model of health care that delivers high-quality services to slum residents with chronic conditions

THIS chapter focuses on an initiative by the African Population and Health Research Center (APHRC) to improve the quality of health care for cardiovascular disease (CVD) conditions available to residents of two slum settlements in Nairobi, Kenya. First, there is a general description of Nairobi City, with emphasis on living conditions in slum settlements where the majority of its residents live. The chapter then describes a research-to-policy initiative by APHRC that aims to provide evidence on the impractical nature of existing Kenyan government guidelines for the management of CVD conditions and why a policy shift is needed to enhance access to CVD care in countries with limited human resources for health capacity and an emerging noncommunicable diseases epidemic. It discusses the current status of access to health care by slum residents, the role played by the private sector, and concludes with the policy implications for chronic disease management in resource-constrained countries in general, and the health of slum dwellers in particular.

## OVERVIEW OF NAIROBI CITY

Nairobi is a typical African city facing an urbanization crisis. Over the last sixty years, its population has increased more than 25 times—from about 120,000 residents in 1948 to more than 3 million by 2002 (UN-HABITAT 2003). This rapid urbanization has occurred amid poor economic performance, especially in the last two decades, poor governance, and poor urban planning. Rapid urbanization has therefore resulted in the mushrooming of informal settlements across the city, commonly referred to as slums. By some estimates, Nairobi has about seventy-eight areas that can be classified as slum settlements, and it is estimated that up to 60 percent of Nairobi's residents live in slum or slumlike conditions (UN-HABITAT 2003). Slum settlements are often characterized by pervasive poverty, overcrowding, social marginalization, poor environmental conditions (UN-HABITAT 2003; Matrix Development Consultants 1993), insecurity, and few or no basic social services (APHRC 2002). Economic insecurity, high levels of unemployment, and high levels of mobility result in social fragmentation and compound residents' vulnerability to catastrophic expenditures in times of serious illness, death, or job loss.

Data and health indicators for Nairobi City are the same as those for Nairobi Province. National survey data are usually aggregated at the provincial level. Although Nairobi Province has relatively good health indicators compared to the rest of the country, there is evidence of large intraurban inequities in health. Slum residents have health outcomes that are in some instances worse than those of their rural counterparts. The indicators in Table 10.1 illustrate how slum

TABLE 10.1 Selected Health and Demographic Indicators in Nairobi Slums, Nairobi Province, and Kenya

| Indicator | Nairobi Slums[b] | Nairobi Province[c] | Kenya[c] |
|---|---|---|---|
| Children fully vaccinated (%; 2003) | 44 | 73 | 57 |
| Children with diarrhea in last 2 weeks (%) | 31 | 13 | 17 |
| Delivery assisted by skilled birth attendant (%) | 54 | 76 | 42 |
| Infant mortality rate (per 1,000 live births) | 96 | 67 | 77 |
| Under-five mortality rate (per 1,000 live births) | 139 | 95 | 115 |
| Neonatal mortality rate | 27 | 32 | 33 |
| Post-neonatal mortality rates | 69 | 35 | 44 |
| HIV prevalence (males and females) | 13.0[d] | 9.9 | 6.7 |
| Maternal mortality ratio (per 100,000 live births) | 631[e] | — | 414 |
| Contraceptive prevalence rate | 46[a] | 51 | 39 |
| Unmet need for contraception (%) | 23 | 13 | 24 |
| Mistimed and unwanted pregnancies (%) | 47 | 34 | 48 |

Sources: (a) APHRC and World Bank (2006); (b) APHRC unpublished data (2003); (c) CBS, MoH, and ORC Macro (2004); (d) APHRC unpublished data (2006); (e) Ziraba et al. (2009).

residents in Nairobi exhibit poorer health outcomes than the average for residents of Nairobi as a whole and for the country.

## GOVERNANCE AND HEALTH SERVICE PROVISION

Nairobi City is administered by the City Council of Nairobi (CCN) under the authority of the Ministry of Local Government. The CCN is headed by a mayor elected by an electoral college comprising fifty elected councilors representing wards—lower-level administrative units—and eighteen nominated councilors. While the CCN has the mandate to provide social services to all Nairobi residents, central government line ministries (such as health, education, and environment) also have a responsibility to provide services specific to their ministries to all Kenyans, including those in Nairobi City. There are two ministries of health: the Ministry of Public Health and Sanitation, responsible for service delivery at primary health care facilities (Levels I to III), and the Ministry of Medical Services, responsible for service delivery in hospitals (Levels IV to VI). Recently, a new ministry, the Nairobi Metropolitan Ministry, has been created to oversee the strategic growth and expansion of the city into a modern metropolis. A recent report suggests that the parallel governance structures in the city, coupled with an inefficient bureaucracy in CCN and insufficient funding, have led to dismal service delivery (OXFAM 2009).

In the health sector, the Nairobi Health Management Board (NHMB) was created to serve as a bridge between the CCN, the central Ministries of Health, and the Ministry of Local Government (before the Nairobi Metropolitan Ministry was created). The NHMB is chaired by the Provincial Director of Public Health and Sanitation for Nairobi Province, and the head of the CCN Department of Public Health is its secretary. The NHMB has representation from other departments in the CCN, the Provincial Directorate of Public Health and Sanitation, and the Provincial Directorate of Medical Services. In terms of service delivery, the CCN operates mostly Levels II and III health facilities in the city, but these are staffed by health personnel recruited and paid by the central ministries of health through the provincial directorates of health, based on the service delivery level. For instance, nurses who run dispensaries would be recruited through the Provincial Directorate of Public Health and Sanitation, while nurses who work in district hospitals would be recruited through the Provincial Directorate of Medical Services. Much of the funding for curative and preventive programs in the city is from the ministries of health, and health programs are implemented in line with the current National Health Sector Strategic Plan. The CCN Department of Public Health plays a marginal role in actual health service provision and in enforcing various Public Health Acts due to chronic underfunding. In 2003–2004, for instance, CCN spent close to 75 percent of its annual budget on wages for bureaucrats, 21 percent on operations and maintenance and a meager 4 percent directly on service delivery (UN-HABITAT 2006). Personnel engaged in the provision of critical social services, such as health and education, are in most instances paid by the central government through the concerned line ministry.

Although the CCN operates health facilities in the city, none of them are located within any slum settlement. Those that serve slum residents are located either on the outskirts of the slums or a few kilometers away. The informal nature of slum settlements is often used as justification for the failure of government to provide adequate health and social services. The few public health facilities that serve slum residents are often overwhelmed by the large numbers of users, because they were built to serve the population in the formal settlements where they are located. Infrastructure development has not kept pace with the high rate of the city's growth, so the existing public health facilities are not even sufficient for the population in formal settlements. Often, these facilities are understaffed, and they run out of essential drugs and commodities. For the majority of slum dwellers, these facilities are also geographically inaccessible either because of transport costs, limited hours of operation (health centers open from 08.00 to 17.00 hours on weekdays only), or insecurity in the slums that precludes movement at night for long distances, even in emergencies.

As a result of the near absence of public health facilities, there has been a proliferation of private health providers who cater to the needs of the majority of slum residents. These include providers who are private-not-for-profit (PNFP), including faith-based organizations, and those who are private-for-profit (PFP). A health service provision assessment survey conducted by APHRC in two large, informal settlements in Nairobi in 2008 showed that out of the 326 health facilities surveyed, there were only three (1 percent) public (government) facilities. Among the 323 private facilities, the majority (88.9 percent) were private-for-profit and the rest (11.1 percent) not-for-profit. The majority of the facilities were clinics (Level II) that accounted for close to 83 percent of all facilities (APHRC unpublished data). The sheer number of private health facilities (323) suggests that there is a large but unregulated health care market, because this number is much higher than the number of facilities registered with the respective district health offices. According to the Health Management Information Systems (HMIS) reports for Nairobi Province, until July 2009, only 405 health facilities (188 of them private) were registered with the respective health district authorities in the whole province (MMS–Kenya 2009). Yet, the APHRC survey, which covered only two of the close to eighty slum settlements, identified almost 50 private health facilities, more than the administrative records show for the entire city.

Though in numeric terms, public health facilities are outnumbered, they provide services to a large proportion of slum residents. Studies conducted by the African Population and Health Research Center in two Nairobi slum settlements showed that 35 percent of households with a sick child seek care from public providers and that 28 percent of pregnant women deliver in public facilities including those far away from the slums. However, private facilities are the first source of health care for childhood illnesses in 51–54 percent of households and for 72 percent of deliveries (APHRC unpublished data). Other studies in the same area have shown that 51 percent of women deliver in what can be described as "inappropriate" health facilities—facilities too ill-equipped to offer many of the signal functions of basic emergency obstetric care—and these are almost exclusively PFP (APHRC and The World Bank 2006; Fotso, Ezeh, and Oronje 2008).

## SERVICE PROVISION FOR NCD IN KENYA

The provision of health services in Kenya is guided by the second National Health Sector Strategic Plan (NHSSP II), which was formulated in 2005 (MoH–Kenya 2005). The NHSSP II details national health priorities and cost-effective interventions and provides guidelines for implementation plans. At the operational level, national Annual Operational Plans (AOP) are generated by a bottom-up approach from districts to provinces to the national level to define national health targets, strategies and indicators for each year, within the limits and confines of the NHSSP II. Since most of the personnel running health services are employed by the central ministries of health and therefore report directly to the Provincial Directorates, the CCN is marginally involved in the formulation and implementation of district AOP. It is only through the NHMB that CCN is involved in the review and monitoring of district AOP.

The NHSSP II defined the Kenya Essential Package of Health (KEPH), which contains priority interventions (curative, preventive, and promotive) for age cohorts over the life course. These cohorts are (1) mothers and newborns, (2) early childhood (2 weeks to 59 months), (3) late childhood (5–12 years), (4) youth and adolescence (13–24 years), and (5) adulthood (25–59 years), and (6) old age (60+ years). Six levels of health service delivery are defined to implement the KEPH. A set of interventions—whether curative, preventive or promotive—have been defined for each level of service delivery, together with the appropriate staffing. The levels are illustrated in Table 10.2.

In NHSSP II guidelines for KEPH, the interventions against noncommunicable diseases (NCD) are rather generic and are not specified in great detail. For example, for the adulthood lifecycle cohort, preventive and promotive interventions are aimed at "diseases of affluence" and include annual screening and medical examinations and promotion of healthy lifestyles (exercise, recreation, nutrition, and so on), while curative interventions are described as "overall treatment and care." For the old age cohort, the curative interventions are described as "access to drugs for degenerative illnesses."

For other lifecycle cohorts like mothers and newborns, interventions are elaborated well, since they mostly deal with communicable diseases and conditions associated with pregnancy and childbirth. Looking at the levels of care where NCD interventions are offered, curative services are only offered at Levels IV to VI while the preventive/promotive interventions are offered at all levels, depending on the

TABLE 10.2  Levels of Health Service Delivery for the Kenya Essential Package of Health

| Level of Care | Type of Health Facilities at This Level | Services Offered | Most Qualified Staff Cadre |
| --- | --- | --- | --- |
| I | None, this level is the community and informal structures that may be present to improve the health of the population | Health promotive and preventive | Not applicable |
| II | Dispensaries, clinics | Promotive, preventive, basic curative | Registered comprehensive nurse |
| III | Health centers, maternities, nursing homes | Promotive, preventive, basic curative | Clinical officer[1] |
| IV | District and sub-district hospitals | Curative, minimal preventive, and promotive | Medical officer[2] |
| V | Provincial hospitals | Curative, minimal preventive, and promotive | Medical specialists |
| VI | National referral hospitals | Curative, minimal preventive, and promotive | Medical super-specialists in various fields |

[1] Clinician with three years medical training, lower cadre than doctor.
[2] Doctor with basic medical training (five to six years), usually without further specialization.

capacities of staff at those levels. This implies that patients may only access curative service for NCDs, such as cardiovascular diseases, at subdistrict or district hospitals or beyond. Preventive and promotive services at the lower levels are limited to group health education sessions and advice given during hasty consultations by cadres of health workers whose training rarely covers management of NCDs.

## CVD CLINICS PROJECT IN TWO NAIROBI SLUMS

Two CVD clinics were set up to operate in the slums of Korogocho and Viwandani, located less than 10 kilometers from the city center of Nairobi—the commercial and political capital of Kenya. The clinics were set up by APHRC to run parallel to a research project to assess the levels of risk factors (both behavioral and physiological) for CVD among the adult population (18 years and older, no upper limit) residing in the geographic area covered by the Nairobi Urban Health and Demographic Surveillance System (NUHDSS). Data collection started in April 2008 and ended in April 2009. The research project targeted 5,000 respondents randomly selected through stratified sampling, but 5,190 were interviewed by the end of the survey. In each of twenty strata, 250 respondents were targeted for personal interviews. As part of the research project, data were collected on alcohol consumption habits, tobacco use, physical activity, and dietary intake (behavioral risk factors) and on weight, height, waist and hip circumference, blood pressure, random blood glucose, total blood cholesterol, and triglycerides (physiological risk factors). Preliminary analysis of the data revealed a high prevalence of the two CVD conditions of interest: hypertension and diabetes.[1]

## The Magnitude of CVD Conditions in the Nairobi Slums

The survey revealed a high period prevalence of hypertension and diabetes as well as risk factors like hypercholesterolemia and obesity. It was also rather striking that most of the people who had the two conditions were largely unaware of them, those who were aware were unlikely to be on treatment, and the few who were on treatment at the time of the survey (that is, who took medication for either high blood pressure or diabetes in the two weeks before the survey) did not appear to be benefiting from the treatment. Blood pressure was measured using professional series digital machines (OMRON® HEM 907), which took three consecutive readings one minute apart. The mean of the second and third readings was used to determine whether someone was hypertensive, using the 140 (systolic) and 90 (diastolic) cut-off points. Hypertension was defined as either a systolic BP $\geq 140$ or a diastolic BP $\geq 90$ or whether someone was on treatment for hypertension (even though their blood pressure was lower than the 140/90 mmHg cut-offs). The crude period prevalence of hypertension was about 20 percent (all prevalence estimates are unadjusted for nonresponse). This translated into 1,048 people out of a sample of 5,190 respondents. After adjustment for sampling to cater for the sex and age distribution in the whole population, the prevalence was 12.3 percent. For diabetes, the crude period prevalence was 6.1 percent (317 respondents), and the adjusted prevalence was 4.3 percent. A diagnosis of diabetes was made based on previous history of being diagnosed with diabetes or random capillary blood glucose >11.1 mmol/dl or an oral glucose tolerance test reading after 2 hours of >11.1 mmol/dl. About 1,238 respondents (crude 23.8 percent; adjusted 15.7 percent) had either of the two conditions, and 108 had both. The awareness, treatment, and control patterns for both conditions after adjusting for sampling probabilities are shown in Table 10.3.

TABLE 10.3  Period Prevalence, Awareness, Treatment, and Control of Diabetes and Hypertension Among Adult Slum Residents, Nairobi, 2008–2009

| | Hypertension | | | | | | Diabetes | | | |
|---|---|---|---|---|---|---|---|---|---|---|
| | (a) Diagnosed during survey n = 1048 | (b) Aware of diagnosis n = 285 | (c) On treatment in last 12 months n = 145 | (d) Currently on treatment n = 100 | Controlled i.e. BP ≤ 140/90 n = 32 | Controlled i.e. BP ≤ 120/80 n = 9 | (a) Diagnosed during survey n = 312 | (b) Aware of diagnosis n = 101 | (c) On treatment in last 12 months n = 72 | (d) Currently on treatment n = 52 | Controlled i.e. RBS* <7.7mmol/dl n = 23 |
| As a % of N (5190) | 20.2% | 5.0% | 2.8% | 1.9% | 0.6% | 0.2% | 6.0% | 1.9% | 1.4% | 1.0% | 0.4% |
| As a % of (a) | NA | 27.2% | 13.8% | 9.5% | 3.1% | 0.9% | NA | 32.4% | 23.1% | 16.7% | 7.4% |
| As a % of (b) | NA | NA | 50.9% | 35.1% | 11.2% | 3.2% | NA | NA | 71.3% | 51.5% | 22.8% |
| As a % of (c) | NA | NA | NA | 69.0% | 22.1% | 6.2% | NA | NA | NA | 72.2% | 31.9% |
| As a % of (d) | NA | NA | NA | NA | 32.0% | 9.0% | NA | NA | NA | NA | 44.2% |

*RBS: random blood glucose.

Definitions for hypertension and glycemic control used in Table 10.3 are rather conservative. For instance, a cutoff of 140/90 to determine blood pressure control is very conservative. Current guidelines for hypertension management advocate reductions in blood pressure to levels even below the 120/80 mark, especially if the patient has a high, ten-year cardiac risk. For diabetes, random blood glucose of 7.7 mmol/dl level is also a rather conservative and rough indicator of glycemic control. Although fasting blood glucose or glycosylated hemoglobin (HbA1c) measurement would have been desirable, the former is not always possible in a survey setting and the latter was not available.

From Table 9.3, it is evident that majority of people in the study area who have a CVD condition are unaware of it; a survey based on self-reported information would miss more than three-quarters of people with hypertension and two-thirds of diabetics. A recent study in Kenya showed that only 21 percent of diabetics in urban settings were unaware of their condition, compared to 48 percent of diabetics in rural settings (Christensen and others 2009). However, the sample selection in this study was not completely random, especially in urban areas, and the high awareness figures could be due to selection bias. A national survey from Cameroon showed that awareness, treatment, and control levels were rather poor. For hypertension, about 23 percent were aware, 46 percent of those were on treatment, and 19 percent of those treated were controlled. For diabetes, only 20 percent of those diagnosed during the survey were aware, 74 percent of those who were aware were on treatment, and about 27 percent of those on treatment were controlled (HoPiT 2004). Compared to urban residents in the only available study from Kenya, limitations notwithstanding, it is evident that awareness levels among the population in the two slums are very low. The low awareness and treatment patterns may reflect the poor access to health services (geographic or financial) or lack of access to right information on the diseases and their management.

A slightly higher proportion of respondents who were aware that they were hypertensive (51 of those who were aware and 14 of all respondents with hypertension) had taken medication in the last 12 months before the survey. This signifies that there are some individuals who know they should be on treatment but, for various reasons, are unable to do it consistently. The poor control among those on treatment may reflect poor adherence to treatment (which may also be linked to poor access), or poor quality of care that reflects lack of skills among health providers, or lack of appropriate lifestyle adjustments to complement therapeutic care. Overall, diabetics are more likely to be aware of their condition than patients with hypertension, and diabetics are also more likely to be on treatment and more likely to be controlled, but only slightly. The medium- and long-term consequences of undiagnosed, untreated, and uncontrolled diabetes and high blood pressure in the community are immense. The risks for CVD endpoints like coronary heart disease, hypertensive heart disease, and stroke are high in the population.

These findings point to a community widely affected by noncommunicable diseases but where the bulk of health efforts are focused on HIV/AIDS and other communicable diseases. This particular community has a prevalence rate of HIV/AIDS 4 percentage points higher than the national average or for either rural or urban areas, manifest both in a high mortality from AIDS and related morbidities (National AIDS and STI Control Programme 2008). The estimated prevalence rate in the population aged 15–49 (females) and 15–55 (males) in the study community is about 12 percent compared to 7.8 percent in the population aged 15–49 years nationally (APHRC 2008; NASCOP 2008). The overall HIV prevalence in a sample with the same age distribution as for the CVD risk factor assessment study (18+ with no upper limit) would be lower than the estimated 12 percent in the study area, since one would expect a lower prevalence in the age groups 55+ years (which are not captured in HIV seroprevalence surveys). This implies that the high HIV/AIDS burden notwithstanding, this population also has a high burden of noncommunicable diseases. Just by looking at two CVD conditions alone, the combined crude prevalence is 24 percent (adjusted: 16.6 percent). Even if other NCDs—such as asthma, chronic obstructive pulmonary disease, cancers, musculoskeletal disorders like arthritis—had a low prevalence (which is unlikely), NCDs among adults are as big a health problem in this community as HIV/AIDS and its related morbidities, if both morbidity and mortality are considered.

The health system is neither prepared nor responsive to this great need for NCD services. Geographic and financial accessibility are not optimal for primary health care facilities (Levels II and III) and are worse for district and subdistrict hospitals (Level IV) where these conditions are supposed to be managed in the current guidelines for service delivery. A recent health service provision assessment of 326 health facilities that serve the two slums settlements in Nairobi, the focus of this chapter, found that there are only two hospitals within the vicinity of the two slums (one public and one private). The majority of health facilities are clinics or Level II health facilities (~82 percent) with neither the staff, nor the equipment, the drugs, or the mandate to handle (prevent, treat, or screen for and refer) chronic diseases. There are three public and eight private health centers (Level III) which are slightly better equipped but are staffed by clinical officers and are not allocated drugs or supplies to diagnose and manage NCDs. Of these eleven, only seven had a functional glucometer and two had a test for urine glucose. Among all facilities surveyed, 82 percent had a blood pressure machine in working order and six of the eleven health centers reported that they offer "lifestyle counseling" for adults.

Given this situation and that there are only two hospitals serving the two slums and also other nonslum areas, it is hard to see how practical current service guidelines are for the management of CVD and other chronic conditions. (The estimated population in the two slums, where the service provision assessment survey was done, ranges from 150,000 to 250,000.) Assuming that adults (18 years and older) account for two-thirds of this population, it means that there are about 12,300 people with hypertension and 4,300 with diabetes in the two slums alone. It is inconceivable that two hospitals can handle such a patient load, because the numbers alone are simply overwhelming. If the two hospitals did, they would not be in a position to offer the intensive counseling and follow-up that such patients need.

## A More Practical Model for Managing CVD Conditions in the Slums

Since May 2008, the African Population & Health Research Center, together with other partners, has been running clinics to manage the two main CVD conditions of diabetes and hypertension in the two slum communities. The clinics were started to offer a way that respondents from the research project referred to earlier that had either or both CVD conditions could access quality health care. Given the dire economic conditions in the study areas and the near absence of appropriate health facilities, it was initially thought that a voucher system could facilitate patients' obtaining treatment at the nearest hospital. This, however, proved unworkable since most patients had serious financial constraints and could not even afford transport to the hospitals on a regular basis despite having their hospital bills covered. Most people also found it difficult to take days off work or to forfeit a day's earning (most people in the two slum settlements work in the informal sector, and those working in factories are usually given work—and paid—on a daily basis). A new strategy was formulated in consultation with the City Council of Nairobi and a reputable nongovernmental organization, Provide International, which runs health centers that offer subsidized health services to residents in five Nairobi slums. This new strategy entailed bringing services nearer to communities—to facilities within walking distance of most patients—and offered on a day when most patients do not have to forgo a day's earning. Though the research project ended in April 2009, the clinics are still running because there is need to further understand the impact of the service delivery model used in these clinics on health outcomes among the beneficiaries.

## Clinic Setup: A Shift in Chronic Disease Care Guidelines

The clinics are run on an outreach basis every fortnight on Saturdays from seven o'clock in the morning until the last patient leaves. Patients are given either bimonthly or monthly appointments to report either to a health center (Level III) run by the City Council of Nairobi on the outskirts of Viwandani slum or to a health center run by an NGO, Provide International, located right in the middle of Korogocho slum.

First, patients are registered, their records are retrieved (if they have previously attended), and then their measurements are taken, that is, weight, blood pressure, and fasting blood glucose (for diabetics only). These measurements are taken by lay community members who were drawn from a team of field assistants involved in the research project described earlier and given some basic training in using the various pieces of equipment. Clinicians (mostly clinical officers) examine the patients and review their treatment history and their blood glucose and blood pressure measurements on that day to decide on the appropriate treatment.

Clinical officers at the clinic have undergone a four-day training on diabetes and hypertension care, the pathophysiology of the two conditions, complications, and treatment and management to supplement their pre-service training. They also have wide experience in managing diabetes and hypertension garnered through participating in free medical camps that focus on screening for and managing diabetes. The medical camps have taken place throughout the country and are usually organized by another local NGO and project partner—the Kenya Diabetes Management and Information Centre (DMI). The clinical officers work with trained clinical nutritionists to offer more comprehensive care to patients. The clinicians focus on the therapeutic management of the patient while the nutritionists offer nutrition advice in a cascade manner. Nutrition education is given to the whole group at the beginning of each clinic session, followed by group sessions that target groups of patients with similar disease conditions (hypertension alone, diabetes alone, both diabetes and hypertension). Then one-on-one counseling for patients follows, especially those whose clinical outcomes are poor. These one-on-one sessions target patients with either poor glycemic control, based on the previous and current fasting blood glucose readings, or fluctuating or increasing or unchanging blood pressure, based on the previous and current readings. Measurement of glycosylated hemoglobin (HbA1c) as an indicator of long-term glycemic control will be introduced in the near future.

Hard-to-manage patients, that is, those who do not improve with therapeutic management coupled with nutrition counseling, are identified for management by medical officers from the nearest district hospital who participate in the clinics every four weeks. Patients who do not improve after three consecutive consultations with the medical officers, despite their compliance with treatment and nutrition advice, are referred for specialist management at the district hospital.

All patients are screened for complications and are either referred or managed by specialists who participate in the clinics once every quarter. Consultation and treatment fees are waived but patients contribute to the cost of the glucose test and patients bear their own transportation costs.

During clinic intervals, patients interact with lay educators, who include former field workers in the research project, community health workers, and other patients. The lay educators provide support and information to the patients and their family members. The educators also act as a link to the clinic, providing information on hospitalization, death, and acute complications among patients within their area. They are also responsible for identifying patients within the community who are currently not on treatment and for referring them to the clinics.

## Building Partnerships

The project is run in two health centers, one owned and operated by the local government and another by an NGO. The project is led by the African Population & Health Research Center (APHRC), an Africa-led regional research institute. One of the partners is the Diabetes Management and Information Centre (DMI), a local NGO; through its networks, it identifies volunteer clinicians trained by its various training programs to run the clinics. Clinical nutritionists are from another local NGO, Nutritionists without Borders (NWB), and are also volunteers. Therefore, the partnership brings together local government, a regional research institute (APHRC), and three local NGOs whose mandates range from health service provision for the urban poor (Provide International), advocacy and public education on diabetes prevention and management (DMI), to advocacy for nutrition as a means of effectively managing illnesses (NWB). Funding is provided by APHRC and the World Diabetes Foundation. Such public-private partnerships are essential if residents of slum areas are to access high quality health care. Private providers need to be brought on board to support government initiatives, and they need access to the same training opportunities as workers in the public sector. Since it is unlikely that government will build health facilities any time soon that are easily accessed by slum residents, reputable private providers who are already on the ground are better placed to offer much needed health and social services in these underserved areas—with government support.

# INTERIM OUTPUTS AND IMPROVED CLINICAL OUTCOMES

Since the clinics opened in April 2008, a total of 783 patients have attended the clinic at least once, but currently about 400 patients attend the clinic on a regular basis. Since all respondents to the survey having either of the two conditions (a total of 1,238) were referred to the two APHRC clinics, and since many more patients who were not part of the research project have started coming to the clinics, it is evident that compliance with referral was very poor. Of the 783 patients who have ever attended, about half have dropped out (have not attended a clinic for at least three months), and these include about 200 patients who did not return after their first visit. On average, 130 patients in Korogocho and 80 in Viwandani are seen every two weeks.

A first look at the clinical outcomes shows there have been improvements in the blood pressure and/or blood glucose measurements for patients who have not dropped out and have attended *at least* three times (the number of clinic attendances for this group ranges from three to fifteen). A 10 mmHg or more reduction in systolic blood pressure from the first clinic attended to the last has been observed in at least 51 of such patients. For 22 patients there has been no perceptible change in the systolic blood (either less than 10 mmHg reduction or less than 10 mmHg increase), and for 28, the systolic blood pressure has increased by more than 10 mmHg. For diastolic blood pressure, a reduction of at least 5 mmHg has been observed in 45 patients, while for 21 there has been no significant change. For 34, the diastolic blood pressure has increased by more than 5 mmHg. However, these estimates do not take into account the length or regularity of attendance, since only the first and last readings were used in the analysis. For some patients, these readings were one year apart, but for others they were only three months apart. All patients are being followed up and more detailed measures of clinical outcomes, changes in behavioral risk factors, and changes in quality of life are being collected so a more comprehensive assessment of outcomes will be done at a later stage.

The strategy adopted in the implementation of the project demonstrates a fundamental shift from the current guidelines for chronic diseases management in the country. This shift is reflected both in the level of the health facilities where these conditions are being managed and the cadre of health workers that are managing the conditions. In the project clinics, therapeutic care is mostly provided by clinical officers instead of medical officers, as stipulated in the guidelines. Care is also being provided in health centers rather than hospitals since the centers are more accessible. Complicated and hard-to-manage cases are referred for care by medical officers. Interim findings suggest that patients who adhere to treatment and nutrition advice see improvements in their clinical outcomes.

Apart from a shift in the actual guidelines, an attempt has been made to use the existing service guidelines to manage the two conditions by involving clinical nutritionists in patient care. The involvement of lay community members in patients' care not only ensures continuity of the research-to-program process, but also ensures that patients are followed up regularly in their homes and that they have access to information and support from sources close to home during the interval between clinics. The capacity of community members to offer advice and support to patients and their families has also been greatly enhanced through this project. But the poor adherence to referral needs to be investigated further and addressed.

## FUTURE PLANS AND POLICY IMPLICATIONS

In this chapter, we present a project targeting an urban-poor population in Nairobi, Kenya, with health problems and needs that are not sufficiently met by the current health service delivery system. The population is not only affected by HIV/AIDS and other communicable diseases, but it also has a large burden of NCDs. It is evident that a shift in current guidelines for the management of NCD is needed in Kenya, given the apparent high disease burden and infrastructural shortcomings, especially in urban-poor areas. The situation in rural areas may not be any better, especially given many rural communities' geographic inaccessibility to district hospitals. Research is still ongoing to explore whether a different model of health care could enhance geographic access and use lower-cadre health workers to manage some NCDs. Preliminary findings from the research show that intermediate health outcomes among those adhering to treatment are much better than the status quo. Further research is needed to establish whether the benefits to patients managed under this model are sustained and translate to improved health outcomes, such as improved quality of life and reduction in mortality at population level. Ongoing research will address some of these questions by comparing long- and medium-term outcomes of patients attending the two clinics with those of patients attending district hospitals. However, in the two slum populations, there is a need for more research about factors that determine adherence to treatment and how they can be harnessed to improve patients' compliance with treatment.

If proven successful, the proposed model may have far-reaching implications for heath care delivery for disease conditions that require long-term care in informal settlements in Nairobi, in rural areas in Kenya, and in other sub-Saharan African countries with similar restrictive guidelines, human resource shortages, and high NCD burdens.

## SUMMARY

This chapter describes a project that aims to demonstrate the huge burden of noncommunicable diseases among the urban poor in one of Africa's fastest urbanizing cities, Nairobi. It also attempts to highlight the shortcomings in the current Kenyan government guidelines for the management of chronic diseases and how a shift is needed in the policy if (1) the health needs of the urban poor are to be met and (2) the existing health services are to be more responsive to the needs of people with NCD conditions, such as diabetes and hypertension.

The burden of NCD, as shown by the prevalence of these two CVD conditions, may be far too great to be handled by the existing infrastructure and personnel if current service guidelines in Kenya remain in place. Though a more comprehensive assessment of the impact of the project has not yet been done, interim findings indicate that qualified clinical officers with additional training and strong referral networks can successfully manage these two conditions and generate clinical outcomes that are better than the status quo. Under the current policy framework, we can assume that the few patients with hypertension and diabetes who are on treatment are being managed by medical officers and/or at hospitals, and we can conclude that this is less effective than the outcome achieved under the project. Therefore, a policy shift is needed if the country is to cope with the apparent high burden of NCDs in the face of a high burden of communicable diseases, especially HIV/AIDS and malaria. There is also a need for meaningful partnerships between the public and private health sectors that will increase access to high quality social services, such as health care, to marginalized populations like those in the ever-increasing slum settlements in Nairobi and perhaps other cities in sub-Saharan Africa that are facing similar urbanization challenges.

## REFERENCES

African Population & Health Research Center (APHRC). 2002. *Population and health dynamics in Nairobi informal settlements.* Nairobi: APHRC.

African Population & Health Research Center (APHRC). 2008. *The economic, health, and social context of HIV infection in informal urban settlements of Nairobi 2006.* Nairobi: APHRC.

African Population & Health Research Center (APHRC) and The World Bank. 2006. *Averting preventable maternal mortality: Delays and barriers to the utilization of emergency obstetric care in Nairobi's informal settlements.* Nairobi: APHRC and the World Bank.

Central Bureau of Statistics (CBS), MoH, and ORC Macro. 2004. *Kenya demographic and health survey 2003.* Calverton, Maryland: Central Bureau of Statistics [Kenya], Ministry of Health [Kenya], and ORC Macro.

Christensen, D. L, H. Friis, D. L. Mwaniki, B. Kilonzo, I. Tetens, M. K. Boit, B. Omondi, L. Kaduka, and K. Borch-Johnsen. 2009. Prevalence of glucose intolerance and associated risk factors in rural and urban populations of different ethnic groups in Kenya. *Diabetes Research and Clinical Practice* 84:303–310.

Fotso, J.-C., A. Ezeh, and R. Oronje. 2008. Provision and use of maternal health services among urban poor women in Kenya: What do we know and what can we do? *Journal of Urban Health* 85(3):428–442.

Health of Populations in Transit Research Group (HoPiT). 2004. *CAMBoD baseline survey report.* Yaoundé, Cameroon: HoPiT.

Kyobutungi, C., A. Ziraba, A. Ezeh, and Y. Yé. 2008. The burden of disease profile of residents of Nairobi's slums: Results from a demographic surveillance system. *Population Health Metrics* 6(1).

Matrix Development Consultants (MDC). 1993. *Nairobi's informal settlements: An inventory.* Nairobi, Kenya: USAID.

Ministry of Health (MoH)–Kenya. 2005. *Reversing the trends: The second national health sector strategic plan-NHSSP-II, 2005–2010.* Nairobi: Ministry of Health.

Ministry of Medical Services (MMS). 2009. List of health facilities in Kenya. http://www.medical.go.ke/index.php?option=com_docman&task=cat_view&Itemid=44&gid=15&orderby=dmdate counter&ascdesc=DESC.

National AIDS and STI Control Programme (NASCOP), Ministry of Health-Kenya. 2008. *Kenya AIDS indicator survey (KAIS): Preliminary report 2007.* Nairobi: NASCOP.

OXFAM. September 2009. *Urban poverty and vulnerability in Kenya.* Nairobi: OXFAM.

United Nations Human Settlements Programme (UN-HABITAT). 2003. *The challenge of slums: Global Report on human settlements.* Nairobi: UN-HABITAT.

United Nations Human Settlements Programme (UN-HABITAT). 2006. *Nairobi urban sector profile.* Nairobi: Regional Office for Africa and the Arab States, UN-HABITAT.

Ziraba, A. K., N. Madise, S. Mills, C. Kyobutungi, and A. Ezeh. 2009. Maternal mortality in the informal settlements of Nairobi City: What do we know? *Reproductive Health* 6:6.

# CHAPTER ELEVEN

# CRIME, VIOLENCE, PUBLIC HEALTH, AND URBAN LIFE

## RICHARD H. SCHNEIDER

---

### LEARNING OBJECTIVES

- Understand that crime and violence are now considered much more than just law enforcement concerns but rather as fundamental public health issues

- See connections between selected socioeconomic, demographic, and environmental design and planning variables in cities relative to crime/violence incidence, impacts and public health outcomes

- Compare the incidence, impacts, and outcomes of homicides and burglaries relative to public health in the developed and developing world

- Understand some of the impacts of the fear of crime, especially relative to homicides and burglaries, on individuals, on neighborhoods, and on public health

- See crime and public health relative to scales of urban environmental design and development

- Identify some proposed interventions to mitigate and prevent urban crime

- Appreciate the growing connections between crime prevention theory and practice and public health research and practice approaches

THIS chapter explores key theory and evidence at global, national, and local levels that connect social and physical factors with crime,[1] violence,[2] public health, and urban life. Crime and the fear of crime and violence have been linked largely (but not exclusively) with urban life and especially with large, dense, and heterogeneous cities (Wirth 1957). Cities are venues of high levels of crime and violence by virtue of the concentration of motivated offenders, opportunities, and rewards. It is only relatively recently, however, that urban crime and violence have been acknowledged as *sociopathologies* with transnational significance and have been characterized as *epidemiological* phenomena (Dahlberg and Mercy 2009).

In this context, the Forty-ninth World Health Assembly declared the prevention of violence to be a public health priority (World Health Organization 1996), and UN-HABITAT devoted the first section of the *2007 Global Report on Human Settlements* to crime and violence as fundamental threats to human security (UN-HABITAT 2007). The United Nations Office on Drugs and Crime stated the point succinctly in 2006: "What was once seen as a matter of law enforcement is now recognized as a social, public health, and good governance issue that can be tackled proactively."

Spurred by these initiatives, criminologists, social scientists, urban designers, planners, and crime prevention practitioners are increasingly using the language and methodologies of public health to monitor and assess (map) incidents, identify risk factors (as distinct from "causes"), including physical and social vulnerability, determine intervention strategies, and evaluate results (UN-HABITAT 2007). Moreover, modern views of human security threats—including those from natural hazards, disasters, disease, and crime—are that they are largely predictable processes (as distinguished from isolated events), based on a convergence of generally localized risk factors that often can be foreseen and managed. Thus, while crime incidence in cities throughout the globe is extraordinarily variable, there are consistent and predictable themes relative to physical, social, and public health issues. This is significant relative to designing interventions and public policy.

To explore these issues, we will look at three constellations of variables related to crime, health, and cities: (1) socioeconomic characteristics, including culture, poverty, and inequality; (2) demographic characteristics, including gender, age, and employment; and (3) environmental (physical) design and planning characteristics. We also discuss the fear of crime as a distinct but related issue linked to all three variables. Within the discussion of each of these variable sets, we look at selected incidence and impacts of two types of personal and property crimes—homicide and burglary per 100,000 population.

A wealth of studies demonstrate the above sets of variables to be primary sources of risks associated with criminal and violent acts and associated crime fear, affecting the sustainability of large and growing urban communities across the globe (WHO 2002; World Bank 2003). They are also inextricably linked to urban and local community health in complex and often subtle ways.

## SOCIOCULTURAL AND ECONOMIC VARIABLES

### Culture

Many studies connect social-cultural and economic factors with crime, fear of crime, and health. These include research on the power of official institutions to change attitudes and behavior as well as the impacts of informal codes of conduct embedded in civil society and social norms and mores. There is little debate that good governance can impact crime and community health. Informal, widely accepted standards of conduct may be even more important.

Modern medicine has recognized the significant impacts that informal codes and cultural norms have on patient conceptions of health, disease, and treatments and has developed theory and practice specializations aimed at understanding the connection between cultural diversity and appropriately sensitive health care intervention approaches (Bigby 2003). Although crime theory has long dealt with community structural and compositional issues through social disorganization and related theories (Shaw and McKay 1942; Sampson 1993), crime prevention theory and strategies have only recently begun to take into account the influence of local culture, context, and informal norms on intervention and mitigation strategies relative to urban crime.[3]

The role of physical disorganization and related design and planning factors in crime prevention is newer still, based on environment-behavior research and practice generated since the mid-1960s in terms of defensible space theory, crime prevention through environmental design (CPTED), "broken windows theory," environmental criminology, and situational crime prevention (Newman 1973; Jeffrey 1977; Wilson and Kelling 1982; Brantingham and Brantingham 1991; Clarke 1997).

The data suggest that much crime takes place within informal contexts, especially in transitional and developing economies, and that environmental design and planning variables can play important aggravating or mitigating roles relative to some types of crime and violence. There also is a growing recognition that violence can be so intertwined with local cultures that they become part of the "structure of society" and in some cases, as in the Hudood Ordinances in Pakistan (which criminalized the *victims* of rape) can become codified into law (Moser 2004).

An example of the power of cultures can be seen through a broad-brush comparison of murder rates. As depicted in Figure 11.1, International Crime Victimization Survey (ICVS) data show homicide rates to be highest in Southern

**160**  URBAN HEALTH

FIGURE 11.1 Comparison of Recorded Homicide per 100,000 inhabitants

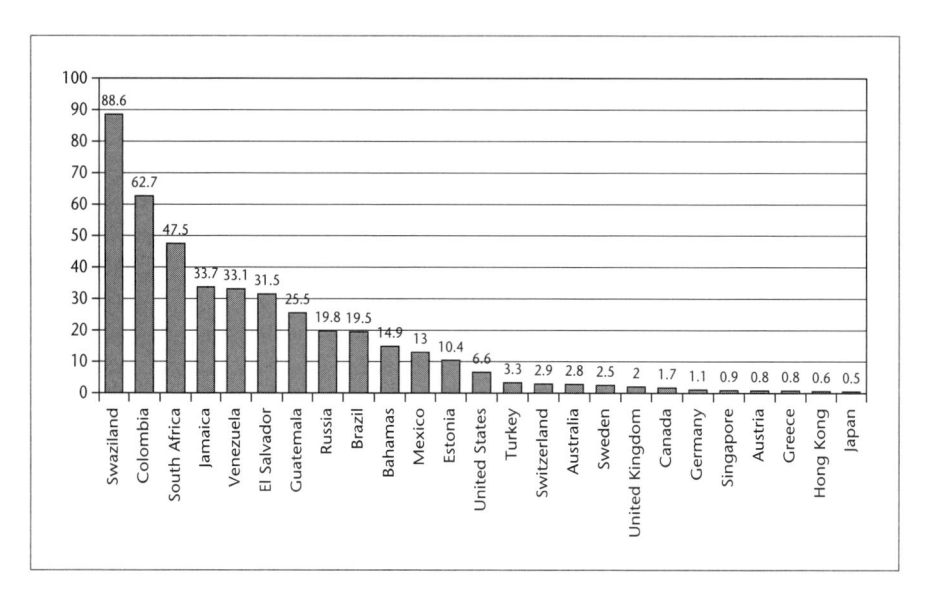

|  |  |
|---|---|
| Swaziland | 88.6 |
| Colombia | 62.7 |
| South Africa | 47.5 |
| Jamaica | 33.7 |
| Venezuela | 33.1 |
| El Salvador | 31.5 |
| Guatemala | 25.5 |
| Russia | 19.8 |
| Brazil | 19.5 |
| Bahamas | 14.9 |
| Mexico | 13 |
| Estonia | 10.4 |
| United States | 6.6 |
| Turkey | 3.3 |
| Switzerland | 2.9 |
| Australia | 2.8 |
| Sweden | 2.5 |
| United Kingdom | 2 |
| Canada | 1.7 |
| Germany | 1.1 |
| Singapore | 0.9 |
| Austria | 0.8 |
| Greece | 0.8 |
| Hong Kong | 0.6 |
| Japan | 0.5 |

*Sources:* International Report on Crime Prevention and Community Safety: Trends and perspectives (2008); estimate based on data collected by ICVS (1998–1999; 2000–2001; 2002–2003; 2004–2005).

Africa, Central America, and South America and lowest in West and Central Europe and in East Asia.

Although many factors affect homicide rates, there is little argument that sociocultural factors play a significant role. For instance, at national levels we find that homicide and property crime rates (including burglary) are generally much lower in parts of Southeast Asia than in North America and the United Kingdom. Figure 11.2 illustrates trends for Japan, the United States, and the United Kingdom over a multiyear period.

These national differences are also reflected at urban levels where crime rates for "pro-social" family and group-focused cities (such as Hong Kong, Seoul, Jakarta, and Tokyo) are consistently lower than for cities of comparable size and density elsewhere. In general, however, cities everywhere have higher crime rates than their rural countrysides. ICVS data show, for instance, that approximately two-thirds of city dwellers globally have been a crime victim over a recent five-year period, with significantly higher rates of victimization in cities in the developing world.

To be sure, culture interacts with other risk factors linked to "high concentrations of poverty and unemployment, high levels of residential instability, family

# CRIME, VIOLENCE, PUBLIC HEALTH, AND URBAN LIFE

FIGURE 11.2  Murder and Property Crime (including burglary) Rates in Japan, the United States, and the United Kingdom

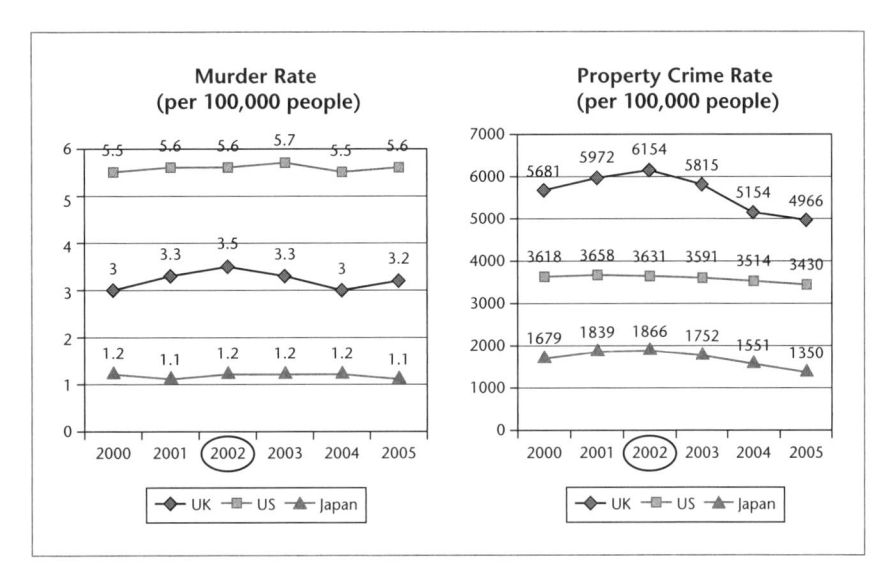

**Murder Rate (per 100,000 people)**

| Year | UK | US | Japan |
|---|---|---|---|
| 2000 | 3 | 5.5 | 1.2 |
| 2001 | 3.3 | 5.6 | 1.1 |
| 2002 | 3.5 | 5.6 | 1.2 |
| 2003 | 3.3 | 5.7 | 1.2 |
| 2004 | 3 | 5.5 | 1.2 |
| 2005 | 3.2 | 5.6 | 1.1 |

**Property Crime Rate (per 100,000 people)**

| Year | UK | US | Japan |
|---|---|---|---|
| 2000 | 5681 | 3618 | 1679 |
| 2001 | 5972 | 3658 | 1839 |
| 2002 | 6154 | 3631 | 1866 |
| 2003 | 5815 | 3591 | 1752 |
| 2004 | 5154 | 3514 | 1551 |
| 2005 | 4966 | 3430 | 1350 |

*Source:* Courtesy of Dr. Kimihiro Hino, Japanese Building Research Institute.

disruption, crowded housing, drug-distribution networks, and low community participation" (Centers for Disease Control 2008, 2). These risks (also characteristics of social disorganization) tend to be associated with high crime and violence rates throughout the world, although there are exceptions within poor and distressed urban neighborhoods, with low rates of serious crime constrained by overarching cultural values and informally enforced norms and rules.

## Poverty

Crime has long been connected with poverty and has been termed both its "consequence and cause" by the United Nations Office on Drugs and Crime (UNODC 2005b). At the global scale homicide and burglary rates are higher for lower-income populations than for higher-income populations (WHO 2002). The urban poor in Africa are much more likely to be victims of burglaries than residents of other regions of the world, and their expectations of being burgled are also higher than people elsewhere (UNODC 2005a). The connection between income and homicide is illustrated by recent Brazilian research where a sample of urban residents was asked how many of them had relatives murdered. The results, plotted against minimum wage (about $175 per month in 2007) are depicted in Figure 11.3. Clearly, murder is associated with income levels for these cohorts.

**FIGURE 11.3  Family Income and Relatives Murdered, by Minimum Wage**

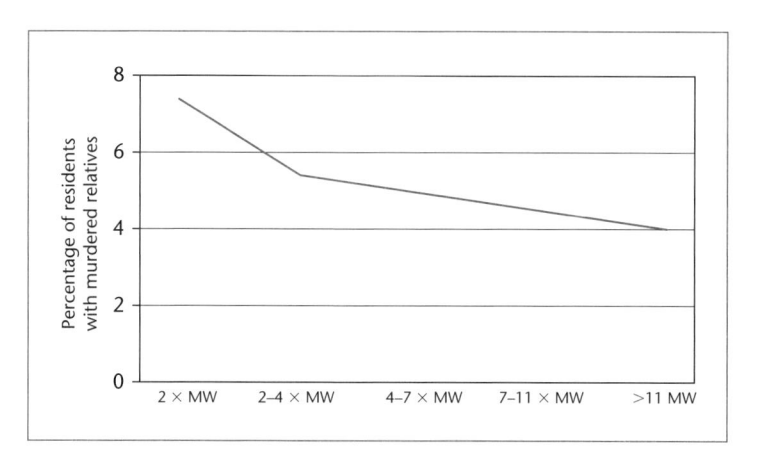

[Line graph: Percentage of residents with murdered relatives vs. income bracket. Values approximately: 2 × MW: 7.5; 2–4 × MW: 5.4; 4–7 × MW: 4.7; 7–11 × MW: 4.1; >11 MW: 4.0]

*Source:* Zaluar (2007).

The cycle connecting poverty, violent crime, and health can be vividly seen in some regions of Africa, where rapid urbanization channels millions of people into burgeoning slums adjacent to or within existing cities. Violent crime here has a negative multiplier effect since victims often cannot afford treatment for injuries from sources other than traditional healers. That, combined with poor physical access to modern medical care, can be devastating since a wound resulting from, say, an attempted murder or interrupted burglary, may not properly heal and can become far more serious, even life threatening.

Where the victim is the breadwinner, there are serious economic implications for families, for the community, and ultimately for society generally. Dependency ratios (the numbers of those for whom the breadwinner is the economic mainstay) are higher in Africa and in slums generally, and insurance and public supports are virtually nonexistent. Therefore, family and community resilience is extremely fragile relative to homicide. Impacts for burglaries are equally significant, especially for slum dwellers. Although they have less to steal than wealthier neighbors, the value of what they do have is proportionally greater since it cannot be replaced by insurance and may be instrumental in eking out an existence. So a stolen cooking pot can be central to survival for a slum food vendor, though it would be easily restored elsewhere.

Residential burglary also contributes to poor health outcomes in direct and indirect ways in cities. First, there are obvious risks to residents who may be physically injured during the course of a break-in. Beyond that, there is evidence that burglaries contribute significantly to psychological burdens such as stress, anger, depression, and heightened fear for victims as well as neighbors (Beaton and others 2000; Skogan 1986). This is especially relevant to repeat victims and vulnerable populations—the elderly, the poor, and women—who often suffer lingering effects.

Therefore, the impacts of homicides, wounding, and property crimes such as burglaries have a stronger ripple effect in poorer communities than would be the case in more affluent neighborhoods in the developed world. The outcomes are often significant depletions of family, community, and national resources, which also sap trust in justice and health systems and in governance generally (UNODC 2005a).

## Inequality

Heightened crime rates have also been predicated, based on the relative distance between the richest and the poorest members of society. In this sense, wide divisions between income sectors breed social tensions that encourage crime against vulnerable individuals, of whatever class. These tensions are especially evident in cities, since this is where people are most concentrated and where affluence distinctions

**FIGURE 11.4   Income Inequality: Income Ratio of the Richest and Poorest Deciles (unweighted averages), 2002 or Most Recent Year**

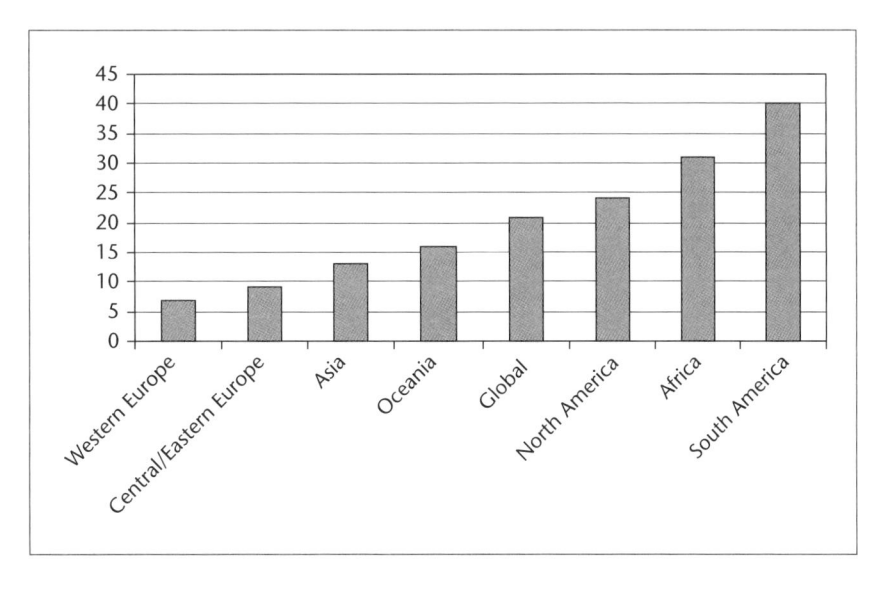

*Note:* The higher the number, the greater the income inequality based on the GINI coefficient.

*Source:* UNDP, adapted from *Human Development Report 2004*, 188–191.

are most visible. According to this theory, societies with the largest gaps between classes tend to exhibit the most pronounced crime rates. Moreover, as Wilkinson and Pickett (2007) argue, income inequality is related to a range of fundamental social problems, including "morbidity and mortality, obesity, teenage birth rates, mental illness, homicide, low trust, low social capital, hostility, and racism, poor educational performance among school children, the proportion of the population imprisoned, drug overdose mortality and low social mobility" (1966).

Figure 11.4 illustrates a comparison of relative deprivation between world regions that generally corresponds to the global homicide distribution shown in Figure 11.1. It is important to note, however, that there is significant variation of crime rates within regions, within nations, and within cities.

Within cities, both homicides and burglaries tend to be focused in areas characterized by low income, low property values, and high environmental risk (UN-HABITAT 2007). In the United States, New Orleans is a prime example of convergence of these risk factors associated with violence and especially homicide. Hurricane Katrina's impacts exacerbated existing high homicide rates.

# DEMOGRAPHIC CHARACTERISTICS

## Age, Gender, and Employment

International research consistently demonstrates that crime and violence are strongly associated with the growth and proportion of youthful populations, especially unemployed or underemployed young males. In terms of homicides, a transnational review of population cohorts between the ages of 15 and 24 years old shows that the percentage of young people in populations was significant in explaining the variability of homicide rates from one nation to the next (Lafree and Tseloni 2006). WHO data reveal that violence is a major cause of death for people between the ages of 14 and 44. For African American males in the United States, violence is among the highest causes of death and is twelve times the rate for white males in the same age category (15–24 years old) (WHO 2002).

World Bank (2003) estimates suggest that about 41 percent of all unemployed people in the world are between 15 and 24 years old. Many of these individuals are urban dwellers, and many will likely remain unemployed for years, with the result that abilities and work motivations atrophy. Consequences include the increased likelihood of resorting to crime for survival, especially through gang affiliations, and the concomitant inability to obtain health insurance or access to decent medical care.

Relative to gender, WHO data also show that boys are almost three times more likely than girls to get involved in fighting, and males aged 15 to 29 account

FIGURE 11.5 Age and Gender as Key Determinants of Vulnerability to Small Arms Violence, 2000: Firearm Mortality Rate per 100,000

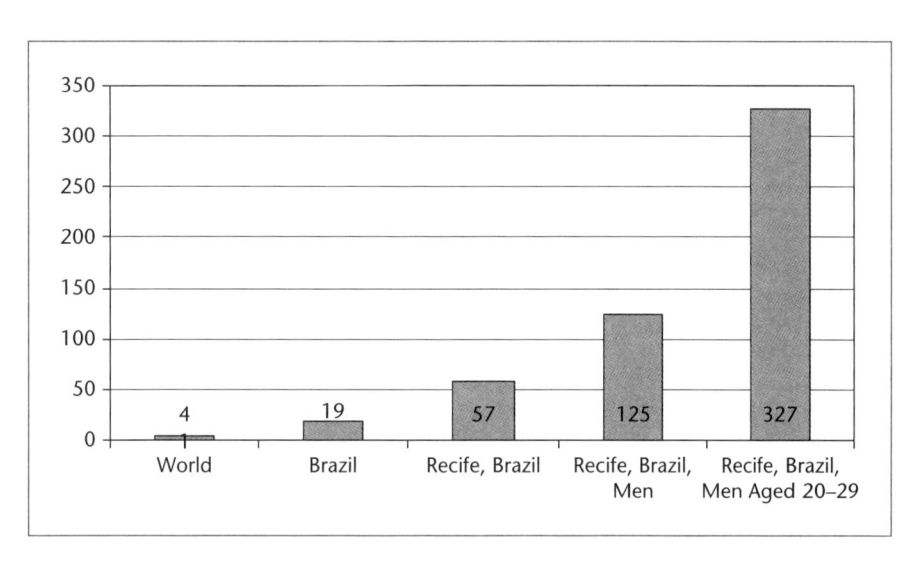

*Sources: World*: Small Arms Survey calculations based on Richmond, Cheney, and Schwab (2005, 348, using 229,000 annual non-conflict-related firearm deaths estimate) and UN Population Division (2005). *Brazil and Recife*: Peres (2004, 129, 130, 132).

for half of global firearm homicide victims, or 70,000 to 100,000 deaths annually (WHO 2002). Figure 11.5 from the 2003 Small Arms Survey illustrates the role of gender and age relative to gun deaths in one Brazilian city compared to the nation and the world.

For growing cities, especially those between 500,000 and one million population in developing and transitional nations, this is sobering data since these urban areas tend to contain a disproportionate number of young, unemployed males—a perfect storm for crime, violence, and associated health impacts and outcomes. One such outcome is illustrated by the near collapse of the Brazilian health care system in the 1980s due to the overwhelming burden of gunshot injuries and psychological trauma associated with urban gang violence and street crime (Zaluar 2007).

## Crime Fear

Young, unemployed urban males are more likely to be perpetrators of violence and crime, but they are more likely to be crime victims as well, even though women, the poor, the elderly, and children suffer significant direct and indirect impacts. For the latter groups, this is especially true relative to the fear of crime.

Crime fear affects urban and suburban children whose parents worry over risks of their being abducted or molested while walking or riding bicycles to school or even within their neighborhoods. From a health perspective, these concerns translate into decreased physical activity, obesity, diminished physical and cognitive functioning, negative impacts on psychological health, and increased risks of cardiovascular disease (Lauer 2005; Stafford, Chandola, and Marmot 2007). Looking at this from a geographic vantage point, Chandola (2001) suggests that fear of crime could be a significant factor in explaining differences in health inequalities from one area (neighborhood) to the next.

## Environmental Design Characteristics: Urban Design and Planning

The physical fabric of the community also has a bearing on violence, crime, and community health. This is so because the variable sets overlap, and physical and environmental elements can help predict the likelihood that citizens will become victims of violence and crime in cities and also suffer health problems.

In this sense, some researchers argue that crime and community health tend to track each other, so that "the same social environmental factors which predict geographic variation in crime rates may also be relevant for explaining community variations in health and wellbeing" (Kawachi, Kennedy, and Wilkinson 1999, 719). The authors suggest that understanding why crime varies within and across nations may help answer "why some communities are healthier than others," a basic mystery in the field of public health.

## Macro, Meso, and Micro Levels of Analysis

For analytic and illustrative purposes relative to crime, violence, and public health, we divide the urban fabric into three general environmental and urban design levels: the macro scale, which includes the overall community layout, land uses, and transportation patterns; the meso scale, which contains neighborhoods, parks and plazas; and the micro scale, whose elements include sites and structures, pathways, and street corners. (This is a nonexhaustive list, to be sure.) Some important descriptive characteristics that span the scales include urban density and massing, structural age and quality (especially housing quality), and infrastructure design (especially lighting) and layout.[4] Taken together at all scales, environmental and urban design elements and characteristics are estimated to play a role in 10–15 percent of all crime incidents (UN-HABITAT 2007; Schneider and Kitchen 2002). This equates to millions of crimes in cities annually.

At the macro urban level, research has linked land use, transportation networks, offender travel patterns, and "routine activities" with crime risks (Brantingham, and Brantingham 1991; Beavon, Brantingham, and Brantingham 1994).

At the meso scale, research on refugees in Africa points to the lack of safety in the design and location of public spaces as a risk factor in sexual and gender-based violence, largely directed against girls (UN Secretary-General's Study on Violence against Children 2006). Hembree and others (2005) have demonstrated that physical neighborhood characteristics in New York City, such as deterioration of the built environment, is significantly associated with the increased probability of fatal, accidental drug overdoses.

Evidence at the micro scale shows connections between building and site design and the potential for crime and violence. Miles (2008) notes that physical disorder (characterized by litter, graffiti, traffic volume, and landscape problems) and perceived security in neighborhoods has a bearing on adults' willingness to encourage children to use local playgrounds and on women's involvement in sports and exercise.

Homicides are well documented and may be widely dispersed throughout urban areas since they often involve troubled intimate partner relationships that occur throughout the general population. However, many homicides are the byproducts of drug deals, bungled robberies, assaults, or burglaries that are geographically concentrated. These are best visualized in macro and meso physical (geographic) contexts using GIS crime maps where incident densities reveal consistent concentrations in certain neighborhoods as well as covariance with other crimes. For instance, in a 2005 GIS-based study of the covariance of drug arrests and murders in Jacksonville, Florida, a multi-year compilation of data (2000–2005) found that 43.5 percent of murders took place in drug arrest hotspots. This is far higher than the distribution that one would expect to see by chance.

Both murders and drug arrests are clearly concentrated within relatively small areas of Jacksonville's impoverished inner city neighborhoods. In a two-year time frame (2004–2005) homicides clustered within Jacksonville's downtown neighborhoods, though there are some outlying hotspots within or adjacent to other outlying low-income areas. Again, this aggregation is much more pronounced than one would expect by mere chance and is connected to and influenced by other factors, including socioeconomic variables and the locations of related and adjacent sociopathologies, including other crimes.

In sum, it is clear that crime and violence, such as burglaries and homicides, and the fear of such offenses are associated with both social and physical characteristics of cities and that they occur at various environmental and urban design scales. Moreover, we know that certain types of offenses tend to re-occur in a relatively limited number of places that provide niches for offending. These places also tend to be associated with poor health outcomes.

# INTERVENTIONS

Many crime prevention interventions in cities around the world focus on changing public policy and practice as well as informal norms and individual behaviors. Most efforts target a wide range of offenses, including homicides and burglary, although some (such as women's groups in Jamaica that focus on reducing gun-crime) aim at specific offenses and outcomes (for example, mortality rates among young men). By necessity, this is only a small sample of policies and programs associated with the vast and overlapping fields of urban violence, crime, and health, and we encourage readers to follow up with the sources provided as intervention strategies evolve and change over time.

### International Level

International efforts to combat crime and violence have expanded greatly since the 1996 declaration of the Forty-ninth Health Assembly that violence is a public health hazard. One example of this is UN-HABITAT's Safer Cities Program which was instituted at the behest of mayors of African cities overwhelmed by crime, violence, and the associated loss of social and human capital. Initiatives, including policy proposals and strategies associated with this program relative to urban planning, design, and municipal service delivery, include interventions aimed at addressing physical and social urban elements as well as formal institutions (for example, planning and local-level municipal governance) and informal, street-level economic activities and groups, including neighbors and street traders (hawkers). (For a description of the Safer Cities Program, see http://www.unhabitat.org/categories.asp?catid=375.)

### National Level

National governments have key roles to play relative to local urban institutions, since this is the level where, in most countries, the power and resources are centralized and can be used to support on-the-ground crime and violence prevention and public health interventions.

An example of national level programs and policy may be seen in Britain, where attempts to fully engage the planning system in crime and violence prevention have been underway since 1994. These efforts have dovetailed, more or less, with the promulgation of national law (specifically Section 17 of the Crime and Disorder Act of 1998); the evolution of national-level (quasi-public), police-initiated guidance relative to local crime prevention strategies (for example, Secured by Design [SBD], http://www.securedbydesign.com); and the creation of a class of local officials beginning in 1989—architectural liaison officers (ALOs)—whose responsibilities include reviewing local planning applications for conformance with SBD and national design guidance. Together, these initiatives have sought to span the broad gaps among policing, planning, and local authorities (councils) and incorporate crime prevention policy and strategy into the planning, review and in some cases, certification of local development (Schneider and Kitchen 2002, 2007). (See also Canada's significant national and international efforts in crime prevention at http://www.crime-prevention-intl.org and especially *International Compendium of Crime Prevention Practices* [2008].)

### Local (Urban) Level

An example of local intervention strategies emerged from a Safer Cities–related survey of people aged 15–35 in Port Moresby, Papua New Guinea. Considered one of the most violent cities in the world—almost half of reported crimes are personal or contact-type offenses—the city is also characterized by a high growth rate (3.6 percent per year), many squatter settlements made up of recent immigrants from the countryside, and a high reliance on the informal sector for employment.

The survey results provide guidance relative to law enforcement and justice, community development, urban management and planning, and culture and family, and pay direct special attention to the importance of traditional and informal norms. They also address many of the social and physical variables that have been discussed in this chapter as key elements relative to crime and violence prevention, and associated public health improvements. (See http://www.preventionweb.net/english/professional/publications/v.php?id=2585 for more details about this initiative.)

## CONNECTIONS BETWEEN CRIME PREVENTION AND PUBLIC HEALTH

The connections between design and management of urban space and crime is new ground for many planners, architects, and urban designers, and the empirical base is fragile. Newer still are connections between crime prevention planning and design *and* public health. Relative to public health researchers, scholars have suggested as recently as 2003, that, "With a few notable exceptions, [they] have not applied these principles or related crime prevention strategies . . . to reduce violence" (Mair and Mair 2003).

This is changing. Researchers employing theory and tools from public health and urban planning and design (and especially crime prevention planning) have begun to conceptualize crime in ways that open up new avenues of inquiry. For example, turning "crime causes" into "risk factors" much more accurately describes the complex and interconnected nature of crime processes. In the same sense, describing "crime prevention" in terms of "interventions" is a much more realistic approach to a sociopathology that, in reality, can be reduced and not prevented.

Therefore, while cities will always be venues for crime and violence, some offenses—even homicides and burglaries—may be mitigated, given the research synergies and strategies that are emerging. A major task will be to reinforce connections among urban designers, planners, and the public health community at professional and academic levels with a focus on the development of integrated intervention strategies to address crime and violence in urban places.

## SUMMARY

This chapter discusses connections among crime, violence, and public health in urban settings. It stresses that crime and violence are significant threats to human security and are no longer the sole province of law enforcement but are now acknowledged as broad public health concerns. Three interrelated constellations (sets) of variables are used to illustrate the linkage, incidence, and impacts of urban crime and violence on public health. These include

- Socioeconomic characteristics (culture, poverty, and inequality)
- Demographic characteristics (gender, age, and employment)
- Environmental (physical) design and planning characteristics (at macro, meso, and micro scales)

Homicides and burglaries per 100,000 population are used to illustrate two of the many types of crimes that affect urban dwellers. Relative to these and other crimes, research has made the following findings:

- There is great variability among nations and cities in homicide and burglary rates, some being ascribable to the strong influence of informal cultures, norms, and social expectations. Poverty and income inequality are significant risk factors for crime and violence, including homicide and burglary. Both poverty and income inequality are also risk factors for poor health outcomes.
- Marginalized, unemployed young males in urban settings are at disproportionate risk of becoming perpetrators and victims of crime and violence.

The chapter also focuses on issues related to fear of crime in terms of impacts on neighborhoods, individual and public health, and national economic sustainability in some countries. The connections between crime and public health issues are strong enough to lead some scholars to suggest that they predict each other (obviously true for homicides and wounding). Crime risks are associated with urban environmental and design elements at different geographic scales.

A range of intervention (crime prevention) approaches and strategies are discussed at the international, national, and local levels. However, the local (city or urban) level is where these strategies must be applied.

## REFERENCES

Beaton, A., M. Cook, M. Kavanagh, and C. Herrington. 2000. The psychological impact of burglary. *Psychology, crime and law* 6(1):33–43.
Beavon D.J.K., P. L. Brantingham, and P. J. Brantingham. 1994. The influence of street networks on the patterning of property offenses. http://www.popcenter.org/Library/CrimePrevention/Volume%2002/06beavon.pdf.
Bigby, J. A., ed. 2003. *Cross-cultural medicine*. Philadelphia: American College of Physicians.
Brantingham, P. J., and P. L. Brantingham. 1991. *Environmental criminology*. Prospect Heights, IL: Waveland Press.
Centers for Disease Control and Prevention, National Center for Injury Prevention and Control. 2008, June 23. Using environmental design to prevent school violence. http://www.cdc.gov/ncipc/dvp/CPTED.htm.
Chandola, T. 2001. The fear of crime and area difference in health. *Health Place* 7(2):105–116.
Clarke, R. V. 1997. *Situational crime prevention: Successful case studies*, 2nd ed. Albany NY: Harrow and Heston.
Dahlberg, L. L., and J. A. Mercy, 2009. *History of violence as a public health problem*. AMA Virtual Mentor 11(2):167–172.
Felson, M. 2002. *Crime and Everyday Life*. Thousand Oaks, CA: Sage.
Hembree, C., S. Galea, J. Ahern, M. Tracey, T. Piper, J. Miller, D. Vlahov, and K. J. Tardiff. 2005. The urban built environment and overdose mortality in New York City. *Health Place* 11(2):147–156.
International Centre for the Prevention of Crime (ICPC). 2008a. International compendium of crime prevention practices. http://www.crime-prevention-intl.org/.
International Centre for the Prevention of Crime (ICPC). 2008b. International report on crime prevention and community safety: Trends and perspectives. http://www.crime-prevention-intl.org/.
Jeffrey, C. R. 1977. *Crime prevention through environmental design*, 2nd ed. Beverly Hills, CA: Sage.
Johnson, S. 2006. *The Ghost Map*. New York: Riverhead.
Kawachi, I., B. P. Kennedy, and R.G. Wilkinson. 1999. Crime: Social disorganization and relative deprivation. Social Science and Medicine 48(6):719–31. Also available online at http://www.ncbi.nlm.nih.gov/sites/entrez.
Lauer, J. 2005. Driven to extremes: Fear of crime and the rise of the sport utility vehicle in the United States. *Crime, Media, Culture* 1:149–168.

Lafree, G., and A. Tseloni. 2006. Democracy and crime: Multilevel analysis of homicide trends in forty-four countries, 1950–2000. *The Annals of the American Academy of Political and Social Science* 605:25–49.

Mair, J., and M. Mair. 2003. Violence prevention and control through environmental modifications. *Annual Review of Public Health* 24:209–225.

Miles, R. 2008. Neighborhood disorder, perceived safety, and readiness to encourage use of local playgrounds. *American Journal of Preventive Medicine* 34(4):275–281.

Moser, C. O. 2004. Urban violence and insecurity: An introductory roadmap. *Environment & Urbanization* 16(2).

Newman, O. 1973. *Defensible space: Crime prevention through urban design.* New York: Macmillan.

Peres, M.F.T. 2004. Firearm-related violence in Brazil (*Violencia por armas de fogo no Brasil*). Geneva: Small Arms Survey.

Richmond, T. S., R. C. Cheney, and C. W. Schwab (2005). The global burden of non-conflict related firearm mortality. *Injury Prevention* 11:348–352.

Sampson, R. J. 1993. The community context of violent crime. In *Sociology and the public agenda*, ed. W. J. Wilson, 267–274. Newbury Park, CA: Sage.

Schneider, R., and T. Kitchen. 2002. *Planning for crime prevention: A Trans-Atlantic perspective.* London: Routledge.

Schneider R., and T. Kitchen. 2007. *Crime prevention and the built environment.* London: Routledge.

Shaw, C. R., and D. D. McKay. 1942. *Juvenile delinquency and urban areas.* Chicago: University of Chicago Press.

Silver, C. 2008. *Planning the megacity: Jakarta in the twentieth century.* London: Routledge.

Skogan, W. 1986. Fear of crime and neighborhood change. *Crime & Justice* 203:203–230.

Small Arms Survey. 2003. *Small Arms Survey: Development denied*, p. 132. Oxford: Oxford University Press. Quoted in UN Office on Drugs and Crime (UNODC). 2005, June. Crime and development in Africa. http://www.unodc.org/pdf/African_report.pdf.

Small Arms Survey. 2006. Few options but the gun: Angry young men. http://www.smallarmssurvey.org/files/sas/publications/year_b_pdf/2006/2006SASCh12-full_en.pdf.

Stafford, M., T. Chandola, and M. Marmot. 2007. Association between fear of crime and mental health and physical functioning. *American Journal of Public Health* 97(11):2076–2081.

United Nations Development Program (UNDP). 2004. *Human development report: Cultural liberty in today's diverse world.* New York: UNDP. Also available online at http://hdr.undp.org/en/media/hdr04_complete.pdf.

UN-HABITAT. 2007. *Enhancing urban safety and security: Global report on human settlements 2007.* Sterling, VA: Earthscan. Also available online at http://www.unhabitat.org/content.asp?typeid=19&catid=555&cid=5359.

United Nations Office on Drugs and Crime (UNODC). 2005a. Crime and development in Africa. http://www.unodc.org/pdf/African_report.pdf.

United Nations Office on Drugs and Crime (UNODC). 2005b. Working to promote "global alliance" to eliminate criminal behaviour. http://www.unis.unvienna.org/unis/pressrels/2005/gashc3817.html.

United Nations Office on Drugs and Crime (UNODC). 2006. Strategic programme framework. http://www.unodc.org/pdf/brazil/final2.pdf.

United Nations Office on Drugs and Crime (UNODC). 2008. International homicide statistics (IHS). http://www.unodc.org/documents/data-and-analysis/IHS-rates-05012009.pdf.

UN Secretary-General's study on violence against children. 2006. Presented to the Third Committee of the General Assembly, October 11, in New York. http://www.violencestudy.org/r25.

van Dijk, J., J. van Kesteren, and P. Smit. 2007. *Crime victimization in international perspective: Key findings from the 2004–2005 ICVS and EU ICS*. Tilburg University, UNODC. http://rechten.uvt.nl/icvs/pdffiles/ICVS2004_05.pdf.

Wilkinson, R. E., and K. E. Pickett. 2007. The problems of relative deprivation: Why some societies do better than others. *Social Science and Medicine* 65(9):1965–1978.

Wilson, J. Q., and G. Kelling. 1982. Broken windows: The police and neighborhood safety. *Atlantic Monthly*, March: 29–37.

Wirth, L. 1957. Urbanism as a way of life. In *Cities and society*, P. K. Hatt and A. J. Reiss, Jr. (eds.) 46–83. New York: Free Press.

World Bank. 2003. The global crisis of youth unemployment. http://www.worldbank.org.

World Health Organization (WHO). 1996. Prevention of violence: A public health priority. Resolution WHA49.25 of the 49th World Health Assembly. http://www.who.int/violence_injury_prevention/resources/publications/en/WHA4925_eng.pdf.

World Health Organization (WHO). 2002. *World report on violence and health*. Geneva: WHO. Also available online at http://www.who.int/violence_injury_prevention/violence/world_report/en/.

World Health Organization (WHO). 2005. Mortality database. http://www3.who.int/whosis/mort.

Zaluar, A. 2007. Conditions and trends in urban crime and violence: The case of Rio de Janeiro, Brazil, Unpublished case study prepared for the Global Report on Human Settlements 2007.

# CHAPTER TWELVE

# A GLOBAL PERSPECTIVE ON DISASTERS AND THEIR CONSEQUENCES IN THE URBAN ENVIRONMENT

**MARIA STEENLAND**

**GODFREY MBARUKU**

**SANDRO GALEA**

## LEARNING OBJECTIVES

- Identify characteristics of the urban environment that contribute to disaster vulnerability
- Identify approaches to mitigation of disasters in urban settings
- Discuss approaches to disaster preparedness in urban settings

**DISASTERS** impose a tremendous health and economic burden annually worldwide (Noji 1997). There is some evidence that the number of disasters that occur each year has been increasing in the past couple of decades. The most recent report from the Center for Research on the Epidemiology of Disasters (CRED) suggests an increasing trend in the number of disasters reported globally (EM-DAT 2007). Specifically, the number of reported disasters worldwide increased from 201 in 1988 to 414 in 2007 (EM-DAT 2007). The majority of the increase in identified disasters was a result of the greater number of hydrometeorological disasters (floods and storms) during this time period. Much of the variation in the human and economic impact of disasters reported in the CRED database is driven by "mega-disasters" which have caused billions of dollars of damage and the loss of millions of lives, including for example, the Asian tsunami in 2004.

Definitions of disaster vary. CRED defines a disaster as "a situation or event which overwhelms local capacity, necessitating a request to a national or international level for external assistance; an unforeseen and often sudden event that causes great damage, destruction, and human suffering." For a disaster to be entered into EM-DAT, the CRED database, one of the following criteria must be fulfilled: 10 or more people reported killed, 100 or more people reported affected, declaration of a state of emergency, or a call for international assistance. The United Nations International Strategy for Disaster Reduction (UN ISDR) approach is similar to CRED's, defining a disaster as "a serious disruption of the functioning of a community or a society involving widespread human, material, economic or environmental losses and impacts, which exceeds the ability of the affected community or society to cope using its own resources" (UN ISDR 2009). The simultaneous development of disaster research in different fields also has resulted in coexisting definitions of the concept (Thywissen 2006). For the purpose of this chapter, we will largely use the definition adopted by the UN ISDR.

The published literature typically differentiates between natural and human-made disasters. Natural disasters have been defined as the rapid instantaneous or profound impact of the natural environment on the socioeconomic system (Alexander 1993, 4). Natural disasters arise from forces of nature, such as earthquakes, volcanic eruptions, hurricanes, floods, fires, tornadoes, and extremes of temperature (Norris 2002, 7). Human-made disasters include industrial/technological, transportation, deforestation, material shortages, complex emergencies such as war and civil strife, and armed aggression (Norris 2002, 7). This chapter will be concerned primarily with natural disasters, building on recent work that has established urban disasters as a distinct area of research that has focused particularly on natural disasters (Pelling 2003; Kreimer 2003; Mitchell 1999).

Increasingly, scholarship in the area is recognizing that a disaster does not result from a hazardous event alone, but rather is the result of both a hazard and an existing vulnerability. Hazards are defined by the UN ISDR (2009) as "a dangerous phenomenon, substance, human activity or condition that may cause loss of life, injury or other health impacts, property damage, loss of livelihoods and services, social and economic disruption, or environmental damage." Consistent with this emerging direction, disasters should be understood as the result of the interaction between a hazard, be it natural or technological, and the context for the occurrence of hazards. In other words, a disaster occurs when a hazardous event exposes the vulnerability of individuals and communities in such a way that it threatens human life, or the economic and social structures that are vital for survival (Thywissen 2006).

Largely building on these perspectives, emerging research suggests that disasters in urban areas may well be a distinct area of inquiry, principally due to the unique features of the urban environment that intersect with hazards to shape population health. This chapter will focus on disasters in the urban context, adopting a global perspective. Throughout the chapter we will describe how the particular characteristics of the urban environment, both physical and social, shape the way that hazards affect health in cities. The chapter will also present disaster preparedness and management strategies that, through lessening physical and social vulnerability, can reduce the adverse health effects of disasters in urban areas.

There is tremendous heterogeneity in the consequences of disasters across countries worldwide. The health consequences of disasters are typically more dramatic in less wealthy countries, because smaller economies and weaker infrastructure are more vulnerable to particular hazards (UN ISDR 2008). For example, in 2007, Asia experienced the greatest disaster, human loss accounting for 90 percent of all reported victims and 46 percent of economic damage worldwide (EM-DAT 2007). In the same year, Europe's 65 disasters accounted for 27 percent of the world's economic loss but only 1 percent of human lives lost (EM-DAT 2007). The disproportionate relationship between the economic loss incurred by disasters and lost lives can be explained by variation in the strength of country economies, preparedness, and the social and physical context of the hazardous event. In this chapter, we will explicitly compare and contrast the impact of disasters on health in wealthier versus less wealthy countries to highlight shared characteristics of the urban environment that ultimately shape the health consequences of hazards.

# THE HEALTH EFFECTS OF DISASTERS

Disasters affect societies in many ways and have both immediate and long-term consequences for human health. These health effects include deaths, physical injury, and psychiatric morbidity.

Mortality is often used as a measure of a disaster's severity. According to the CRED database, in 2007, natural disasters were responsible for the death of 16,847 people. Disaster-related mortality is not evenly distributed among geographic regions. In 2007, the 10 most affected countries accounted for 76.5 percent of disaster mortality, although these countries make up only a little over 50 percent of the world population (EM-DAT 2007).

Disasters also often result in physical injuries and psychiatric morbidity. Physical injuries following disasters include the experience of being crushed under building debris, burns from fires, and inhalation of toxic fumes following an earthquake (Sever, Vanholder, and Lameire 2006) and cyclone-related injuries including lacerations, blunt trauma, and puncture wounds (Shultz, Russell, and Espinel 2005). There is also ample evidence of the burden of psychopathology after disasters (Norris 2002). Post-traumatic stress disorder is the mental health disorder most commonly associated with disasters; however, depression and anxiety are also commonly observed after disasters (Norris and Elrod 2006).

Aside from their direct health consequences, disasters can destroy local health infrastructure, create unhealthy environmental conditions that increase the risk of communicable disease, and lead to food shortages, causing malnutrition. In some cases, disasters may cause population displacement, which often results in crowding, poor sanitation, and contaminated water (Noji 1997).

## DISASTERS IN URBAN AREAS

Several features of the urban environment set cities apart and influence vulnerability to disasters. Key features of the urban environment that are frequently cited as contributing to disaster vulnerability include denser settlement patterns, increasingly sophisticated and technical physical infrastructure, and a higher concentration of economic activity. Some authors have suggested that the urban environment or urbanization explicitly increases disaster risk. Pelling (2003), for example, proposed a theory of the co-evolution of urbanization and risk. He suggests that urbanization results in environmental risk as well as inequality, which increase the vulnerability of urban areas to disaster. Building on this work, we suggest that although urbanization has the potential to increase vulnerability, urban risk is not inevitable; by decreasing social and physical vulnerability, urban areas can become more resilient. In the next section, we discuss specific features of the urban environment that may influence disasters and their consequences, dividing the sections into the physical and social environment for ease of exposition and then discussing their potential joint interaction.

# URBAN ENVIRONMENT FEATURES THAT INFLUENCE DISASTERS AND THEIR CONSEQUENCES

## The Physical Environment

The physical environment includes built roads, buildings, infrastructure, communications, and energy facilities, as well as waterways, soils, topography, geology, and other natural systems (Godschalk 2003).

**How the Physical Environment Affects Disaster Vulnerability** This section focuses on two major features of the physical environment, the built environment and the location of cities and housing settlements. Characteristics of the built environment, such as structures like bridges, are vulnerable to natural and human-made hazards (Galea 2005). More vulnerable infrastructure can lead to greater mortality after a disaster occurs; for example, differences in buildings explain mortality differences between the 1995 earthquake in Kobe, Japan, which killed 5,200 people and the 2003 earthquake in Bam, Iran, which led to 26,000 deaths (Galea 2006). Buildings in Kobe had been reinforced to cope with earthquake tremors, but most of the buildings in Bam were not constructed with that precaution and therefore collapsed during the earthquake. Construction in Bam has traditionally used mud bricks that collapse quickly; although some of the buildings were historic, others were more recently constructed (Murphy 2004).

Buildings are not the only feature of urban infrastructure that can be vulnerable to hazards. Sewage systems, garbage collection, drinking water, and drainage systems can also be damaged or insufficient. For example, in 2005, heavy monsoons in Mumbai resulted in over 200 deaths when makeshift dwellings were washed away by floodwaters. The areas of the city where the urban poor resided in shanties had blocked drains or, in some cases, had no drainage system at all, which resulted in extreme water buildup (Gandy 2008).

Further, the land itself where housing is built can be more vulnerable in particular urban contexts. In many cities worldwide, poor urban residents live on the worst quality land, such as slopes or flood-prone embankments, where they face the possibility of mudslides and other hazards (Sanderson 2000). The placement of housing in areas that are characteristically prone to hazards augments and exacerbates the immediate post-disaster losses, including mortality, injury, and other health impacts as well as long-term impacts related to resultant homelessness (Pelling 2003).

Aside from vulnerable infrastructure and the land where housing is built, a city itself may be located in a geographic region that is vulnerable to hazards. One of the most striking examples of this phenomenon is the proximity of many cities to coastlines and waterways. It is expected that 50 percent of the world's population will live within 100 kilometers of a coast by 2030, substantially increasing our vulnerability to tsunamis, flooding, and hurricanes (Adger and others 2005). In the United States, many of the largest urban areas are situated in coastal regions that are at high risk of natural disasters, such as earthquakes or hurricanes (Stehr 2006). Human commercial activity can also degrade the surrounding environment in ways that make urban areas more vulnerable to hazards. For example, chronic overfishing and declining water quality around coral reefs have made them—and the adjacent cities—more vulnerable to cyclones and global warming (Adger and others 2005).

Although modern architecture has identified ways that modern urban structures can be more disaster-resistant, interestingly, anthropological research on disasters has documented how some traditional societies found ways to mitigate disasters' effects on their urban areas. However, much of this knowledge and practice has been lost through the transformation of societies under the influence of the industrialized world (Oliver-Smith 1996). For example, indigenous groups in pre-Colombian Peru had adapted settlement strategies that decreased their hazard risk to both flash flooding and earthquakes that are very common in the region. When the Spanish arrived, they often placed towns at the meeting places of rivers that were vulnerable to floods and landslides. The Spanish also did not adopt traditional building practices that protected houses, such as tying walls together at the corners. Instead, they built homes with untied walls, which were often two stories, using heavy roofing materials that were much more likely to be destroyed in an earthquake. The placement of towns, housing construction, and more dense settlement patterns in the traditional Spanish design of perpendicular streets arranged around a central plaza all contributed to the hazard vulnerability of Peru, which in 1970 experienced an earthquake that killed over 70,000 people (Oliver-Smith 1999).

## The Social Environment

The social environment has been defined as the groups we belong to, the neighborhoods where we live, the organization of our workplaces, and the policies we create to order our lives (Yen and Syme 1999). Here we consider the social environment to include those factors and also larger, more "'macro-social" factors, such as the political and economic environment (Galea 2007). Urban areas share certain social characteristics, such as high concentrations of political activity and power structures in addition to functioning as centers of economic activity. For this reason, when urban areas are affected by hazards, the loss of life and the economic impact is substantial. Disasters can also change the social dynamics of cities, both by deepening economic or political inequalities and by forming new political groups to cope with disaster impact. Boulle (1997) points out that disasters can result in sociopolitical change in cities by weakening existing power concentrations, which temporarily allows for the emergence of new political groups. In other words, the social environment both affects the way that hazards are experienced in urban areas and is altered by the experience of disaster.

Many aspects of the social environment can make a city more or less vulnerable to hazards, including economic and spatial inequality, economy and development, politics (political change, political advantage), and social capital. The social environment can affect the way that a disaster is experienced, and how cities recover, and the preparedness or resilience of cities. Inequality can lead to increased vulnerability of lower-income urban residents when hazards occur. Although there are notable exceptions, generally wealthier countries have less income inequality than less wealthy countries. However, economic inequality has had a profound impact on vulnerability to hazard in wealthy countries, such as the United States, as illustrated by Hurricane Katrina in New Orleans. Hurricane Katrina disproportionately affected minorities and poor residents. Poorer residents were less likely to evacuate the area prior to the storm because of fewer monetary and social resources, such as a lack of transportation or financial security to afford gas and hotel costs. It has been suggested that the events that occurred in New Orleans after Katrina were the result of decades of Federal disinvestment that left the city more vulnerable to disaster and revealed unacknowledged inequalities, resulting from years of failed social policy (Stehr 2006). In other words, the social and political systems did not address the issue of urban poverty in the area, and when a hazard occurred, those with fewer resources were left substantially more vulnerable.

Spatial segregation—more specifically, the growth of slums in urban areas in low-income countries—has increased hazard vulnerability in these areas. For example, in Kampala, construction of unregulated shelters by the poor in such slums as Kalerwe, Katanga, Kivulu, and Bwaise has reduced infiltration of rainfall, increasing run-off to six times what would occur in natural terrain (Douglas and others 2008). Greater quantities of water make flooding in these areas much more likely. Concentrations of lower-income residents in certain locations can result in less attention by city officials to these areas and isolation from urban resources. Consequently, low-income areas—or in the case of low-income countries, informal housing—have weaker built environments and fewer social services, making them more vulnerable.

The political representation of a community and political interest in disaster mitigation may dramatically influence the way that hazards affect urban areas. The interest of governments and lawmakers in creating legislation to fund disaster risk reduction can play a role in the vulnerability of urban areas. Local and state government's political will to invest resources in disaster preparedness is in large part determined by interest groups instead of evidence-based risk assessments. It is much more likely that politicians will focus on disasters if they receive persuasive signals from their constituents (Godschalk 2003). Political will at the level of national government can also affect the vulnerability of urban areas to hazards. Project Impact, a hazard-mitigation program started during the Clinton administration to provide grants to cities, was eliminated in 2001, although it cost only about $20 million per year, leaving local governments the responsibility of funding projects. This decentralization of responsibility demonstrates national policy that expects city governments to plan and fund their own initiatives to protect citizens from hazard risk (Stehr 2006).

Disasters can alter the political environment when government leaders fail to adequately respond to the event. Recovery from large-scale urban disasters can also reveal local political dynamics that may have been obscured prior to the event (Semenza 1996). In some cases disasters provide the opportunity for political organization and transform preexisting political structures. The 1985 Mexican earthquake stimulated neighborhood and student political movements that changed government control over relief (Oliver-Smith 1996). This change in relief allocation represented a major threat to the ruling party during the event. In the case of the Mexico City earthquake, when the government was not able to provide sufficient relief, citizen groups mobilized recovery and rebuilding efforts to fill this void. These civic groups continued to function and remained prominent political actors after recovery was over (Foweraker and Craig 1990).

Social capital, the access to resources and information that households have by virtue of their noneconomic social relations with other people (Kreimer 2003), also may drastically influence the vulnerability of cities. Social capital can have a protective effect during hazard events. Semenza and colleagues (1996) found that during the 1995 heat wave in Chicago, variables related to social contact and networks strongly predicted mortality in addition to factors such as location and access to air conditioning. Individuals who participated in church and social groups had a significantly lower risk of death during the heat wave.

In Guyana, it has been shown that social and political assets play key roles in shaping access to local, national, and international resources for environmental management—all factors that shape vulnerability to flood hazards (Pelling 2003). Pelling notes that because those most likely to experience flooding have been excluded from involvement in local decision making, efforts to reduce community vulnerability to flooding have been less effective.

Social capital can also influence relocation following disasters. Mileti (1999) noted that pre-disaster social capital influences where people relocate after a disaster; those who have weaker social networks are more likely to use public shelters. Other factors, such as differences in income and household resources, home ownership, and access to affordable housing, also impact housing options after a disaster (Mileti 1999).

### Interaction of the Physical and Social Environment

Although we have presented how the physical and social environment separately may contribute to disasters in cities, in reality, social and physical attributes of urban areas function together to influence hazard vulnerability.

To demonstrate the ways that physical and social environments interact to create vulnerability, we will use the example of land use. During rapid urbanization with little city planning, migrants with few resources may be forced to settle in areas vulnerable to landslides and flood plains, resulting in spatial segregation of social classes within urban areas. Therefore, it is a combination of poor city leadership and planning capacity, wealth inequality, and the geographic location of physical vulnerabilities that results in greater vulnerability to hazards for the residents on the peripheries of cities (Pelling 2003). In less wealthy countries, poorer residents are often excluded from formal housing markets. Therefore, migrants settle on the outskirts of urban areas. For example, in Bogotá, 60 percent of the population live on steep slopes that are at high risk of landslides (Pelling 2003), and in Calcutta 66 percent of the population live in squatter settlements at risk from flooding and cyclones (Wisner 2004).

The consequences of this spatial location of vulnerable groups can be devastating. For example, in 1999 heavy rains in Vargas, a coastal Venezuelan state with a population of about 300,000, swept over 5,000 homes into the ocean. This disaster affected between 80,000 and 100,000 people and resulted in the death of up to 30,000 people. Although many were evacuated after the landslides, after eight months, 33,000 homeless people were left living in shelters in the areas (International Red Cross and Red Crescent Societies 2001). In the case of Vargas, the homes were vulnerable because they were located on flood plains. The people living on the hillsides were residing in this vulnerable area because they lacked the resources to purchase homes in safer areas, but were dependent on the urban economy to earn a living.

# DISASTER MANAGEMENT

## Mitigation

The first step in disaster preparedness and the phase that will be emphasized most in this chapter is disaster mitigation. Mitigation can be defined as "a sustained effort undertaken to reduce hazard risk through the reduction of the likelihood and/or the consequence component of the hazard's risk" (Coppola 2006, 175). Mitigation is the management strategy that offers the greatest possibility of reducing vulnerability through measures that focus on features of the social and physical environment.

Mitigation strategies that affect the physical environment include both structural (relocation, construction of barriers, deflection, or retention systems, land use) and nonstructural (regulatory measures, protective resource preservation) sustained efforts undertaken to reduce a hazard risk. Burby and colleagues (1999) identified several development management tools that can be used by local governments to carry out hazard mitigation plans. These tools include development regulations, public facility policies (for example, location of school and other public facilities at hazard-free sites, location of street and public utilities to minimize disruption from hazards), land and property acquisition, taxation and fiscal policies, and information dissemination. It has also been suggested that hazard mitigation activities should be linked to efforts to control and ultimately reverse environmental degradation by combining hazard reduction efforts with natural resource management and environmental preservation (Godschalk 2003).

Other important tools for hazard mitigation that relate to the physical environment are building codes and standards. Building codes establish minimum acceptable standards necessary for preserving the public health, safety, and welfare and also the protection of property in the built environment (Mileti 1999). For codes to reduce vulnerability, it is essential that they are created in conjunction with government mandates at both the federal and state level, which serve to ensure that both planning and building codes are well enforced (Mileti 1999).

Mitigation efforts also can focus on social factors. Management activities and strategies that intervene on the social environment include relocation, community awareness and education programs, behavioral modification, community knowledge, and economic diversification.

One example that illustrates how mitigation can function on many levels to reduce disaster vulnerability is the difference in the effect of major natural hazards in the United States compared to less-prepared countries, such as Bangladesh. Adger and others (2005) note that Hurricane Andrew, a category 5 storm that hit Florida in 1992, caused $26.5 billion dollars in devastation, and 23 deaths. A similar tropical typhoon that hit Bangladesh in 1991 caused over 100,000 deaths, and millions of people were displaced. The reason for these different outcomes was that Florida had a higher capacity to manage the storm, thanks to its stronger institutions and early warning systems.

This is not to say that only countries with tremendous resources can achieve effective mitigation efforts. In the late nineteenth century, for example, Colombia banned the use of colonial building technology that resulted in a shift to a wall-building bahareque technique, based on wooden elements and local bamboo. Therefore, cities such as Manizales, which are vulnerable to earthquakes because of their physical location, did not experience much damage during the earthquakes that occurred throughout the second half of the twentieth century. These materials are locally available, require fewer resources than advanced Western technology, and provide protection to urban residents (UNDP 2004).

## Preparedness

Preparedness is the second phase of disaster management. It involves precautionary measures that are implemented once it is known that a hazardous event will occur. The management activities that are a part of preparedness include regionalization of resources, training, statutory authority, public education, and emergency operations plans (Coppola 2006). The purpose of preparedness is to ensure the readiness of a society to forecast, take precautionary measures, and respond to an impending disaster (Christoplos, Mitchell, and Liljelund 2001, 186). The goal of preparedness is also that households, businesses, and government develop response strategies for when disasters occur (Tierney 2001). Preparedness also ensures that resources that will be needed to effectively respond to a disaster are in place before the disaster occurs (Tierney 2001).

Another way that preparedness can reduce vulnerability of cities is through advanced warning systems. The considerable interest in implementing early warning systems is reflected in the UN ISDR's focus on improvements in early warning effectiveness (Zschau and Küppers 2003). Warning systems have achieved some success. China, for example, has 1,300 professional and local stations at the national, regional, and provincial levels to predict the seismic precursors of earthquakes. However, these warning systems can only predict some earthquakes and their reliability is limited (Zschau and Küppers 2003).

Community-based disaster preparedness is emerging as an approach that builds on our understanding of how social factors influence hazard vulnerability and applies this insight to disaster management. An example from Senegal illustrates the advantages of this approach. A combination of the physical environment and the social environment created hazard vulnerability in the Senegalese city of Rufisque. Much of the residential areas of the city are below sea level and in the past, the ground water was polluted by sewage from pit latrines. Flooding of the areas further worsened the sanitation in the city and, as a consequence, there were high rates of diarrhea and dysentery, particularly among children. In the 1980s, a joint government and NGO-led project began to reinforce the coast and prevent housing losses from soil erosion. This project was designed to build twelve parallel dikes to break the current and allow sand buildup on the eroding coastline. During project implementation, it was noted that the community was very capable of contributing and also that the level of sanitation along the coastal area was very bad. After the conclusion of this project, another was established which focused on removing waste and water purification. Horse-drawn carriages were used to collect waste, and a water purification and recycling center was constructed to treat water. Local management committees that are democratically elected ran this project, and all of the technical aspects are managed by local people. Most of the funding for the project came from the community itself (Gaye and Diallo 1997). As this program was entirely managed by the local community, it takes advantage of existing social capital and community members who were invested in the area. It also promoted equality of access by electing leaders of the management groups rather than leaders coming from traditional elites.

## Response and Recovery

The final stages of disaster management are both response and recovery. While these two phases are distinct in some ways, they tend to overlap in practice. Management activities of these phases include warning and evacuation; positioning of supplies and resources; search and rescue; first aid and medical treatment; health and sanitation; economic recovery; provision of food, water, and shelter; and recovery of the housing sector (Coppola 2006). The purpose of response is to limit injuries, loss of life, and damage to property and the environment prior to, during, and immediately after a hazard event. Recovery has a different purpose that is more oriented towards long-term outcomes. One way that recovery can be completed in a manner that reinforces the health system's capacity to manage future hazards is to implement emergency services following a disaster (Razzak and Kellermann 2002). In the past, emergency medical services were not considered an important part of the international health agenda; however, there is a growing understanding that implementing emergency services in resource-poor countries should be a part of basic health services (Razzak and Kellermann 2002).

There are a number of different ways that recovery efforts can be influenced by the social environment. For example, after the 1995 Kobe earthquake in Japan, the city formed town development organizations called Machizukuri in some areas. These organizations were based on existing community organizations, such as neighborhood associations. Machizukuri organizations allowed community members to take part in the rehabilitation process and also served as a link between the community and city planning officials (Nakagawa and Shaw 2004).

Work in the city of Bam in Iran provides an example of how recovery processes can reduce the vulnerabilities of cities. Iran is a country that is highly susceptible to disasters. In December 2003, an earthquake was responsible for the death of one-quarter of the city—30,000 people—and left 70,000 people homeless (UNDP 2006). Following the earthquake, the United Nations Development Program (UNDP) began a crisis prevention and recovery intervention in the region. The work of the UNDP project took into account two of the factors described above in their reconstruction plans. First, one of their goals was to mobilize the participation of local communities in their reconstruction work and the second was to construct environment-friendly and earthquake-resistant housing, decreasing physical vulnerability. To accomplish their goals, UNDP used a reconstruction model that was earthquake-resistant and adapted to the traditional housing design of Bam. They also engaged 430 local building workers, 70 engineers, and 70 reconstruction managers, both to consult about the design and to assist in the reconstruction itself. They formed a group of local authorities, responsible for identifying families who had the greatest need for aid, which ensured greater equity in the reconstruction process (UNDP 2006).

## SUMMARY

This chapter is based on the assumption that most disasters do not arise unexpectedly; instead, they are predictable events that result from the interaction of physical and social factors described above. Urban areas create a particular set of interactions that affect the vulnerability of urban residents. Disasters may be the result of interrelated components of urban poverty, including insufficient incomes and assets, poor quality housing, lack of basic infrastructure providing water and sanitation, and a lack of civil and political rights (Bull-Kamanga and others 2003). This suggests that disasters cannot be prevented in isolation from the broader social context. If we seek to more effectively mitigate disasters, our management strategies will need to take into account the reasons why disasters occur, bringing to the forefront the importance of the urban context.

It is clear that a focus on mitigation as the most important part of disaster planning is both cost-efficient and effective. It is equally apparent that effective mitigation should take into account many levels of society, from communities to national governments. However, it is necessary to recognize that implementing these concepts at a practical level will face serious challenges, particularly in less wealthy countries. These countries are faced with other critical issues, such as internal conflicts and economic crisis, which compound the risk of hazards experienced. So disasters themselves are not isolated from other crises, and the relationship between economic problems and disasters may be more reciprocal than linear. How then can a country experiencing ongoing severe drought, food shortages, and economic crisis be expected to implement changes to the social and physical environment that can mitigate the potential consequences of disasters? The examples presented above show how social capital and hazard-resistant housing can be a part of sustainable disaster planning, even in the context of low-income countries. Other measures, such as income distribution or decreasing spatial segregation, will require fundamental societal change. The challenge for future mitigation efforts will be how to incorporate social change into management strategies in the context of weak institutions and struggling economies and how to generate the political will to make social change a major focus of disaster mitigation.

# REFERENCES

Adger, W. N., T. P. Hughes, C. Folke, S. R. Carpenter, and J. Rockstrom. 2005. Social-ecological resilience to coastal disasters. *Science* 309(5737):1036–1039.

Alexander, D. E. 1993. *Natural disasters.* Dordrecht, the Netherlands: Kluwer.

Boulle, P. 1997. Vulnerability reduction for sustainable urban development. *Journal of Contingencies and Crisis Management* 5(3):179.

Bull-Kamanga, L., K. Diagne, A. Lavell, E. Leon, F. Lerise, H. MacGregor, and others. 2003. From everyday hazards to disasters: The accumulation of risk in urban areas. *Environment and Urbanization* 15(1):193.

Burby, R. J., T. Beatley, P. R. Berke, R. E. Deyle, S. P. French, and D. R. Godschalk. 1999. Unleashing the power of planning to create disaster-resistant communities. *Journal of the American Planning Association* 65(3):247.

Christoplos, I., J. Mitchell, and A. Liljelund. 2001. Re-framing risk: The changing context of disaster mitigation and preparedness. *Disasters* 25(3):185–198.

Coppola, D. 2006. *Introduction to international disaster management.* Oxford: Butterworth-Heinemann.

Douglas, I., K. Alam, M. Maghenda, Y. Mcdonnell, L. Mclean, and J. Campbell. 2008. Unjust waters: Climate change, flooding and the urban poor in Africa. *Environment and Urbanization* 20(1):187.

EM-DAT: The OFDA/CRED International Disaster Database. 2007. *Annual disaster statistical review: The numbers and trends 2007.* Brussels, Belgium: Center for Research on the Epidemiology of Disasters (CRED).

Foweraker, J., and A. L. Craig. 1990. *Popular movements and political change in Mexico.* Boulder: Lynne Rienner Publishers.

Galea, S. 2005. Urban health: Evidence, challenges, and directions. *Annual Review of Public Health* 26(1):341.

Galea, S. 2006. Social context and the health consequences of disasters. *American Journal of Disaster Medicine* 1(1):37.

Galea, S., ed. 2007. *Macrosocial determinants of population health.* New York: Springer.

Gandy, M. 2008. Landscapes of disaster: Water, modernity, and urban fragmentation in Mumbai. *Environment and Planning* 40(1):108.

Gaye, M., and Diallo, F. 1997. Community participation in the management of the urban environment in Rufisque (Senegal). *Environment and Urbanization* 9(1):9.

Godschalk, D. R. 2003. Urban hazard mitigation: Creating resilient cities. *Natural Hazards Review* 4(3):136–143.
International Red Cross and Red Crescent Societies. 2001. Chapter 4 summary: Trapped in the gap—post-landslide Venezuela. In *World disasters report 2001*. http://www.ifrc.org/publicat/wdr2001/index.asp.
Kreimer, A. 2003. *Building safer cities: The future of disaster risk*. Washington, DC: World Bank.
Mileti, D. S. 1999. *Disasters by design: A reassessment of natural hazards in the United States*. Washington, DC: Joseph Henry Press.
Mitchell, J. K. 1999. *Crucibles of hazard: Mega-cities and disasters in transition*. Tokyo: United Nations University.
Murphy, C. 2004, January 2. Starting from scratch in Bam. BBC. http://news.bbc.co.uk/2/hi/middle_east/3363125.stm
Nakagawa, Y., and R. Shaw. 2004. Social capital: A missing link to disaster recovery. *International Journal of Mass Emergencies and Disasters* 22(1):5–34.
Noji, E. K., ed. 1997. *The public health consequences of disasters*. New York: Oxford University Press.
Norris, F. H. 2002. 60,000 disaster victims speak: Part I. An empirical review of the empirical literature, 1981–2001. *Psychiatry: Interpersonal Biological Processes* 65(3):207.
Norris, F. H., and C. L. Elrod. 2006. Psychosocial consequences of disaster. In *Methods for disaster mental health research*, ed. F. N. Norris, S. Galea, M. J. Friedman, and P. J. Watson, 20–42. New York: Guilford.
Oliver-Smith, A. 1996. Anthropological research on hazards and disasters. *Annual Review of Anthropology* 25(1):303.
Oliver-Smith, A. 1999. Peru's five-hundred-year earthquake: Vulnerability in historical context. In *The angry earth: Disaster in anthropological perspective*, ed A. Oliver-Smith, and S. Hoffman, 74. New York: Routledge.
Pelling, M. 1998. Participation, social capital and vulnerability to urban flooding in Guyana. *Journal of International Development* 10(4):469–486.
Pelling, M. 2003. *Vulnerability of cities: Natural disasters and social resilience*. London: Earthscan.
Razzak, J. A., and A. L. Kellermann. 2002. Emergency medical care in developing countries: Is it worthwhile? *Bulletin of the World Health Organization* 80:900–905.
Sanderson, D. 2000. Cities, disasters and livelihoods. *Environment and Urbanization* 12(2):93.
Semenza, J. C. 1996. Heat-related deaths during the July 1995 heat wave in Chicago. *New England Journal of Medicine* 335(2):84.
Sever, M. S., R. Vanholder, and N. Lameire. 2006. Management of crush-related injuries after disasters. *New England Journal of Medicine* 354(10):1052–1063.
Shultz, J. M., J. Russell, and Z. Espinel. 2005. Epidemiology of tropical cyclones: The dynamics of disaster, disease, and development. *Epidemiologic Reviews* 27(1):21–35.
Stehr, S. D. 2006. The political economy of urban disaster assistance. *Urban Affairs Review* 41(4):492–500.
Thywissen, K. 2006. *Components of risk—A comparative glossary*. New York: United Nations University.
Tierney, J. K. 2001. *Facing the unexpected: Disaster preparedness and response in the United States*. Washington, DC: Joseph Henry Press.
United Nations Development Programme (UNDP). 2004. *Reducing disaster risk: A challenge for development*. New York: United Nations Development Programme.

United Nations Development Programme (UNDP). 2006. Sustainable housing reconstruction in Bam through community mobilization and participation. http://www.undp.org.ir/project.aspx?projectID=5.

United Nations International Strategy for Disaster Reduction (ISDR). 2008. *Towards national resilience: Good practices of national platforms for disaster risk reduction.* New York: United Nations Secretariat of the International Strategy for Disaster Reduction (UN/ISDR).

United Nations International Strategy for Disaster Reduction (ISDR). 2009. UNISDR terminology of disaster risk reduction. http://www.unisdr.org/eng/library/lib-terminology-eng%20home.htm.

Wisner, B. 2004. *At risk: Natural hazards, people's vulnerability and disasters.* London: Routledge.

Yen, I. H., and Syme, S. L. 1999. The social environment and health: A discussion of the epidemiologic literature. *Annual Review of Public Health* 20(1):287–308.

Zschau, J., and Küppers, A. N. 2003. *Early warning systems for natural disaster reduction.* New York: Springer.

# CHAPTER THIRTEEN

# URBAN TERRORISM

### ROBERT J. BUNKER
### PAMELA L. BUNKER

## LEARNING OBJECTIVES

- Define terrorism
- Describe the global distribution of terrorism
- Identify characteristics of cities which make them targets for terrorist acts
- Consider the public health impact of terrorism on cities
- Discuss responses to terrorism

TERRORISM is a major issue in the modern world, and cities with large aggregations of people are the most frequent and likely targets. Modern forms of terrorism come in many varieties, including those derived from nationalism, revolutionary (far left) or far-right extremism, single-issue groups, and religious extremism. While terrorism from governmental perspectives is traditionally defined as either containing a political component or itself represents a political act, this is too narrow a perspective for urban health concerns. High levels of street criminality, such as violent acts conducted by the majority of less-evolved street gangs (Sullivan 1997), while devoid of political elements, must also be included as a form of urban terrorism as must some of the coercive activities of organized crime and other illicit groups. Distinctions between domestic and international forms of terrorism, state versus nonstate basis of terrorism, and even rural versus urban terrorism are also made. The distant roots of urban terrorism can be found in the early days of the city-state when one organized political body engaged in the use of indiscriminate force against another. Terrorist acts taking place in wars, revolts, insurgencies, and other conflicts have been chronicled for thousands of years. Cities are where people concentrate, social movements gather, commerce and communication focus; therefore, cities can be the source and target of terrorist acts. Perspectives on urban terrorism and a discussion of its roots, identifying its effects, health issues, and the response strategies to mitigate it within the context of the developed and developing world, are reviewed here.

# PERSPECTIVES AND ROOTS

## Definition of Urban Terrorism

A major encyclopedia series on terrorism defines it as "the indiscriminate use of force to achieve political aims" (Crenshaw and Pimlott 1997). This definition accepts that both states and nonstate groups may engage in this practice. For this chapter, then, the focus is on terrorist acts rather than the more contentious issue of terrorist actors (that is, one person's terrorist is another's "freedom fighter"; one person's counterterrorism is another's "state terror").

For the purposes of this chapter, the definition must also include an urban context. Cities, with their built environment, their economies of scale for providing human goods and services, and their role in national development, are targets for terrorist attacks. Cities absorb much of the impact, but they are also vital for rebuilding society after such attacks.

While a political element is contained in all traditional definitions of terrorism, such as the preceding one, organized groups promoting criminal aims, such as street gangs and other illicit groups, have now grown in size and numbers, much like a spreading cancer; they are literally terrorizing the communities where they have entrenched themselves. From a mental health perspective, the effects of these groups on urban communities is no different than that of traditional terrorist activities. Therefore, urban terrorism will be defined as "the indiscriminate use of force directed at urban populations to achieve political and organized criminal aims." This broader definition is of immense importance for urban health needs, because how you define a problem shapes how, or even if, you will recognize and respond to it. Such a perspective is also in line with the thinking of many security and defense scholars. These individuals are concerned that global conflict has shifted into a new pattern where irregular and unconventional warfare now dominates. One scholar has gone so far as to say:

> In the future, war will not be waged by armies but by groups whom we today call terrorists, guerrillas, bandits and robbers, but who will undoubtedly hit on more formal titles to describe themselves. Their organizations are likely to be constructed on charismatic lines rather than institutional ones, and to be motivated less by "professionalism" than by fanatical, ideologically based loyalties. (Van Creveld 1991)

This shift in war and conflict is attributed to the weakening of the nation-state-based international system through globalization of communication, transportation, and technology. As these forces of globalization are concentrated in cities, cities become targets of attacks.

Another element for defining terrorism is the means of action. Terrorism is less about the physical (destructive) act and more about the disruptive effects within communities, cities, and peoples. This makes terrorism a form of disruptive targeting. The actual act of violence is comparable to throwing a rock into a tranquil pond. While the initial impact only affects a small part of the pond, much like that of a shooting or bomb blast, the ripples that it creates spread across the urban community instilling fear in the populace. For example, New York City and Washington, DC, in 2001 were disrupted for weeks with twenty-three cases of anthrax. Of concern is the fact that weaponry and informational technology advances have increased terrorist disruptive potentials manyfold over the last half-century. At the same time, more and more people are living in urban zones: in the developing world, people are concentrated in mega-cities with teeming slums, making them increasingly vulnerable to incidents of terrorism.

## Roots of Urban Terrorism

For the modern period, works such as *Mini-manual of the Urban Guerilla*, published in 1969, delineate older perspectives of rural insurgency with the emergence of urban guerrillas. This new guerilla subclass became identified as the ideologically motivated terrorists of the 1960s and early 1970s who engaged in a theatrical form of terrorism, primarily based on hostage-taking. A second wave of terrorists, less professional and more extreme in their views derived from their religious fervor, emerged in the 1980s and 1990s. These groups were far less constrained in their use of violence and willing to cross the older, self-imposed ban on the use of weapons of mass destruction. As a result, a focus on mass killing and body counts took precedent over terrorist stage plays. These newer groups also did not share the earlier notion of simply gaining statehood or achieving their limited-issue cause as the desired end state. Rather, many of these groups sought to challenge the existing international system based on the nation-state form and destroy it.

Palestine is a case illustration of the transformation of urban terrorism in recent decades. The traditional and so-called terrorist group Fatah (the PLO) was secular in orientation and motivated to achieve a political end—a Palestinian state next to the Israeli state—within the context of the state-based international system of the modern world. However, Hamas, the newer and more radicalized terrorist group, as some have labeled it, is religious in orientation and motivated to achieve a political end—an Islamic caliphate and the destruction of the Israeli state—incompatible with the norms and values of the modern international system. A power struggle is now taking place between these two groups with Hamas preeminent in 2009.

Along with these trends in terrorist groups themselves, a whole host of other nonstate entities that participate in terrorist acts have been emerging during the last four to five decades. These included street gangs, drug cartels, warlords, mercenaries, and even more guerrilla and insurgent groups. While many of these groups remained just that—groups—others were able to take control of state areas, forming para-states and entire states themselves that resulted in their criminalization. In many cases, this takeover progressed street by street and block by block, as the institutions of the legitimate state were defeated and replaced by the norms and values of the local street thugs. The victors of this trend are also those entities whose values are increasingly incompatible with the values of the modern international system.

## THE GLOBAL DISTRIBUTION OF URBAN TERRORISM

Urban terrorism is global in terms of events and impact. Much of the attention focused on urban terrorism since September 11, 2001, has been on the Global North. Although spectacular attacks have taken place—the infamous 9/11 attacks, principally in New York and Washington (2001), train bombings in Madrid (2004), and the subway bombings in London (2005)—the threat to the physical safety of this group overall has been negligible to date. Only terrorist groups, most importantly those belonging to Al Qaeda and its affiliates, are currently of major concern. While physical threats may be limited, the potential for damage to the national economy due to terrorist acts is real, as are feelings of anxiety and concern among the populace.

The larger threat of terrorism in the Global North is to those living in more marginal and unsafe communities, focused to a larger extent on street gang activity. While politically motivated terrorism is of general concern overall, the more marginal segment of the urban population is struggling with high unemployment levels, lack of educational and jobs skills, broken families, alcohol and drug abuse, and low incomes conducive to the growth of street gangs and their culture of violence. Drive-by shootings represent random acts of violence that generate ambiguity in the minds of local populations, and gang graffiti serves as a constant reminder that the gangs and not the community own the local turf. Children growing up in gang territories witness death at a young age and typically have lost multiple loved ones, neighbors, and schoolmates to gang violence. For many children in these enclaves diagnoses of post-traumatic stress disorder (PTSD) have been made, which equates to soldiers in war zones suffering combat stress.

While organized crime is evident in the developed world, it is almost invisible in its more affluent areas. Its reach and activities are predominately found in more marginal locales and neighborhoods, older industrial areas and ports, and occasionally in some service industries such as waste disposal and those tied into labor unions. Terrorist-like acts undertaken are generally discriminate and symbolic in nature and simply viewed as an adjunct to illicit business activities, such as the threatening of beatings, rapes, and killings to facilitate overdue money collections.

The Global South, even excluding the Middle East, experiences a high number of terrorist attacks, injuries, and fatalities (Tables 13.1 and 13.2). Terrorist activities take on a whole different perspective to the mass of humanity living in the urban slums of the developing world. Those living within the domain of criminal and para-states may find themselves terrorized by the state as a tool of political control. The rest face the threat of violence and brutality from any combination of terrorists, insurgents and guerrilas, gangs, drug cartels, warlords, mercenaries, and the organized crime group that controls their neighborhood, city block, or immediate cluster of slum shanties. Some try to eke out low-paying livings in service industries or scavenging in trash dumps. Many times, the locals are forced to band together to protect themselves, creating new gangs or seeing the wisdom of joining already established and well-armed groups.

TABLE 13.1  Global Incidents of Terrorism by Year, 1998–2007

| Year | Incidents | Fatalities | Injured |
|---|---|---|---|
| 1998 | 1,286 | 2,172 | 8,202 |
| 1999 | 1,172 | 847 | 2,534 |
| 2000 | 1,151 | 783 | 2,570 |
| 2001 | 1,732 | 4,571 | 6,403 |
| 2002 | 2,648 | 2,763 | 7,349 |
| 2003 | 1,899 | 2,346 | 6,200 |
| 2004 | 2,647 | 5,066 | 10,860 |
| 2005 | 4,976 | 8,192 | 15,269 |
| 2006 | 6,660 | 12,071 | 20,991 |
| 2007 | 3,479 | 8,763 | 18,694 |
| Total | 27,669 | 47,596 | 99,072 |

Source: MIPT (domestic and international). Adapted from Alex P. Schmid (director of the Centre for the Study of Terrorism and Political Violence), "The Trajectory of Terrorism 1990–2030" (presentation at Netherlands Institute for International Relations "Clingendael," Prinses Juliana Kazerne Conference Challenging Uncertainties: The Future of the Netherlands Armed Forces, December 16–17, 2008. http://www.clingendael.nl/cscp/events/20081216/20081216_presentatie_schmidt.ppt).

TABLE 13.2  Terrorist Incidents by Region: 1998 Through March 3, 2008

| Region | Incidents | Injuries | Fatalities |
|---|---|---|---|
| Africa | 572 | 8,639 | 2,694 |
| East and Central Asia | 128 | 393 | 164 |
| Eastern Europe | 1,455 | 5,127 | 2,010 |
| Latin America and the Caribbean | 1,834 | 2,648 | 1,688 |
| Middle East/Persian Gulf | 13,865 | 54,707 | 28,248 |
| North America | 120 | 2,408 | 2,996 |
| South Asia | 4,881 | 17,953 | 7,744 |
| Southeast Asia and Oceania | 1,738 | 5,552 | 1,748 |
| Western Europe | 3,087 | 1,787 | 401 |
| Total | 27,680 | 99,214 | 47,693 |

Sources: MIPT, at http://www.tkb.org, as of 03/03/2008. MIPT (domestic and international). Adapted from Alex P. Schmid (director of the Centre for the Study of Terrorism and Political Violence), "The Trajectory of Terrorism 1990–2030" (presentation at Netherlands Institute for International Relations "Clingendael," Prinses Juliana Kazerne Conference Challenging Uncertainties: The Future of the Netherlands Armed Forces, December 16–17, 2008. http://www.clingendael.nl/cscp/events/20081216/20081216_presentatie_schmidt.ppt).

The lower visibility of terrorism in the Global South is because it is one among many forms of violence. Cities are also sites of battles for access to space and resources in the form of political violence, civil wars, and communal riots. These occur in settings that also have criminal violence and gang warfare. All of this happens in the context of grinding poverty, limited infrastructure, poor service delivery, and ineffectual government. Those urban dwellers in the developing world that live in marginal areas to some extent mimic the experiences of those less fortunate populations of the developed world. While the threat of violence posed by street gangs may be a burning issue, other groups, including insurgents and cartels, also may be of concern—including the state itself.

Those select few who form the urban elite of the developing world have a very different and almost surreal perspective on terrorism. Either they may be part of the problem and are important members of the criminal-state or para-state, terrorizing others, or are successful professionals who hunker down in their gated cities fearful of kidnappings and robberies. Quite a few developing world elites now travel by helicopter rather than car in urban areas to stave off the threat of kidnapping and send their families off to safe and affluent regions of the developed world to vacation, be educated, and even to reside.

The Global South is not isolated from the North. Local attacks may be designed to have global repercussions. Attacks on cities are not necessarily a deliberate attack on the city itself. A number of attacks on busy urban tourist locations in the Global South (for example, Bali) were not aimed at the cities themselves, or the governments of their countries, but were used to make statements that would reverberate around the world. The London subway bombing in 2005 suggests a different trend with global implications; it involved attackers who were British of Pakistani descent with the attack organized from Pakistan, and with the intention to support a broader Arab cause. Burning issues in one part of the world can be felt in another part.

Criminal gangs are a special form of terrorism, and they can have a global network. While early forms of street gangs are viewed as only promoting criminal aims, in their later and more mature stage of development, they are found to develop political agendas, like the criminal and para-states that are now in direct conflict with the dominant international order. Group formation and growth occurs frequently in cities. One example is Mara Salvatrucha-13, or MS-13, which was formed by immigrants who fled the civil war in El Salvador in the 1980s. The number 13 relates to the thirteenth letter of the alphabet, or M, a known to reference La Eme, or the Mexican Mafia, a California-based prison gang that exercises control over MS-13 members and other street gangs whose members pay taxes in exchange for protection. This group of immigrants found discrimination, virtually no access to benefits, and little opportunity for advancement in the U.S., which was followed by engaging in criminal activity. Prisons provided networking for the development of MS-13, which has operated for the past fifteen years in areas of Los Angeles including, but not limited, to Rampart, Wilshire, Olympic, and Hollywood. The gang is estimated to have several thousand members in multiple U.S. cities and also throughout Central America and Mexico, and it is known for its brutality.

# IMPACT OF URBAN TERRORISM

## Physical Health Issues

The main difference between conventional warfare and politically based terrorism is that in warfare, physical destruction is commonly the main threat to urban environments. Physical destruction, be it to infrastructure or urban populations, is less of a concern from all forms of political terrorism, short of those using weapons of mass destruction (WMD). Even then, only certain forms and thresholds of WMD use—specifically nuclear devices and certain biological agents, such as smallpox—meet the criteria needed to create wide-scale killing within an urban environment. The 9/11 attack is the closest terrorist incident to a traditional WMD event with the deaths of approximately 3,000 people, environmental pollution and health threats, and the loss of 13 million square feet of Class A office space in Manhattan, which is equivalent to all of the Class A space in Atlanta or Miami (Fullilove 2006).

Physical health issues stemming from non-WMD forms of political terrorism are principally derived from shootings and bombings. These are based on the use of point and area-influencing weaponry that kill and injure in ranges from 1s to 10s for point weaponry (for example, semiautomatic guns and small booby traps) to 10s and 100s for area weaponry (for example, suicide bombers and car bombs). Death and bodily injury are common outcomes of these forms of attacks, with higher percentages of injuries over fatalities. Such attacks can shut down public urban spaces and roadways while consequence management operations take place, crime scene investigations are conducted, and facilities and infrastructure repairs are implemented. This results in area denial and nonuse of these places and spaces for hours to days for small-scale incidents, such as shootings and days to months for large-scale incidents such as a mall or facilities bombings. As seen with the 9/11 attacks, the urban space once occupied by the World Trade Center has been shut down for years now, and it will be over a decade before it has been rehabilitated for economic and public use because of the sheer magnitude of the incident and HAZMAT (hazardous material) concerns. Further, specific infrastructure targeting, such as the destruction of power lines and generating plants, key bridges, oil and gas pipelines and storage tanks, and hospital trauma centers, can create denial-of-service attacks, which negatively influence the physical health of urban populations.

For criminally based terrorism, guns and, to a lesser extent, bombs are the weaponry of choice. Deaths and injury are in line with political terrorism at the 1s (single or few) and 10s (dozens) level but rarely go above it except for unique cases derived from narco-terrorism, such as during the fighting between the Colombian state and the Medellín cartel in the 1980s and early 1990s. Even current strife in Mexico between the federal government and the various drug cartels and among the cartels themselves typically sees incidents in the 1s and 10s, though that widespread conflict at aggregate levels of incidents is now seeing total deaths and injuries well into the 1,000s on a yearly basis. In retrospect, such high levels of physical casualties is no different than the endemic gang wars on American streets that are also in the 1,000s of injuries and deaths on a yearly basis in poor and marginalized urban communities.

In tandem with the street gang strife in the poorer sections of American cities is the inability of local residents to safely walk to and attend school and participate in activities in public venues, such as playing in the park, taking a stroll down the street, or even shopping in a neighborhood controlled by a rival street gang. This threat of violence is much like that experienced in parts of Iraq and in other insurgency-type situations where the use of improvised explosive devices and suicide bombers, illegal checkpoints manned by armed gunmen, and random sniper attacks result in area denial of public spaces.

## Mental Health Issues

Data on population mental health following terrorist attacks are limited. After the World Trade Center disaster in 2001, studies were done to estimate the rate of post-traumatic stress disorder (PTSD) in the general population. The essential feature of PTSD is the development of certain characteristic symptoms after direct personal exposure to an extreme stressor, involving actual or threatened death or serious injury, or learning about the same regarding a family member or close associate. The immediate emotional reaction includes intense fear, helplessness, or horror. Characteristic symptoms that subsequently emerge cluster in three domains: persistent re-experiencing of the event (dreams, nightmares or intrusive recollections); persistent avoidance of stimuli associated with the event and generalized numbing of emotional responsiveness; and persistent symptoms of increased arousal (insomnia, irritability, exaggerated startle response, poor concentration, or hypervigilance). The presentation of symptoms after such an event can vary markedly from one individual to another, ranging from immediate symptoms resolved within a short period to delayed onset that can last for years.

While studies of earlier disasters have focused on learning about PTSD among direct victims, rescue workers and their families, including children, data on the effect of disasters for the general population showed that those not directly affected also experienced elevated rates of PTSD. In one report (Galea and others 2003), three random-digit-dial telephone surveys of adults in progressively larger portions of the New York City metropolitan area were conducted 1–2 months, 4–5 months, and 6–9 months after September 11, 2001; 1,008, 2,001, and 2,752 demographically representative adults were recruited in the three surveys, respectively. The past-30-day prevalence of probable PTSD related to the September 11 attacks in Manhattan declined from 7.5 percent 1–2 months after September 11 to 0.6 percent 6–9 months after September 11. Although the prevalence of PTSD symptoms was consistently higher among persons who were more directly affected by the attacks, a substantial number of people who were not directly affected by the attacks also met criteria for probable PTSD. These data suggest a rapid resolution of most of the probable PTSD in the general population of New York City in the first nine months after the attacks. Factors associated with developing PTSD included directly affected (exposed to event), experienced loss (person or property). Whether directly affected or not, factors associated with PTSD included female gender, lower socioeconomic status, previous and current life stressors, and panic attacks around the time of the event. Presumably, PTSD among those not directly affected may be due to word of mouth, watching the events in person or on television, and the disruption of services that was ubiquitous in NYC. Persistence of PTSD can last for years among those who were most directly affected by the disaster, but among those not directly affected, it was relatively infrequent. Reasons for persistence of PTSD among those indirectly affected included ongoing stressors (for example, job loss) following the event. These studies showed that the psychological consequences of a large-scale terrorist attack in a densely populated urban area may extend beyond people directly affected by the disaster to people in the general population.

The March 11, 2004, train bombings in Madrid, Spain, provide another example of the impact of a terrorist attack on an urban population. Using a cross-sectional random-digit-dial survey of Madrid residents to assess the prevalence of PTSD and major depression in the general population of Madrid one to three months after the March 11 train bombings, 2.3 percent reported symptoms consistent with PTSD related to the March 11 bombings, and 8.0 percent of respondents reported symptoms consistent with major depression (Miguel-Tobal and others 2006). The prevalence of PTSD was substantially lower, but the prevalence of depression was comparable to estimates reported after the September 11 attacks in Manhattan. The findings suggest that across cities, the magnitude of a terrorist attack may be the primary determinant of the prevalence of PTSD in the general population, but other factors may be responsible for determining the population prevalence of depression.

Data on population mental health following terrorist attacks in the Global South are sparse. In one study, a self-report questionnaire which assessed potential risk factors and identified symptoms matching DSM-IV criteria for post-traumatic stress disorder was answered by 2,883 Kenyans, one to three months after the bombing (Njenga and others 2004). Results showed that 35 percent of respondents reported symptoms approximating to the criteria for post-traumatic stress disorder.

The examples reported here reflect general population surveys for probable PTSD following a single event. PTSD represents one diagnosis. Studies of depression and other psychiatric diagnoses as well as rates and clinical course for those exposed to ongoing attacks show that terrorist attacks do more than cause physical damage. Mental health issues are not limited to those most directly affected. Broad population health perspectives, assessment, and response are needed to address terrorist attacks.

# RESPONSE STRATEGIES

## Political-Based Terrorism Response

The response strategies to politically based forms of urban terrorism are intertwined with the following trends. The first is that groups engaging in terrorism have become more network-like in their organizational structures. This newer form of organization is superior in its informational and operational capabilities vis-à-vis older industrial and hierarchical models used by nation-states and their coercive arms, such as police and military forces. As a result, legitimate states, to counter network-based groups engaging in terrorism, must create their own network-based security structures. These security structures need to go beyond traditional governmental structures and encompass private sector and nongovernmental organizations as active allies within threatened operational areas.

The second trend is derived from the fact that local and federal governmental responses to the effects of sustained, and even sporadic, incidents of terrorism in urban centers have been typically inadequate. The focus of effort from a consequence management perspective has been on emergency transport of the wounded, cleaning up the incident scene (which includes removal of the dead), and the repair of physical damage to the infrastructure. Far fewer resources have been allocated to mitigating the disruptive effects of terrorism on an urban population's mental health, because the damage is invisible (nonphysical).

Both of these trends and governmental response need to focus on the rise of network organizational forms—to use them as part of a structural response and to mitigate the effects of network disruptive attacks on civil society. The integration of governmental and nongovernmental response and a hybrid organizational structure response, incorporating hierarchical and network forms, has been discussed since at least the mid-1990s in Los Angeles. These discussions developed in tandem with the rise of the Los Angeles Terrorism Early Warning (TEW) Group model in 1996 and its subsequent spread to over two dozen other cities within the United States over the course of a decade. Specific components of this bottom-up network response included law enforcement, public health, and fire responders working together alongside academic and research institutions to ward off group think and myopic thinking. National Guard personnel, military personnel, in an advisory role only, and federal personnel complemented these groups, along with select private sector members.

Of significance was the establishment of the first domestic fusion effort to integrate public health disease surveillance and disease early-warning into an ongoing indications and warning framework for terrorism. The Epidemiological Intelligence (Epi-Intel) Cell worked as an integrated component of the TEW's net assessment architecture. It relied upon syndromic surveillance, disease reporting, OSINT (open source intelligence) such as Promed and Epi-X, and conducted assessments. A key component of this capability was the use of Biological Terrorism, Food, and Water Surety Playbooks (Sullivan 2005).

These early gains have been severely eroded with the loss of Department of Homeland Security (DHS) funding for the TEW Group national expansion program and the creation of state fusion-centers across the United States that have reverted to a top-down federal model, emphasizing criminal intelligence procedures. Another area of consternation has been the fact that very little thought or program implementation has existed concerning the mitigation of network disruptive attacks on civil society. Terrorism is still viewed from the perspective of physical destruction and death. Its disruptive basis, which is organic to how networks engage in conflict, is still overlooked in the governmental consequence management sector. This represents a significant societal protection capability gap and also has resulted in missing the opportunity to create a new and important capability to engage in offensive disruptive targeting against opposing force (OPFOR) networks.

## Criminal-Based Terrorism Response

Response strategies to criminal groups, such as street gangs, drug cartels, and organized crime, with actions that mimic the effects of terrorist acts on urban populations, are also required to use a network structural response and to mitigate the effects of network disruptive attacks. Each of these threat areas of concern, such as street gangs, are being responded to in a vacuum separate from counterterrorism, counternarcotics, and other governmental response disciplines. Since endemic criminal acts within an urban population zone, such as a neighborhood or a section of a city, are not typically viewed from the perspective of urban terrorism, little is being done to address public health issues generated by the cumulative effects of disruptive societal targeting. The end result is that urban terrorism is being addressed in a piecemeal and ad hoc fashion within the United States. Many times, the affluence of a community, its political clout, and decision-maker perspectives on the intractability of the problem within some neighborhoods influences the level of resources that will be allocated towards addressing the perceived threat.

The response is also dictated by what the perpetrator group has been designated as—terrorist group, street gang, or drug cartel—because this signifies which discrete governmental agency should respond to the problem. The entire response protocol ignores the blending and evolving aspects of these groups, and more importantly, is not being conducted as an integrated strategy to mitigate a range of armed and dangerous nonstate groups threatening the urban health of a besieged city's populace.

## Developed World and Developing World Differences

The United States's experience with response to terrorism is not unique to the developed world. The more developed countries typically stovepipe perpetrator group response, because this is in line with the hierarchical nature of their governmental structure from the national down to the local community level.

The case of response to terrorism in developing countries is more complex. Response to politically based terrorism is a hit-and-miss proposition and usually results in the blanket use of oppression against ethnic and other suspect peoples and groups. Many times, it is the government itself—especially those representing illegitimate states and para-states—that is the cause of the repression and terrorism.

Response to criminally based terrorism in the developing world is even more dismal. If the criminal groups are not viewed as threatening the state and its elites, they become designated as a second tier problem. Rampant crime in urban slums committed by street gangs is an accepted norm within the developing world. As long as "those people" prey upon each other, the state has little interest in exerting limited resources to attempt to suppress the problem. Alliances between corrupt members of governmental institutions and local gangs are not uncommon and may also help to perpetuate ongoing conditions in the slums and other marginalized areas. It may not be surprising that one of the self-help measures of slum dwelling populations is to form their own private militia or street gang to provide local neighborhood protection.

One approach in response to terrorism (or acts) within the developing world is the deployment of peacekeeping and peace enforcement troops by the United Nations into failed and failing state environments. These deployments are typically reactive in nature and are only made after much global outcry concerning issues of genocide, ethnic cleansing and mass displacements of peoples, rapes, torture, and other crimes against humanity visited by one side on another and sometimes reciprocated. These deployments are primarily responses to politically motivated forms of urban terrorism but outright community failure, as seen in Port-au-Prince, Haiti and Mogadishu, Somalia, could conceivably be considered just as much a response to criminally motivated forms of urban terrorism, since the perpetrators of violence were nothing more than heavily armed street gangs. These UN peace operations are sporadic in nature because of the international politics involved and many times have proven ineffectual, so their benefit to the developed world is still somewhat questionable.

Large private security and mercenary corporations, with exotic names like Executive Outcomes (now defunct) and Blackwater (now Xe), have existed for over two decades and also have to be factored into the equation when responses to urban terrorism are now being formulated. For some urban populations, private forces can be considered godsends, like the wealthy communities that employed them in post-Katrina New Orleans. For other urban populations, the benefits of their deployments are more questionable. For some communities, such as some of those in Iraq, their status at one point of being above the law and accountable to no one, made them recognized as part of the problem.

## SUMMARY

Urban terrorism has existed since the emergence of the first city-states thousands of years ago. Definitions and perceptions concerning it have naturally changed and evolved over the course of history with current concerns over both politically based and criminally based forms of urban terrorism evident today. Urban terrorism has been exacerbated by the massive increase of urban populations over the last half-century and the emergence of sprawling slums in most of the larger cities within the developing world. A shifting pattern of global conflict, based on unconventional and irregular warfare waged by non-state entities and illegitimate states and para-states, has further brought about heightened levels of terrorist and terrorist-like incidents. On one level, much of this conflict can be attributed to a "war over social and political organization" now taking place between the nation-state and nonstate challengers over its position of primacy in the international system (Bunker 1997).

On another level, much of this global conflict has been brought about by societal inequalities, with economically marginalized tribes, ethnic groups, minorities, and communities either being subjected to urban terrorism as a form of repression—utilized by both the state and local thugs or criminals—or nonstate groups and communities engaging in it as a result of political or criminal activities to further their access to economic and material goods. This situation is unlikely to change well into the future because the international political economy and state-based system is structurally founded on the acceptance of huge differences in the social-economic classes ranging from the very rich to the very poor. As a result, terrorism has now to some extent become a tool of the social classes and is being used in urban environments against competing peoples. This is especially true within economically marginalized communities of the developed world and throughout much of the developing world.

# REFERENCES

Bunker, R. J. 1997. Epochal change: War over social and political organization. *Parameters* 27( 2):15–25.
Crenshaw, M., and J. Pimlott, eds. 1997. *Encyclopedia of world terrorism*. Vols. 1–3. Armonk, NY: M E. Sharpe.
Davis, M. 2006. *Planet of slums*. New York: Verso.
Fullilove, M. T. 2006. Fifty ways to destroy a city: Undermining the social foundations of health. In *Cities and Public Health*, ed. N. Freudenberg, S. Galea, and D. Vlahov, 176–193. Nashville: Vanderbilt University Press.
Galea, S., D. Vlahov, H. Resnick, J. Ahern, E. Susser, J. Gold, M. Bucuvalas, and D. Kilpatrick. 2003. Trends of probable post-traumatic stress disorder in New York City after the September 11 terrorist attacks. *American Journal of Epidemiology* 158(6):514–524.
Miguel-Tobal, J. J., A. Cano-Vindel, H. Gonzalez-Ordi, I. Iruarrizaga, S. Rudenstine, D. Vlahov, and S. Galea. 2006. PTSD and depression after the Madrid March 11 train bombings. *Journal of Trauma Stress* 19(1):69–80.
Njenga, F. G., P. J. Nicholls, C. Nyamai, P. Kigamwa, and J. R. Davidson. 2004. Post-traumatic stress after terrorist attack: Psychological reactions following the U.S. embassy bombing in Nairobi: Naturalistic study. *British Journal of Psychiatry* 185:328–333.
Sullivan, J. P. 1997. Third generation street gangs: Turf, cartel, and net warriors. *Transnational Organized Crime* 3(3):95–108.
Sullivan, J. P. 2005. Terrorism early warning and co-production of counterterrorism intelligence. Presented at the Canadian Association for Security and Intelligence Studies (CASIS) 20th anniversary conference, October 21, in Montreal, Quebec, Canada.
Van Creveld, M. 1991. *The transformation of war*. New York: Free Press.

# CHAPTER FOURTEEN

# THE CULTURE OF PEACE AGAINST VIOLENCE IN ZAGREB

## STIPE ORESKOVIC

### LEARNING OBJECTIVES

- Understand the social background, historical roots, and behavioral patterns of urban youth violence
- Describe how a specific public health action was organized by the city of Zagreb to change social climate, address key factors, and prevent youth violence
- Learn how communication and social interaction among media, nongovernmental organizations (NGOs), and community can help prevent urban youth violence

**THIS** chapter will introduce readers to the variety of public health projects in the city of Zagreb, which created broad partnerships to address the growing problem of urban youth violence. After providing some general demographic and descriptive information about Zagreb, its population and public health policies, this chapter explains how a strategy was developed engaging city government, NGOs, media, and the private sector in a comprehensive action to promote a culture of peace and tolerance.

## OVERVIEW OF THE CITY

Zagreb has been a member of the Healthy Cities movement from the very beginning and was the host for 2008 Healthy Cities Conference commemorating 20 years of the movement. Zagreb is also the place where Andrija Stampar, a founding father of the World Health Organization, established the second oldest school of public health in Europe in 1927.

Today, Zagreb is the only Croatian city whose metropolitan population exceeds one million people. There were 1,088,841 people in the Zagreb metropolitan area in 2008, which included the smaller cities of Samobor, Velika Gorica, and Zaprešić. A total of 784,900 lived in the city proper in 2008. With 640 square kilometers of land and a city budget of US$1.56 billion, Zagreb is a mid-size urban Central European city. Compared to the Croatian average, Zagreb is more likely to become an "old city" with 15.8 percent inhabitants less than 15 years old, 65.8 percent between 15 and 65, and 14.9 percent over 65. Most citizens are Croats, making up 91.9 percent of the city's population (2001 census). The same census records 40,066 residents belonging to ethnic minorities (Republic of Croatia, Central Bureau of Statistics 2001). On average, citizens of Zagreb enjoy good health as compared to the Croatian or Southeastern European data. The average life expectancy for someone born in 2006 is 73.6 years for men and 79.9 years for women. The death rate of 11.0 per 1,000 has been stable for the past five years. By far, the single largest cause of death is heart disease (49.4 percent), followed by cancers (28.3 percent), intestinal disease (4.5 percent), and respiratory system disease (4.5 percent) (City of Zagreb 2008). The latest public health policy plan for Zagreb identifies several priorities directly or indirectly connected to groups that are involved in acts of youth violence: psychosocial health (including depression and anxiety disorders, behavioral problems among the youth like social isolation), and drug abuse (including tobacco and excessive alcohol use, but also cannabis and club drugs).

No country or community is untouched by violence. It is among the leading causes of death for people aged 15–44 years worldwide. Concerning violence, Zagreb is not a special case or exception when examined within the trends documented for Southeastern and Eastern Europe. In the last decade of the twentieth century, the rates of violent deaths were increasing dramatically in countries experiencing rapid social and economic change and moving from dictatorship to democracy, particularly in the countries of Central and Eastern Europe and the newly independent states. In some countries, the homicide rate increased by over 150 percent in the period of separation and declaration of independence. In addition, the rates of child abuse, violence by intimate partners, and abuse of elderly people rose considerably during the last decade. Suicides also increased during this period. Populations in urban areas and cities in transition countries suffer from interpersonal violence, child maltreatment, intimate partner violence, elder abuse, sexual violence, and growing youth violence.

## THE HISTORY OF VIOLENCE IN ZAGREB

Zagreb is also an old Central European city, dating back to 1094, when the Hungarian King Ladislaus (1040–1095) founded the Zagreb bishopric, a Roman Catholic diocese. During the course of history, Zagreb has been many times an object of violence, conflicts, and aggression. That is why it was fortified in the thirteenth century to defend against the Tartars, and again in the sixteenth century against Ottoman Turks. Fighting ensued also inside the walls, between the Zagreb diocese and the free sovereign town of Gradec for land and mills, and sometimes also for political reasons. The period from the fifteenth to the seventeenth century was marked by bitter struggles with the Ottoman Empire. In the twentieth century, Austria attempted a germanization of the Croatian homeland. During the Croatian national revival in the nineteenth century, both the pan-Yugoslav and Croatian independence movements were centered in Zagreb.

In World War II (1939–1945), Zagreb became the capital of the Nazi puppet Independent State of Croatia, with the Croatian radical right Ustase in power. The Ustase enacted racial laws and formed eight concentration camps targeting minority Serbs, Romas, and Jewish populations. Partisans under Josip Broz Tito (1892–1980) liberated the city in May 1945. After World War II, Croatia belonged to the six-part Socialist Federative Republic of Yugoslavia.

During the 1991–1995 Croatian War of Independence, the city was the scene of some sporadic fighting surrounding its Yugoslav Federal Army barracks, but it escaped major damage. In May 1995, it was targeted by Serb rocket artillery, which killed seven civilians. Zagreb was once part of the wealthiest of the Yugoslav republics, but its economy suffered during the 1991–1995 war as its output collapsed and missed the early waves of investment in Central and Eastern Europe, which followed the fall of the Berlin Wall. Since 2000, Croatia's economic fortunes have begun to improve, led by a rebound in tourism and credit-driven consumer spending.

## Alcohol, Drugs, and Violence

There is strong association between the use of alcohol, drugs, and other addictive behavior and violence. Some strong evidence links masculine social identity and heavy group drinking, and the importance of issues of male honor in the social interaction that leads to much violent behavior (Tomsen 1997). In such a context, it is not surprising that results of The European School Survey Project on Alcohol and Other Drugs from 2007 shows that alcohol consumption among students in Croatia is above the European average in all categories (Sakoman, Raboteg Šarić, and Kuzman 2002). Surveys conducted among school boys and school girls of the sixth grades of Zagreb County elementary schools shows that 11 percent of respondents tried to smoke cigarettes, 60 percent of respondents tried to drink alcoholic beverages, and 22 percent of respondents tried to take drugs. Ten percent of respondents smoked occasionally or on a regular basis, 35.3 percent of respondents drank occasionally or on a regular basis. About half of the medical students reported regular alcohol consumption on a monthly (37 percent), weekly (9.5 percent), or daily (3.4 percent) basis (Kruzić-Lulić, Delfin, and Gajnik 2008). Furthermore, 15 percent reported regular monthly, and 2.8 percent regular weekly, drunkenness. The prevalence of students reporting regular drinking or regular drunkenness was significantly higher in men than in women (Trkulja and others 2003).

The findings of a survey conducted by the Child Protection Centre Zagreb in 2003 showed that one out of every fourth child was exposed to some form of abuse (verbal or physical; each can include sexual, economic, and emotional abuse) on a daily basis. Also, the survey showed that the amount of violence among children increases with age. The types of aggressive behavior to which children are exposed daily include exclusion from games and isolation (33 percent), daily threats (25 percent), bullying (35 percent of boys and 31 percent of girls), and 17 percent had been badly hurt by someone (Poliklinika za zaštitu djece grada Zagreba n.d.).

The UNICEF study on violence in schools shows that no gender differences were identified in the quantity of experienced violence, with 10 percent of students of both sexes exposed daily to aggressive behavior (UNICEF 2009). This survey also suggests that in some schools, violence is more prevalent than in others. The tendency to confide in one's parents about exposure to bullying dropped with increasing age among girls but rose among boys, which can probably be explained by the types of abuse to which girls and boys were most frequently exposed, ranging from verbal (name-calling, mocking, demeaning, threatening), social (avoidance, ignoring, exclusion from activities, gossiping, spreading malicious rumors), psychological (damage to property, theft and throwing things, threatening looks, stalking) to physical (pushing, knocking down, punching). Almost anyone can be a target of youth violence behavior.

Unfortunately, for too many adolescents, violence is either the only or the most effective way to achieve status, respect, and other basic social and personal needs. Like money and knowledge, violence is a form of power, and for some youth, it is the only form of power available. When such limited alternatives are combined with a weak commitment to moral norms (internal controls) and little monitoring or supervision of behavior (external controls), violent behavior becomes rational (Barnhart 2009).

Some neighborhoods also provide opportunities for learning and engaging in violence. The presence of gangs and illegal markets—particularly drug distribution networks—not only provide high levels of exposure to violence, but also violent role models and positive rewards for serious violent activity. Single-parent families, ineffective parenting, violent schools, high dropout rates, high adolescent pregnancy rates, substance abuse, and high unemployment rates are all concentrated in such neighborhoods. While these neighborhoods are areas with high rates of concentrated poverty, the critical feature of such neighborhoods that is most directly related to the high rates of violence, crime, and substance use, is the absence of any effective social or cultural organization. It is directly related to the levels of neighborhood discomfort, as determined by an index including unemployment, inflation, and housing conditions. The poor areas of the city with higher incidence of crime and violence (Dubrava, Pescenica, and Sesvete neighborhoods) are the areas of the city with higher incidence of other public health problems, including epidemic diseases related to risk behavior such as hepatitis B or HIV/AIDS (Pyle and others 2000). In the last few years, there were periods of epidemic violence, leading to serious injuries and deaths of young people (Frano Despic, Ivana Hodak) in Zagreb within only a few months (WikiVelv 2009).

There are different answers to the question of links between epidemics of youth violence or violence against youth and the recent war in Croatia during the 1990s. One answer may be the simmering class resentment that is a legacy of the war that caused a deep socioeconomic chasm, left thousands without homes or jobs, yet left a select few who amassed unimaginable fortunes. The children of these families were dubbed the "Golden Generation" in the Croatian media (Bilefsky 2009). There was also violence among those who could be hardly counted as rich—the football fans.

### The "Football" War

Football in Zagreb has special symbolic, social, cultural, and political meaning. Football means the football club, Dinamo, which plays at the stadium near the park Maksimir, first opened May 5, 1912. Over its history, it has gone through many facelifts, but starting in 1997 it received a major rebuilding that lifted its seating capacity to over 40,000. For fourteen years, the Croatian football team had a proud unbeaten record at this stadium in any competitive match.

Although FIFA and UEFA, two international football organizations, invested a lot in the promotion of culture and tolerance and led official campaigns against racism and violence, there are still many football fans who approach football in the same way that Von Clausewitz understood war (that is, war is a continuation of policy by other means). Football and violence were and are still closely connected. There is even a historical example of the "Football" War (*La guerra del fútbol*), also known as the Soccer War: a four-day war fought by El Salvador and Honduras in 1969. It was caused by political conflicts between Hondurans and Salvadorans, mostly concerning the immigration from El Salvador to Honduras.

In the former Yugoslavia, Dinamo Zagreb was the main symbol of Croatian independence and the symbol of the confrontation against Belgrade policy. On many occasions, this confrontation was not only symbolic, but also physical. The infamous "Football Riot" of 1990 is a violent reaction some view as one of the triggers for subsequent wider Yugoslavian conflict. Eighteen years ago, Dinamo had been scheduled to host Serbian rivals Red Star from Belgrade. Some 1,500 members of Crvena Zvezda's fan club, Delije, attended the game from different parts of Yugoslavia. This had been happening in the context of resurgent nationalism and growing fissures in Yugoslavia's federal composition, and the violence appears to have been inevitable and in all likelihood premeditated. Both sides plus the police found themselves engaged in a savage pitched battle. Dinamo Zagreb's Zvonimir Boban, later with AC Milan, attained legendary status and a six-month ban after landing a flying-kick on a member of the police. Key to the fighting were Dinamo's Bad Blue Boys (BBB) and Red Star's Delije fans.

When the Yugoslavian civil war officially began in 1991, members of both groups formed vital components of their countries' forces. Now a BBB statue outside the Maksimir stadium stands as testament of the time with the epitaph: "To the fans of this club, who started the war with Serbia at this ground on May 13, 1990" (Gray 2007). This says a lot about the influence of Dinamo fans on new Croatian history and vice versa. Some authors explain this conflict as rooted only in nationalism and hate between Croats and Serbs, which found a way to express themselves at the football match. However, the violence was more complex and more widely determined than nationalism itself. Two decades after this famous conflict which "started the war," the fans of Dinamo (Bad Blue Boys) were still fighting against the fans of Hadjuk, Torcida. At the last match in Split, it seemed that everyone got what they wanted, as the Dinamo BBB managed to provoke the riot police to enter their bleachers, and a full-blown brawl occurred. After barely a minute into the game, the police were summoned as pockets of Dinamo fans ignited flares, with a fire breaking out in front of the stands (Assis de Moreira 2009). The lyrics of the anthem were written by a popular rock'n roll band, Pips Chips and Video Clips. Bad Blue Boys changed a few words and added the last rhyme to make it a more explicit call to violence and aggression:

> With stakes and chains
> And strikes to the head
> Kick, ruin
> For Dinamo glory
> 
> *YouTube, 2009*

Over the last three years, the Croatian Football Association (FA) has had to pay out more than 200,000 Swiss francs for misbehavior of fans at home and abroad, including fights on Malta and in Hungary and insulting chants during the Euro 2008 quarter-final against Turkey ("Croatia moves to rid sport of violence" 2008). The questions is: How to tackle violence? The history and experience from Zagreb show the need for comprehensive international, national, and local programs, state interventions, and civil society actions.

## INTERNATIONAL PROGRAMS AGAINST VIOLENCE

In March 2003, the WHO *World Report on Violence and Health* was presented in Zagreb. The World Health Organization's global campaign for violence prevention made tackling violence a top priority for the health community. The report stated, "Violence thrives in the absence of democracy, respect for human rights and good governance. We often talk about how a 'culture of violence' can take root. It is also true that patterns of violence are more pervasive and widespread in societies where the authorities endorse the use of violence through their own actions. In many societies, violence is so dominant that it thwarts hopes of economic and social development" (Mandela 2002).

Dr. Andro Vlahusic, minister of health of Croatia at that time, pointed out that "by convening this conference, Croatia demonstrates not only its support for the global anti-violence campaign, but also its readiness to actively contribute to addressing violence as a public health problem. The health sector has a special interest in preventing violence" (WHO 2003). Croatia declared, as many countries of the region did at that time, its support for the campaign by joining with WHO to develop ways to address this priority. In the years that followed, violence has not disappeared from the streets, homes, or families, but fortunately, also not from the agenda of policymakers and civil society. But comprehensive action against violence has started.

Five years after the presentation of the WHO *World Report on Violence and Health* in Croatia, the mayors and senior political representatives of European cities gathered at the 2008 International Healthy Cities Conference in Zagreb, on October 18, 2008. The message of the Zagreb Declaration for Healthy Cities was about changes that will substantially improve the health and well-being of citizens and significantly reduce the social injustice that costs so many lives and is responsible for so much human misery in Europe and beyond. The idea was to build on this learning and address "new and continuing concerns and challenges of health inequalities, social exclusion, and preventing and addressing specific health threats, especially to vulnerable groups, including children, older people and migrant populations" (WHO-EURO 2008). The declaration pointed out that social and health inequities are not only an affront to human dignity but also a risk to social stability and economic performance, creating injuries and violence, which result in premature deaths, disability, suffering and enormous economic costs.

## ACTION OF CIVIL SOCIETY

When Luka Ritz, a young peaceful student and songwriter, was killed by a group of adolescents, a broad anti-violence movement was spontaneously started by youth, artists, and journalists. After the police turned up no evidence about potential killers, young friends of Luka Ritz started their investigation, creating networks, collecting information, and distributing flyers. Jeronim Maric, front man of the group Adastra, wrote a song, "Rough City," to increase the pressure on the police to find the perpetrators (Adastra 2008). The concert was organized at the main city square where thousands took part. The concert began by delivering letters to Luka Ritz's mother, Suzana Ritz. She read them aloud, with the message that the city needed love, tolerance, and focus on young people. She urged social services to start doing their job, because young people need to be addressed directly. One of Luka's friends, also a member of the band, said he felt sadness and pride because of his late friend. The band member sang, "Souls of the innocent victims in our dark apartment, streets, parks and the graves, they cry: Stop the violence!"—this was the message on the posters made by the students of the graphic arts school Luka Ritz attended ("Croatia moves to rid sport of violence" 2008). Finally, the pressure of civil society made an impact: the police arrested a group of five adolescents suspected of the crime, and they confessed to the killing of Luka Ritz.

## GOVERNMENTS OF CROATIA AND CITY OF ZAGREB PROGRAMS AGAINST VIOLENCE

The most important document regulating peer violence in Croatia is the Program of Activities for the Prevention of Violence Among Children and Adolescents, drawn up by the Ministry of Family, Veterans' Affairs and Intergenerational Solidarity and adopted by the government of the Republic of Croatia in 2005. In addition to this program, the Ministry issued the Rules of Procedure in Cases of Violence Among Children and Adolescents. UNICEF and its program For a Safe and Enabling Environment in Schools also played a significant role; this program is aimed at increasing the level of awareness among children, school staff, and parents about the issue of peer violence.

The city of Zagreb, together with the Andrija Stampar School of Public Health, conducted a Rapid Appraisal to Assess Community Health Needs in the development of the City Health Profile and City Health Plan, applying a bottom-up approach for counties selecting public health priorities (Sogorić and others 2005). This led to a consensus conference that selected the priority areas for their Healthy City Project, established the working groups, and developed the City Action Plan for Health. The method proved that communities have the capacity to recognize and deal with their health problems, including prevention of violence as a very important health problem. Several activities were undertaken to prevent youth violence in Zagreb while addressing the key predictors for youth violence.

First, an important message coming out from surveys was that Croatian schoolchildren need education in sport fan behavior to stamp out the hooliganism and racism that have marred the country's image in recent years. Recently, a football tournament was organized by Zagreb's XVIII High School, where the students were joined in the game by Zagreb's Mayor Milan Bandic (Bandic 2008). The tournament promoted zero tolerance of violence among the youth. Citizens sent in three hundred proposals on how to improve security in the city. A great number of these proposals focused on the work of the police. In a separate attempt to tame violence in stadiums, Croatian Deputy Prime Minister Djurdja Adlesic visited London to talk to British officials about how they tackled similar problems. Another project, dubbed The Fans' Etiquette, came from Zagreb schoolteacher

Bozica Uroic, who wrote a handbook on the rules of civilized behavior at sports events, from leaving home to attending a game and returning safely.

Among other actions to prevent violence, the Brave Phone, in cooperation with the Center for Child Protection in Zagreb, conducted research about children's experience while surfing the Internet. The study indicated that most children (82 percent) were always or sometimes alone while surfing the Internet and only 4 percent of children surfed the Internet under parents' control. Twenty-seven percent of children have been exposed to messages with sexual content. Further, 27 percent of children who answered the questionnaire indicated that they would go to meet a stranger alone without any supervision. Based on these results, the Brave Phone started the project Safer Internet—preventing violence against children through the Internet (Hrabri telefon 2009). The focus of Safer Internet is to inform and advise children about safe and positive ways of surfing the Internet. It also involves parents with dilemmas about how to act in case a child is exposed to violence on the Internet or how to set up the rules for surfing the Internet. The main goal of the project is to provide adequate and practical information for children and parents about safe ways and methods for surfing the Internet and effective ways of protecting children from violence on the Internet, using group work and individual counseling. The results of these activities are awareness of children and their parents about available resources, improved protection of children from abuse, modified children's behavior towards using contemporary mass media (especially the Internet), an increasing number of revealed and registered cases of violence through the Internet, and an increasing number of children who feel protected and safe.

In an effort to prevent family violence and provide protection to victims, the government of the City of Zagreb has set up the Child Protection Centre and the Home for Child and Adult Victims of Family Violence–*Duga*. The primary purpose of the Child Protection Centre is to provide psychological, social, psychiatric, special-education, and pediatric assistance to children exposed to various traumatic experiences, and to their parents, to help them cope better and more successfully with the consequences of bad experiences. In addition to diagnostic and forensic processing, professionals provide individual and group consultancy work and support to children and parents.

The Home for Child and Adult Victims of Family Violence–*Duga* also provides shelter and accommodation to children and adult family members exposed to family violence. Shelter is normally provided for up to six months, and in some exceptional cases, for up to one year. In addition to board and lodging, the shelter provides health care and personal hygiene facilities, psychosocial support, and counseling. The Home collaborates with the competent social services centers regarding creation of preconditions for an independent family life. Children and adult family members who have been exposed to family violence are entitled to shelter. Shelter is obtained on the basis of a referral from the Social Services Centre Zagreb, and the person seeking shelter must be accompanied by a medical worker.

The Zagreb police department prevention programs "I can, if I will," MAH 1 and MAH 2, are conducted as part of the health promotion program "I know, I will, I can," which is implemented in 103 elementary schools, including private and special-education schools. During 2007, more than 15,000 students were included in these programs, with 500 lectures and different visits to police stations. For students who took part in these prevention programs, four Opportunity Fairs were provided at the police academy, which were attended by 11,800 students. "No, no, no to drugs" is a group project of the Zagreb police department, the City Office for Education, Culture and Sports, and the City Office for Health, Labor, Social Protection and Veterans. The program comprises three parts designed to educate the target groups about the harmful effects of narcotics consumption for the body and mind and the sanctions stipulated by law for drug abuse. The first part consists of viewings of the documentary, *Ecstasy Kills*, followed by a lecture on the consequences of consumption of addictive substances from the police perspective. The second part puts the prevention theory into context through situation teaching on the topic "Party," with simulations of parties and places where young people usually get an opportunity to consume and buy narcotics. This part of the program is conducted by classroom teachers and school educators, with the assistance of police community support officers who explain the police procedure in such situations. The third part of the project is the Web portal www.hrskole.com, which is operated by the association, Prometej, and provides an option to contact the local police community-support officer through the Internet, allowing students to complain about violence or addiction-related problems at any time of day or night (City Health Report 2009).

## SIGNS OF PROGRESS

Zagreb City has taken key steps considered necessary for policy development in violence prevention. From the "institutional side," there has been positive progress in the areas of national policy development, surveillance, multisector collaboration, and capacity building. A draft national plan has been developed and needs to be ratified. Croatia scores 87 percent of effective interventions reported as implemented out of a total of 69 planned interventions to prevent a range of injuries, in contrast to the regional median of 56 percent and the third quartile of 80 percent. In terms of whether a range of selected effective interventions were implemented, Croatia reported overall implementation of 85 percent of these for injury prevention and 90 percent for violence prevention (WHO-EURO n.d.).

However, the most important contributions to the results came from university and public health institutions, civil society, NGOs, and media organizations in urban areas, specifically in the city of Zagreb.

Although it is not easy to measure long-term change in culture and behavior even statistically, there have been changes. Criminal offenses committed by children have increased by 0.3 percent, while those committed by juveniles have dropped by 4.9 percent (City Health Report 2009). Juveniles have committed fewer offenses related to drug abuse (a 12.8 percent decline between 2006 and 2008) and fewer serious thefts and car thefts, while criminal acts such as robbery, bodily harm, extortion, and violent behavior increased.

In 2008, a total of 839 offenses were committed against minors. Of the total number of committed offenses, 321 were offenses related to child and minor abuse and neglect, which is 7.2 percent less than 2006. In 2007, a total of 1,515 drug seizures were made, which is 11.7 percent less than 2006. Compared to 2007, 4.0 percent fewer criminal offenses against minors were reported.

Since most of violent behavior is learned behavior, the general strategy for prevention and treatment interventions was to reduce the modeling and reinforcement of violence by including all of the primary institutions that serve youth, families, health agencies, schools, employment, and justice, as well as a broad coalition of civil society ad-hoc initiatives, NGOs, media, and politics in an integrated, coordinated effort. It looks like it is beginning to work.

## SUMMARY

Violence, especially violence among youth, is a major public health problem in cities throughout the world. Zagreb, while not a special or exceptional case, provides a relevant case study because of its context. Over the centuries, Croatia has been at the center of major conflicts, from the invasion of the Tartars through the German and then Soviet occupations. Furthermore, Croatia is a transitional country undergoing the challenges of the post-Soviet era along with the movement for independence from the Yugoslav confederation. This history suggests a culture of violence that in recent times has played out most dramatically in loyalties to and clashes between fans of regional football (soccer) teams. One incident in particular, the death of Luka Ritz, created a platform that galvanized citizens to call for a response to youth violence. The local government and citizens developed a multicomponent approach that included services, outreach, and social media to reshape norms against violence at sporting events and in the community. This approach has been associated with a decrease in violent crimes and may serve as a model for addressing youth violence in other cities.

# REFERENCES

Adastra. 2008. Svačije je pravo živjeti! Prosvjedni koncert za Luku Ritza. http://www.youtube.com/results?search_type=&search_query=adastra+surovi+grade&ag=f.
Assis de Moreira, R. 2009. Football violence: Hadjuk Split, Dinamo Zagreb fans incite riots in stands. Bleacher report. http://bleacherreport.com/articles/128277-football-violence-hadjuk-split-vs-dinamo-zagreb.
Bandic, M. 2008. Zagreb's mayor: We are not city of violence. dalje.com, November 13. http://www.javno.com/en-croatia/zagrebs-mayor—we-are-not-city-of-violence_203589.
Barnhart, E.T. 2009. The criminal youth inmate subculture. corrections.com, May 11. http://www.corrections.com/news/article/21533.
Bilefsky, D. 2009. Arrest in Croatia murder doesn't erase all doubt. *New York Times*, April 25. http://www.nytimes.com/2009/04/26/world/europe/26croatia.html?_r=1&scp=1&sq=Hodak&st=cs.
City Health Report. 2009. Gradska slika zdravlja. Gradski ured za zdravstvo, rad socijalnu. http://www.zagreb.hr/UserDocsImages/zdravlje/gradska%20slika%20zdravlja/Gradska%20slika%20zdravlja.pdf.
City of Zagreb. 2008. The city health development plan: Zagreb, September 2008. http://www.zagreb.hr/Userdocsimages/dokument.nsf/52e5cbe929e7b66fc125696500452b27/aca541f1c 92616d1c1256a0d0049db58/$FILE/City%20Health%20%20Development%20 Plan.pdf.
Croatia moves to rid sport of violence. 2008. Dalje.com, October 10. www.javno.com/en-sports/croatia-moves-to-rid-sport-of-violence_190895.
Dinamo Ja Volim (anthem of soccer club Dinamo Zagreb). 2006, September 27. http://www.youtube.com/watch?v=o4uk00nVgM4&feature=PlayList&p=DDB1F561AFB9FAD5&playnext=1&playnext_from=PL&index=1.
Gray, D. 2007. War memorials. *When Saturday comes*. http://www.wsc.co.uk/content(view/1243/29.
Hrabri telefon. !Dijete na internetu (Child on the Internet!). http://www.hrabritelefon.hr/adminmax/file/dijete%20i%20internet_iddd%20(1).pdf?PHPSESSID=0e94bf25192545d2f47b94316337695c.
Kruzić-Lulić A., D. Delfin, and D. Gajnik. 2008, October. Smoking and alcohol drinking habits in high school students of Zagreb County. *Croatian Journal of Public Health* 4(16):7.
Mandela, N. 2002. Foreword to *World report on violence and health*, ed. E. G. Krug, L. L. Dahlberg, J. A. Mercy, A. B. Zwi, and R. Lozano. Geneva: WHO. http://whqlibdoc.who.int/publications/2002/9241545615_eng.pdf.
Poliklinika za zaštitu djece grada Zagreba (Child Protection Center of Zagreb). n.d. http://www.poliklinika-djeca.hr/index.php?option=com_content&task=category&sectionid=16&id=65&Itemid=133.
Pyle, G. F., S. Oreskovic, J. Begovac, and C. Thompson. 2000. Hepatitis B and HIV/AIDS in Zagreb: A district level analysis. *European Journal of Epidemiology* 16(10).
Republic of Croatia, Central Bureau of Statistics. 2001. Population by ethnicity, by towns/municipalities. Census 2001.

Sakoman, S., Z. Raboteg Šarić, and M. Kuzman. 2002. The incidence of substance abuse among Croatian high school students. *Drustvena Istazivanja* 11(2–3):58–59.

Sogorić, S., T. V. Rukavina, O. Brborović, A. Vlahusic, N. Zganec, and S. Oresković. 2005. Counties selecting public health priorities: A "bottom-up" approach (Croatian experience). *Collegium Antropologicum* 29(1):111–119.

Tomsen, S. 1997. A top night: Social protest, masculinity and the culture of drinking violence. *British Journal of Criminology* 37:90–102.

Trkulja, V., Z. Livcec, M. Cuk, Z. Lackovic. 2003. Use of psychoactive substances among Zagreb University medical students: Follow-up study. *Croatian Medical Journal* 44(1):50–58.

UNICEF. 2009. Stop violence among children. http://www.unicef.hr/show.jsp?page=55225.

WHO Regional Office for Europe (WHO-EURO). 2003, March 21. Zagreb meeting: Building a bridge between WHO research on violence and national public health policies. Press release EURO/02/03, Copenhagen and Zagreb. http://www.euro.who.int/mediacentre/PR/2003/20030314_1.

WHO Regional Office for Europe (WHO-EURO). 2009. Zagreb declaration for healthy cities. Statement from 2008 International Healthy Cities Conference in Zagreb. http://www.euro.who.int/document/E92343.pdf.

WHO Regional Office for Europe (WHO-EURO). n.d. Progress in the prevention of injuries in the WHO European region: Croatia. http://www.euro.who.int/document/VIP/croatia.pdf.

WikiVelv. 2009. Rat subkultura. http://wiki.velv.hr/wiki/index.php/Rat_subkultura.

Zdun, S. 2008. Violence in street culture: Cross-cultural comparison of youth groups and criminal gangs. *New Directions for Youth Development* Fall(119):39–54.

# CHAPTER FIFTEEN

# URBAN HEALTH SERVICES AND HEALTH SYSTEMS REFORM

## JULIO FRENK
## OCTAVIO GÓMEZ-DANTÉS

### LEARNING OBJECTIVES

- Identify the health challenges faced by urban populations in low- and middle-income countries
- Discuss some potential responses to the health challenges confronted by urban populations and health systems in developing nations
- Discuss the benefits of the adoption of national health policies to improve the performance of local urban health systems
- Illustrate the use of the responses to health challenges in urban settings with examples from the recent Mexican health reform
- Discuss the opportunities offered to urban health systems by the global movement to strengthen health systems and recognize health care as a human right

IN this chapter, we discuss the challenges confronted by urban health systems in the developing world and the response to them through the use of three pillars: a new generation of health promotion and disease prevention strategies, the expansion of social protection in health, and the adoption of innovations in the delivery of health services. In the first part, we examine the health challenges faced by urban populations in low- and middle-income countries, many of them associated with what has been called *maldevelopment*. We then discuss some potential responses to these challenges, building on the lessons of the primary health care (PHC) experience and illustrating them with examples from the recent Mexican health care reform, which made extensive use of these three pillars in urban settings. The main message in this regard is that national health policies can offer alternatives to improve the overall performance of urban health systems. We conclude with some reflections on the opportunities offered by a global movement to strengthen health systems and recognize health care as a human right.

## URBAN HEALTH CHALLENGES

Half of the world's 6.6 billion population is living in urban settlements. This figure will increase to 55 percent in 2015 and to more than 60 percent in 2030, when the world urban population will reach 5 billion (United Nations 2004). Virtually all of this growth will take place in developing countries, especially in Asia, where one billion additional city dwellers are expected before 2020 (ISTED 2009). China and India alone will be home to 500 million new urban inhabitants, but Africa, the Middle East, and Latin America will also witness important increases.

A certain level of urban concentration is desirable and even enjoyable. Cities are centers for economic activity and employment. They are the quintessential niche of modern living, where female labor force participation is now the rule, diversity is common, and alternative ways of living are better tolerated and even promoted. Cities are also social and cultural emporiums that house all kinds of manifestations in the arts, science, religion, and entertainment. Up to a point, increased population density reduces the pressures of human beings on local ecosystems, since this usually implies lower per capita costs of providing infrastructure and basic services (Cohen 2006). Urban residents tend to enjoy better access to education, health care, electricity, water, and sanitation than people in rural areas.

However, rapid and overextended urbanization, in the absence of urban planning and regulatory institutions, ends up producing costs that exceed the benefits of living in urban conglomerates: long commutes, traffic accidents, high levels of air and water pollution, violence, stress, and the squalor of slums.

Developing countries are experiencing both fast and extended urbanization. At the beginning of the twentieth century, sixteen cities in the world had one million inhabitants or more, and almost all of them were located in developed nations. Today, there are close to four hundred cities with one million inhabitants or more, and about 70 percent of them are in the developing world (United Nations 2001). In China alone, there are eighty-nine cities with a population of one million or more, including fifteen of the world's fastest growing cities (Normile 2008).

Mega-cities are also becoming particularly common in low- and middle-income countries. According to UN projections, by 2015, sixteen of the twenty-two cities with more than 10 million people will be located in the South (United Nations, 2004).

However, it is also true that a small proportion of urban residents in developing nations live in mega-cities. In fact, 24 percent of them live in small cities ranging from 100,000 to half a million in size, which tend to have a much lower coverage of basic services than larger conglomerates (Montgomery 2009).

One of the characteristics of urban growth in developing countries is the explosive increase of urban poor. In many developing nations, the proportion of urban poor is increasing faster than the overall rate of urban population growth. Around 72 percent of city dwellers in Africa live in slums (United Nations Human Settlements Programme 2003). The figure is 43 percent for Asia and the Pacific and 32 percent for Latin America. Rapid urban growth throughout the developing world has surpassed the capacity of cities to provide adequate services for their inhabitants.

To the lack of basic services, we should add the problems of social exclusion, spatial segregation, and alienation generated by the large immigration of populations fleeing rural poverty, political oppression, or natural disasters. Johann Gottfried von Herder, an eighteenth-century German philosopher, stated that belonging to a community was an essential need; deprived of the sense of belonging, people feel lonely, diminished, nostalgic, and unhappy (Gardels 1991). Two centuries later, Hannah Arendt, another German philosopher, argued that to live fully and securely, every human being needs "specificity," the social and political status that comes with full membership in a community (Kirsch 2009).

As cities in low- and middle-income countries grow, the effects of urbanization on health and its pressures on health services become increasingly complex. This complexity is due not so much to a lack of resources, which is implicit in the term "underdevelopment," as it is to what the French sociologist Alain Touraine (1992) conceived as "maldevelopment," a qualitative notion that refers to a discrepancy between the needs of a specific population and the responses generated to meet them. Many cities in developing nations are victims of maldevelopment through their poor planning procedures, careless adoption of inadequate urban models, and badly implemented policies.

In our view, the essential characteristic of maldevelopment is the juxtaposition of problems. In contrast with the development model of currently advanced societies, where new problems tended to replace old ones, in maldeveloped societies, old and new problems coexist in a complex present fraught with contradictions and inequalities.

The field of health reflects better than any other this qualitatively different pattern of development. Although rich countries experienced a substitution of old for new patterns of disease, the developing world is simultaneously facing a triple burden of ill health: first, the unfinished agenda of infections, malnutrition, and reproductive health problems; second, the emerging challenges represented by noncommunicable diseases, mental disorders, and the growing scourge of injury and violence; and third, the health risks associated with globalization, including the threat of pandemics like AIDS and influenza, the trade in harmful products like tobacco and other drugs, the health consequences of climate change, and the dissemination of harmful lifestyles leading to the obesity pandemic.

This protracted and polarized health transition is compressed in urban environments, especially in those areas where the very poor tend to live. Limited access to drinking water, inadequate sewer facilities, and insufficient waste disposal favor the dissemination of common infections, which sometimes show higher rates than in rural areas.

At the same time, urban lifestyles expose people to risk factors linked to noncommunicable ailments, like diabetes, cancer, cardiovascular diseases, and chronic respiratory ailments. In their concern for equity, some public health professionals have underestimated a well-documented reality: that problems *only* of the poor, like many common infections, malnutrition, and maternal deaths, are no longer the *only* problems of the poor (Frenk 2006). In fact, urban populations in developing regions show the highest rates of noncommunicable diseases and their associated risk factors.

Injuries are also conspicuous in big cities. It is estimated that 1.2 million deaths and 50 million injuries due to traffic accidents occur annually worldwide, most of them in developing nations (WHO 2004). In Mexico, motor vehicle collisions and homicide and violence are two of the five leading causes of death in Mexico's urban areas (Lozano and others 1999). Pedestrian injuries over a three-year period in Mexico City were three times those of Los Angeles (Hijar, Trostle, and Bronfman 2003). Factors associated with pedestrian injuries in Mexico City included poverty, inattention to risky conditions, insufficient public investment in traffic lights, and the dangerous mix of industrial, commercial, and private traffic.

This clash of the old and the new is further compounded by rural-urban migration. In a sense, these migrants accelerate the health transition. Having been exposed to the risk factors of a pre-transitional rural environment, they then move to a post-transitional urban set of exposures. In the course of their lifetimes, they transit from an intrauterine environment often characterized by undernutrition, through childhood affected by the many risks of infection that haunt rural areas, to adulthood in an urban slum under the threat of injurious lifestyles.

The intensity of migration shows no sign of abating. One of the disappointments of urban planners a few decades ago was that urbanization did not imply de-ruralization. Actually, another paradox of maldevelopment is the simultaneous growth both of urban concentration and rural dispersion. In Mexico, between 1960 and 2000—a period of intense urbanization—rural communities with less than 2,500 inhabitants grew from 95,000 to 196,000 (Reyna-Bernal and Hernández-Esquivel 2007). This means that rural areas in developing countries are not simply urbanizing and solving their service delivery problems. Rather, they continue to supply a stream of urban migrants, further straining the insufficient service infrastructure of cities, while simultaneously increasing their level of dispersion, which limits the access to basic services to those that stay.

The rifts in the social fabric, particularly frequent in socially excluded populations, constitute a fertile soil for the development of mental problems, addictions, and violence. In many middle-income countries, two of the main causes of loss of disability-adjusted life years in poor urban dwellings are major depression in women and alcohol consumption in men. To this we should add the deaths produced through murder and suicide, and the injuries generated by all sorts of violence, including domestic violence. The regions showing the highest rates of violent deaths in the world are Latin America and Southeastern and Central Africa (Worldmapper 2009).

Now, the global environmental problems are posing additional pressures on poor urban centers. Dengue fever, which was an epidemic disease at the beginning of the twentieth century, is becoming an endemic urban phenomenon associated with both slum growth and global warming.

## THREE PILLARS OF URBAN HEALTH SYSTEMS

Urban health systems in the developing world have not been able to keep up with the pressures resulting from this complex coexistence of challenges characteristic of urban maldevelopment. Such complexity can only be addressed through a comprehensive response, which should be built on three major pillars: first, the design of a new generation of health promotion and disease prevention strategies; second, the extension of universal social protection; and third, the adoption of innovations in the delivery of health services that make full use of the various technological, managerial, and policy revolutions of our times.

We illustrate the actual use of these three pillars with examples from the recent reform experience of Mexico, which was initially implemented in urban settings. The aim of this reform was to achieve universal social protection in health in a country where half of the population—50 million people, most of them poor—had been uninsured and had therefore been denied access to comprehensive care. Obviously, this ambitious effort included rural communities, but in a country where close to three-quarters of the population now live in cities, the reform also had a distinct urban flavor to it and was initially implemented mostly in the poor areas of urban dwellings. More importantly, the rural and the urban are not separate realities; rather, they interact in a complex dialectic.

To begin with, a universal health system with portable benefits is the only adequate response to the intense internal migration experienced in low- and middle-income countries. One of the major causes of such migration is the search for health care, particularly for high-specialty services. As the epidemiological transition makes chronic disease more prevalent in rural areas and as high-technology options continue to be deployed in cities, we can expect that this type of health-seeking migration will increase. It should be clear, therefore, that urban health systems care not only for city dwellers but also for rural inhabitants, especially in light of an internal brain drain of health workers.

## Mexican Health Reform

In Mexico, the right to health care was recognized by the Mexican Constitution in the early 1980s. However, not all individuals had been equally able to exercise it. The Mexican health system is a segmented system with three broad categories of beneficiaries: (1) workers of the formal sector of the economy, retired people, and their families; (2) self-employed workers of the informal sector of the economy, the unemployed, and their families; and (3) the population with the ability to pay (Gómez-Dantés 2009).

Workers in the formal sector of the economy and their families are the beneficiaries of social security institutions, which in 2003 covered around 45 million people. The uninsured population was mostly covered by the service network of the Ministry of Health. The third category includes the users of private health services, mostly upper- and middle-class individuals. However, the poor and those affiliated with social security institutions also use private services on a regular basis.

The purpose of the recent health reform was to increase public funding for health to meet the challenges posed by the increasing prevalence of noncommunicable diseases and to extend social protection in health to all Mexicans who lacked health insurance.

Mexican reform drew on extensive research and learning around health system performance assessment in Mexico and internationally and was inspired by the tenets of evidence-based policy making. In this sense, one could say that the drivers of the reform were both ideas and ideals, since it was based not only on the best knowledge available, but also on a set of explicit values predicated around the notion that health care is not a commodity or a privilege, but a social right (Frenk and Gómez-Dantés 2009).

The reform was based on a new law establishing a universal System of Social Protection in Health (SSPH) (Frenk 2006; Frenk and others 2006). The law was passed by a large majority of the Congress in 2003 and came into effect in January 1, 2007. The SSPH will gradually expand to protect over 12 million uninsured families over a period of seven years. The vehicle for achieving this aim is a public voluntary insurance scheme called Popular Health Insurance or *Seguro Popular*.

Through the new law, the right to health care, established in the Mexican Constitution in 1983, was given concrete meaning by defining the entitlements to which the affiliates to the Seguro Popular have access to a package of 266 essential preventive and curative interventions for health conditions of high incidence and relatively low cost, including the respective drugs; and a package of 18 high-cost interventions for health conditions with potentially catastrophic consequences for families, including HIV/AIDS, critical neonatal conditions, cancer in children, and cervical and breast cancer, among others (Seguro Popular de Salud 2009).

The new law also allowed for the expansion of the financial base of the health system to meet the expected expansion in the demand for personal health services, increasingly related to chronic conditions. Public funding will grow by a full percentage point of the gross domestic product over the seven years of coverage expansion. Most of the resources come from federal general taxes supplemented by state-level contributions.

But the changes were not only quantitative. The new law also created a fund for community health services and health-related public goods (first pillar) and a separate fund to finance new insurance for the self-employed (second pillar). This separation was explicitly designed to avoid documented problems of underfinancing of public health activities in reforms based on demand-side subsidies. The new financial architecture also allows for innovation in the delivery of health services (third pillar).

Today, 10 million families (over 30 million individuals) have been affiliated with Seguro Popular; 64 percent live in urban dwellings (Poder Ejecutivo

Federal 2009). The goal is to reach universal coverage (12.5 million families) by the end of 2010.

## First Pillar: New Generation of Health Promotion and Disease Prevention Strategies

Urban health systems in developing countries will not be able to cope with the triple burden of disease without a renewed emphasis on public health. Traditional measures directed to control risks and prevent diseases through health promotion, and epidemiological surveillance and control should be strengthened. However, these systems will also need to mobilize all instruments of public policy to design not just health policy but also *healthy* policies: to expand access to water and sanitation, to improve housing, to increase transportation and road safety, to prevent crime, to combat tobacco consumption and drug-addiction, and to increase physical activity.

Some of these actions (media campaigns to combat tobacco consumption, to stimulate the use of seat belts, or to promote exercise) may be directly implemented by urban health systems themselves. However, the design and implementation of healthy policies require coordination with other sectors of society. Although PHC emphasized the need to act on the determinants of health, in reality, it was involved mainly with the direct provision of clinical and public health services. This is a key function, but to generate major improvements in the health conditions of urban populations, urban health systems must now develop other enabling functions, such as stewardship. To articulate intersectoral interventions that affect social determinants of health at the local level, the regulatory and convening capacities of local ministries of health to promote healthy policies need to be invigorated, especially given the extended process of decentralization witnessed by health services in developing countries in the mid-1990s. Examples of intersectoral interventions include the expansion of water and sanitation networks, road safety measures to prevent traffic accidents, legislation to fight domestic violence, norms to promote occupational health and prevent work-related injuries, and tax increases to combat tobacco consumption.

In recent Mexican reform, four specific public health instruments were developed: (1) a protected financial fund for community health services, targeting health promotion and disease prevention interventions; (2) a scheme of health cards with a gender and life-course perspective which supports highly effective preventive measures for each age and sex group, mostly directed at controlling emerging risk factors prevalent in urban contexts (overweight, hypertension, unsafe sex, tobacco consumption, drug abuse, and domestic violence); (3) a new public health agency, Federal Commission for the Protection Against Sanitary

Risks (COFEPRIS), charged with food safety, definition of environmental and occupational standards, regulation of the pharmaceutical industry, and control of hazardous substances like alcohol and tobacco; and (4) public health investments to enhance human security through epidemiological surveillance and improved preparedness to respond to emergencies, natural disasters, and potential pandemics, to which urban concentrations are more prone and vulnerable.

The National Center for the Prevention of Accidents was also strengthened with the intention of controlling one of the main causes of death and disability in urban Mexico—road traffic accidents. Its mandate is to direct all national policies devoted to the prevention of road traffic and other kinds of accidents, and help coordinate the actions in this regard, developed by public and private agencies and organizations.

## Second Pillar: Universal Financial Protection in Health

Parallel to the first pillar, urban health systems need to mobilize additional resources to provide comprehensive services to respond to exposures that have already occurred and have produced health damages. Traditionally, the federal Ministry of Health, as steward of the national health system, approaches the Ministry of Finance and the Congress and tries to convince them of the need for additional resources to meet the health demands of an increasingly urban population now exposed to risks associated with chronic diseases, which are more complex and costly than common infections and ailments related to malnutrition and reproductive events. These resources, however, should be managed rationally to guarantee the provision of effective and efficient services, and to protect the population against catastrophic health expenditures.

Such expenditures are a common risk in cities in developing nations, where private services, mostly financed out-of-pocket, tend to dominate the supply of health care. Even in the Latin American region, where social security is more inclusive, only 20 percent of the population has access to public insurance schemes (Fay 2005). Financing, in fact, is probably the health system function that has changed the most since Alma-Ata and is thus demanding major changes to adapt PHC to the present situation of health care in urban areas of the developing world.

To protect urban populations from "poverty shocks" caused by health events, risks must be aggregated. However, innovations in this regard should be considered, since, as mentioned above, access to traditional social security schemes is limited because an important proportion of the population in cities of developing countries is either self-employed or earns its living in the informal sector of the economy.

Urban health systems also need to change incentives both for providers and for users. They must introduce payment mechanisms that reward high quality care and responsiveness. Families themselves can benefit from incentives tied to health-promoting behaviors. Conditional cash transfer programs have been implemented successfully in many developing countries. They have reduced poverty while improving educational, nutritional, and health status of vulnerable populations.

Finally, urban health systems should make priorities and entitlements explicit through the design of packages of essential health services. These packages are a powerful instrument for planning and quality assurance. Explicit entitlements also empower people to exercise their right to health care and help strengthen the organization of civil society groups around health goals, a key factor in overcoming the obstacles to access health care.

In Mexico, these packages were devised as a priority-setting tool. However, they have also provided the blueprint to estimate the resources required to strengthen the health system through three master plans for long-term investments in infrastructure, medical equipment, and health personnel. The package of essential interventions has also been used as a quality assurance tool. Every facility has to be accredited to participate in this insurance scheme. Accreditation is based precisely on having the required resources to provide the stipulated interventions. This package has also been used as an instrument for empowering people by making them aware of their entitlements. The new Mexican Health Law states that the Seguro Popular affiliates will have access to all health interventions included in both packages and to the respective drugs. At the moment of registration, all affiliates receive a Charter of Rights and Duties that includes a list of the health interventions to which they are entitled.

Initial evaluations of Seguro Popular have shown significant positive effects on the use of health services and on the prevalence of catastrophic expenditures, among other variables (Gakidou and others 2006; King, Gakidou, and Imai 2009).

## Third Pillar: Innovations in the Delivery of Health Care Services

One of the biggest transformations of the twentieth century is the development of differentiated and specialized systems to care for health. Like so many other areas, this one also led to maldevelopment in poor countries, with a number of problems: segmentation of populations, transformation of PHC into "primitive" health care, overspecialization of health care, lack of responsiveness of health care organizations to populations' needs, and concentration of care in health facilities.

The solution to these problems is integration: of populations through universal systems that bridge the divide between poor and nonpoor, formal and informal, rural and urban; of health and healthy policies through intersectoral strategies; of different levels of care through the creation of networks that guarantee the continuity of care of people now living with a health condition; of formal and informal health care spaces through the extension of the supply of health care and health-promoting activities to a diversity of spheres—homes, schools, workplaces, and recreational areas—to move from *health centers* to *healthy spaces*; and of public and private providers through the design and enforcement of common requirements for quality and public financial protection.

The instruments to build these networks, which constitute the core of the third pillar of urban health systems, lie in a number of revolutions of the twenty-first century: biomedical, communications, and managerial. The new model for delivery of health care services in urban areas should be based on networks that make extensive use of diagnostic and monitoring tools better suited to deal with large populations living with chronic ailments. It should also take advantage of the telecommunications revolution, which is opening vast perspectives for improving access to care by underserved populations. It should also make use of the managerial innovations that emphasize teamwork, total quality, efficiency, and patient satisfaction.

In Mexico, the macro-level financial reform was complemented by a micro-level management reform that is strengthening the delivery capacity of urban health systems. Measures adopted to improve the provision of services include long-term planning of new facilities, technology assessment, efficient schemes for drug supply, human resource development, outcome-oriented information systems, facility accreditation, provider certification, quality assurance, and performance benchmarking among states and organizations. It also included the design of a new health care model that emphasizes the creation of networks for the provision of prompt, effective, safe, and continuous services, centered on the patient and respectful of their human rights (Secretaría de Salud 2006). Through this model, public institutions are gradually incorporating information (electronic medical files), communication (telemedicine), and medical (monitoring devices) and managerial innovations (quality assurance programs, managerial agreements) to the daily operation of their health care services.

Some of the initiatives included in the micro-level management reform were implemented as public-private partnerships (PPPs). Some of the regional specialty hospitals built recently were built as partnerships where contractors paid the construction costs and rented the hospital back to the public sector, allowing the government to expand the health infrastructure without mobilizing big sums of resources. PPPs have also been used to increase the supply of new medical technology. In this case, public hospitals allow the establishment of high-specialty medical equipment, such as MRI units and linear accelerators, in the hospital facilities and pay the private providers for the rendered services, thus avoiding the huge investments associated with the acquisition and operation of specialty medical technology. Several state ministries in Mexico have also strengthened drug supply through collaboration with networks of private drug distributors or local drugstores.

## LESSONS FROM MEXICAN HEALTH CARE REFORM

We can conclude this section by drawing the global lessons of the Mexican reform experience for urban health systems in developing nations as was done for a *Lancet* series (Frenk 2006). These lessons can be summarized as the ABCDE of successful reform:

- **Agenda.** To guarantee success, it is necessary to link health to the broader agenda of development and security. Decision makers in urban health systems must learn to address the larger concerns of heads of government, legislators, ministers of finance, and other policy makers who have to balance the claims of several sectors. In this advocacy effort, they can make use of global evidence showing that health, in addition to its intrinsic value, contributes to the overall welfare of cities by increasing educational abilities, developing human capital, protecting savings and assets, relieving poverty, stimulating economic growth, and enhancing security. They can use national priorities to guide local priority-setting among multiple stakeholders.
- **Budget.** Placing health at the center of the urban agenda enhances the negotiating power of federal, state, or city ministers of health, who can then convince finance authorities to allocate more money for health. However, it is also necessary to develop the capacity to deliver more health for the money, since the focus is increasingly on accountability for results.
- **Capacity.** Long-term investments in capacity building in two areas are crucial. The first refers to the delivery of both personal and public health services through investments in physical infrastructure and human resources. The second is related to the development of institutions that can undertake the necessary research and analysis to generate evidence for policy. Current Mexican reform has benefited from sustained efforts to create and nourish centers of

excellence that have produced relevant research and policy analysis, trained researchers who have occupied key policy-making positions and carried out sound evaluations.

- **Deliverables.** To gain public support for reform, health authorities need to communicate its benefits in a clear and attractive way by focusing on diseases and risk factors that generate concern in urban settings. By doing this, the public can relate abstract financial and managerial notions to concrete deliverables.
- **Evaluation.** The Mexican experience also confirms the need for solid evaluations to adjust the implementation of health programs and services and for accountability purposes. Impact evaluations of health initiatives are also crucial, in the transition from one political administration to another, to guarantee the continuity of the reform efforts.

# OPPORTUNITIES TO STRENGTHEN URBAN HEALTH SYSTEMS

The new health context of urban conglomerates in developing countries is offering a great opportunity to discuss health care delivery in the twenty-first century. Major challenges have always been a force for improvement in public health. After all, modern public health was born in the hostile environment of European cities in the nineteenth century, threatened by cholera (Delaporte 1986; Johnson 2006).

As discussed in this chapter, the biomedical, communications, and managerial revolutions are providing novel tools to address these new challenges. But two other opportunities can also contribute to improving the health conditions of urban populations in the developing world: (1) the new worldwide interest in health systems and (2) what Michael Ignatieff (2000) has called the rights revolution, which is turning abstract declarations into concrete entitlements that people can be empowered to demand.

The current interest of major global health actors—G8, multilateral health agencies, multilateral developments banks, bilateral agencies, and major philanthropic organizations—in strengthening health systems as the way to meet the health-related Millennium Development Goals offers a unique opportunity to develop urban health systems better adapted to the changing needs of residents in cities of the developing world. The vision is to offer high-quality services through schemes that emphasize health promotion and disease prevention, favor the continuity of care, and assure universal social protection in health.

In turn, the global movement to advance health care as a human right is empowering users of health care by making them conscious of their entitlements and facilitating the creation of civil society groups around health and health care goals. This struggle transcends local legislations and the idea of citizenship, since social rights are, by definition, rights that everybody posses as a member of the human race (Postel 2007). This issue is particularly relevant, given the level of international migration that cities of the developing world are witnessing. Finally, the human nature of the right to health care also implies that support for this claim can come from anywhere in the world. This opens an enormous field of action for international advocacy and global solidarity.

# SUMMARY

Developing countries are experiencing fast and extended urbanization, surpassing the capacity of cities to provide adequate services for their inhabitants. As cities in low- and middle-income countries grow, the effects of urbanization on health and its pressures on health services become increasingly complex. This complexity is due to maldevelopment, a qualitative notion that refers to a discrepancy between the needs of a specific population and the responses generated to meet them. The essential characteristic of maldevelopment is the juxtaposition of problems, expressed by the fact that these countries are facing a triple burden of ill health: first, the unfinished agenda of infections, malnutrition, and reproductive health problems; second, the emerging challenges represented by noncommunicable diseases; and third, the health risks associated with globalization.

Urban health systems in the developing world have not been able to keep up with the pressures resulting from this complex coexistence of challenges. Such complexity can only be addressed through a comprehensive response, which should be built on three major pillars: first, the design of a new generation of health promotion and disease prevention strategies; second, the extension of universal social protection; and third, the adoption of innovations in the delivery of health services that make full use of the various technological, managerial, and policy revolutions of our times. In the discussion of these pillars, this chapter reviews some of the lessons of the PHC movement relevant to providing health care in cities of developing nations. The actual use of these three pillars is illustrated with examples from the recent health reform experience of Mexico. The aim of this reform was to achieve universal social protection in health in a country where half of the population had been uninsured and had therefore been denied access to comprehensive care. The main message in this regard is that national health policies can offer alternatives to improve the overall performance of local health systems. The chapter concludes with some reflections on the opportunities offered by a global movement to strengthen health systems and recognize health care as a human right.

# REFERENCES

Cohen, B. 2006. Urbanization in developing countries: Current trends, future projections, and key challenges for sustainability. *Technology in Society* 28:63–80.

Delaporte, F. 1986. *Disease and civilization. The cholera in Paris, 1832*. Cambridge, MA: MIT Press.

Fay, M. 2005. *The urban poor in Latin America*. Washington, DC: World Bank.

Frenk, J. 2006. Bridging the divide: Global lessons from evidence-based health policy in Mexico. *Lancet* 368:954–61.

Frenk, J., E. González-Pier, O. Gómez-Dantés, M. A. Lezana, and F. M. Knaul. 2006. Comprehensive reform to improve health system performance in Mexico. *Lancet* 368:1525–1534.

Frenk, J., and O. Gómez-Dantés. 2009. Ideas and ideals: Ethical basis of health reform in Mexico. *Lancet* 373:1406–1408.

Gakidou, E., R. Lozano, E. González-Pier, J. Abbott-Klafter, J. Barofsky, C. Bryson-Cahn, D. Feehan, D. Lee, H. Hernández-llamas, and C.J.L. Murray. 2006. Assessing the effect of the 2001–06 Mexican health reform: An interim report card. *Lancet* 368:1920–1935.

Gardels, N. 1991. Two concepts of nationalism: An interview with Isaiah Berlin. *New York Review of Books* 38(19):1–11.

Gómez-Dantés, O. 2009. Mexico. In *Comparative health systems. Global perspectives*, ed. J. A. Johnson and C. H. Stoskopf, 337–347. Boston: Jones and Bartlett.

Hijar, M., J. Trostle, and M. Bronfman. 2003. Pedestrian injuries in Mexico. A multi-method approach? *Social Science and Medicine* 57(11):2149–2159.

Ignatieff, M. 2000. *The rights revolution*. Toronto: House of Anansi Press.

ISTED. 2009. *Urbanization in developing countries*. http://www.isted.com/pole-ville/urban_cooperation/coop_ch1.pdf.

Lozano, R., C. Murray, and J. Frenk. 1999. El peso de las enfermedades en Mexico. In *Las consecuencias de las transiciones demografica y epidemiological en America Latina*, K. Hill, J. B. Morelos, and R. Wong. Mexico City: El Colegio de Mexico.

Johnson, S. 2006. *The ghost map. The story of London's most terrifying epidemic and how it changed science, cities, and the modern world*. New York: Riverhead.

King, G., E. Gakidou, and K. Imai. 2009. Public policy for the poor? A randomised assessment of the Mexican universal health insurance programme. *Lancet* 373:1447–1454.

Kirsch, A. 2009. Beware of pity. Hannah Arendt and the power of the impersonal. *The New Yorker* January 12:62–68.

Montgomery, M. R. 2009. Urban health in low- and middle-income countries. In *Oxford textbook of public health*, R. Detels, R. Beaglehole, M. A. Lansang, and M. Gulliford, 1376–1394. Oxford: Oxford University Press.

Normile, D. 2008. China's living laboratory in urbanization. *Science* 319:740–743.

Poder Ejecutivo Federal. 2009. Salud. *Tercer informe de gobierno* [Third Government Report, Mexico]. http://www.informe.gob.mx/informe/pdf/3_2.pdf.

Postel, D. 2007. Caminar sobre la cuerda floja. Una conversación con el filósofo iraní Ramón Jahanbegloo. *Letras Libres* 9(101):22–26.

Reyna-Bernal, A., and J. C. Hernández-Esquivel. 2007. Poblamiento, desarrollo rural y medio ambiente. Retos y prioridades de la política de población. In *La situación demográfica de México*, 191–206. Mexico City: CONAPO.

Secretaría de Salud. 2006. *Modelo integrador de atención a la salud*. Mexico City: Secretaría de Salud.

Seguro Popular de Salud. 2009. http://www.seguro-popular.salud.gob.mx.

Touraine, A. 1992. *Critique de la modernité*. Paris: Fayard.

United Nations. 2001. *World urbanization prospects: The 1999 revision*. New York: United Nations.

United Nations. 2004. *World urbanization prospects: The 2003 revision. Data tables and highlights*. New York: United Nations.

United Nations Human Settlements Programme. 2003. *The challenge of slums: Global report on human settlements 2003*. London: Earthscan XXV.

World Health Organization (WHO). 2004. *World report on road traffic injury prevention: Main messages and recommendations*. Geneva: WHO.

Worldmapper. 2009. Violent deaths. Map No. 291. http://www.worldmapper.org.

# CHAPTER SIXTEEN

# INFORMATION FLOW AND INTEGRATED E-HEALTH SYSTEMS

VERONICA OLAZABAL

TICIA GERBER

BEATRIZ DE FARIA LEAO

CLAUDIO GIULLIANO DA COSTA

KARL BROWN

ARIEL PABLOS-MÉNDEZ

## LEARNING OBJECTIVES

- Learn what e-health is and how it can help improve the efficiency, quality, and affordability of health provisions in urban settings
- Understand the difference between a health information system and an integrated health information system

- See the importance of networks and partnerships in moving health information in cities
- See the potential for an integrated health information system in the developing world, using São Paulo, Brazil, as an example
- Appreciate the growing connections between e-health, public health, and policy

THE provision of health to urban populations is complex and challenging. At the crux of these challenges is the lack of data and information needed by decision makers to manage their cities' limited resources and the lack of data needed by health providers to efficiently serve populations in need. Defined as the use of information and communications technology to improve health systems performance, e-health represents a promising frontier. With its focus on addressing the lack of data on the health status of people, e-health has the potential to transform local health systems by enabling improvements in efficiency, equity, and quality in the provision of health services. The purpose of this chapter is to build on the already rich discussions around health informatics by showing how "integrated" e-health systems can be used to inform urban policy and planning, particularly in the developing world. We begin with a review of e-health in the developed world, what has been learned, and how e-health can be used to improve the efficiency of health systems in low-resourced settings. Next, we review the evolution of integrated e-health systems, discussing select urban models. We then move to e-health efforts in the developing world, highlighting the challenges and lessons learned specifically in the metropolitan area of São Paulo, Brazil. We conclude by addressing some of the policy changes needed to fully enable such systems.

---

The authors thank Robert Buckley, Julie Carandang, and Charlanne Burke for their valuable comments on the manuscript.

All authors contributed to the research, writing, and editing of this manuscript. The authors have no conflict of interest to declare. This work did not require funding or ethics committee approval. The views expressed in this paper are solely the authors' and may not reflect those of their institutions.

## E-HEALTH IN THE DEVELOPED WORLD

Standardized health information systems and the ability to share health data across mixed public and private health systems are essential for monitoring the quality and coverage of populations. While many places may be a long way from such a system, the emergence of e-health applications, such as electronic health records (EHR), telehealth, and mobile health efforts, have added a new potential to the provision of health services throughout the developed world. Many of the lessons learned through these efforts can be transferred to the developing world. Perhaps the most critical lesson is not to build stovepiped, siloed information systems—the United States provides a cautionary example.

In the United States, systems were developed in a decentralized fashion without strong incentives for unifying policy and technical frameworks up front. And now the tough, wholesale retrofitting in America has begun. The United States will need to spend billions of dollars to harmonize disparate local, state, and federal health information systems to allow them to share data. A new process to reach consensus on national e-health policies and interoperability, supported by $19 billion of targeted investment proposed by President Barack Obama, was enacted into law on February 17, 2009. President Obama's efforts build on those of former U.S. Secretary of Health and Human Services Mike Leavitt to advance a health system in which all health records can be linked through an interoperable system that protects privacy as it connects patients, providers, and payers—resulting in fewer medical mistakes, simplified administrative process, lower costs, and better health.

Just as America looks within for important e-health policy change, it is also peering out and integrating the lessons of its neighbors engaging in health technology experiments, such as Canada. Canada's Health Infoway was formed in 2001 to foster and accelerate the development and adoption of compatible electronic health information systems to strengthen Canada-wide health infrastructure and improve quality, access, and timeliness of health services. Health Infoway has provided more than one billion dollars to implement EHR, telehealth, and disease surveillance solutions across Canada with the goal of ensuring an interoperable EHR program is in place across 50 percent of Canada by 2010. Health Infoway has highlighted the importance of coordination among federal, provincial, and territorial deputy ministers of health to develop joint three-year technology and investment plans; align national and provincial e-health strategies; and jointly issue or share requests for proposals (RFPs), thereby benefiting from volume pricing while reducing the time and risk of purchasing new information technology systems. Health Infoway is considered to be the most successful e-health experiment to date.

While it is too early to come to a conclusion about the impact of e-health systems on health outcomes (limited evaluations have been conducted), e-health tools, platforms, and applications can help offset health system costs by strengthening the efficiency of health data collection, improving the quality of the data that are collected, and facilitating access to transfer of needed health data from urban centers to remote localities. For example, the individual medical record of a patient can be used by his or her clinician, but it can also feed into aggregate data stores used by clinic managers to assess health system quality or into data stores used by public health workers to track disease and risk patterns in populations as they move. These types of systems can also decrease the significant reporting burden on underresourced settings when donors increasingly demand evidence and data to support the effectiveness of interventions.

# INTEGRATED E-HEALTH SYSTEMS IN THE DEVELOPED WORLD

There are many examples and models of e-health systems in the developed world but very few that actually connect multiple institutions or organizations; there are even fewer that integrate information technology across a wide group of clinical, research, education, policy, and support applications and across a large geographic region, such as an urban metropolitan area. To better understand the significance of this point, we must first take a closer look at the emergence of what could be noted as the first integrated e-health system.

In the early 1980s, academic health centers began to develop various (integrated) platforms to make necessary health information accessible from a single desktop computer. Integrated data, that is, information collected from various sources, between dissimilar technologies was hypothesized to be the key to reengineering workflows and human systems to create a more effective and efficient academic health care environment (Matheson and Cooper 1982). As funding grew, various academic systems began emerging. Each of these efforts varied and ranged from bringing to reality the concept of information at the point of need, accessible from a single workstation, through an integrated, best-of-breed approach, primarily in a clinical arena, to building institutional architectures to support access to information resources across disparate environments using standard vocabularies and unique institutional assets.

These initial efforts laid the foundation for future e-health initiatives, as subsequent outcomes included the development of several medical informatics programs, the development of a sophisticated information infrastructure for patient care, and networking knowledge-based information resources across an academic health center enterprise. More specific to the purpose of this chapter, while typically relegated to a single institution, these efforts were pivotal in shaping initial ideas for an integrated information architecture that crosses multiple organizations.

In 2001, the Indiana University School of Medicine (IUSM)/Regenstrief Institute for Healthcare began building an integrated health information system that spanned a geographical urban area (McGowan and others 2004). With a strong health informatics program, the Regenstrief Institute built a sophisticated information infrastructure for patient care, supported by the Indianapolis Network for Patient Care and Research (INPCR) and a well-developed network of knowledge-based information resources across the academic health center enterprise, fostered by the IUSM libraries. When the Indiana Department of Health leveraged the INPCR to facilitate the transfer of information among city hospitals, what emerged from this partnership was the next generation of an integrated health information system, "one in which institutions with different missions and organizational priorities [could] work together to improve healthcare delivery across a community" (McGowan and others 2004). The next step for this effort is to build on their established system of health information management and move beyond the hospital to the primary care practice site, connecting with the health department to help inform the development of policy and protocol in response to infectious disease outbreaks and other threats.

The success of the Regenstrief Institute is an example of how developing a common standard, or language, is integral in allowing various streams of information to connect. More important, however, is the development of the right partnerships and necessary strategic alliances. In the Indianapolis example, the success of the initiative can be largely credited to the Regenstrief Institute, which developed the right partnerships through its ongoing work and contributions to both the academic and public sectors; the institute was seen as the credible coordinator among all parties. The Indianapolis example also shows the value of a strong pre-established network, which provided the initial forum for bringing all the relevant decision makers together to discuss the issues.

It is interesting to note that, to this point, these efforts were all academically led and so the ultimate beneficiaries were the academic, medical, and scientific institutes that developed the systems. While leading to better access to clinical data for clinical research, these information management systems were not necessarily built to help guide public policy. And although the Indianapolis system is on its way to doing so, many lessons can be learned from taking a closer look at a publicly driven urban initiative, such as the one in New York City.

The New York City Primary Care Information Project (PCIP) is the nation's largest community EHR extension project, with 148 primary care practices and over 1,000 providers—helping nearly one million underserved patients in the city's poorest neighborhoods (New York City Department of Health and Mental

Hygiene n.d.). The PCIP's goal is to maximize the quality of care through the investment of public funds; it is currently operating on $60 million in city, state, federal, and private funding (Mostashari, Tripathi, and Kendall 2009). This particular program shows the potential for integrating the routine practice of primary care and, in so doing, changing the way health care is delivered. The EHR includes standardized clinical data elements, registry functions for patient recall and anticipatory care, automated clinical quality measurement, decision support tools, and patient self-management tools. Like the Indianapolis example, the program also ensures the exchange of secure standardized electronic data exchange between EHR-enabled primary care providers and laboratories, hospitals, insurers, and public health (immunization registry, school health, and disease reporting).

The PCIP also uses an innovative pay-for-quality program that rewards physicians for providing high quality cardiovascular prevention, with additional incentives for hard-to-control populations. This program, based on standard data collected by the EHR system versus traditional claims data, is currently being rolled out in a trial design, where ninety small, primary care practices are random omized either to receive financial incentives for achieving recommended treatment goals or to receive nothing at all. All practices are measured on their performance in four areas: aspirin therapy for patients with cardiovascular conditions; blood pressure control for patients with hypertension; cholesterol control for patients with hyperlipidemia, diabetes, or vascular disease; and smoking cessation intervention for smokers. By early 2011, PCIP hopes to have demonstrated that quality incentives based on EHR data can improve life-saving patient care, helping urban policy makers understand whether incentive payments, other efforts such as panel management services, or a combination of both would provide the greatest health returns given limited resources (Mostashari, Tripathi, and Kendall 2009). The New York City Department of Health and Mental Hygiene is also well known for its syndrome surveillance system with reporting-form practices and electronic records on selected communicable diseases.

# E-HEALTH IN THE DEVELOPING WORLD

While many questions remain around the challenges for e-health in the developing world, there is rising evidence that the information and communication technologies infrastructure necessary for implementing e-health applications is rapidly coming online; both Internet and mobile phone adoption having grown at over 40 percent annually since 2000. In particular, mobile phones, often cited anecdotally as being ubiquitous in the developing world, are now owned by nearly 30 percent of all inhabitants in the developing world.

With this infrastructure in place, donor and nationally funded e-health projects are being seeded at an increasing rate throughout the developing world. A recent inventory of e-health efforts in the developing world show that there are indeed "a thousand flowers blooming." As a result, many of these efforts are fragmented, spend much time reinventing the wheel, and are sometimes too focused on providing data streams to a particular program or for a particular disease without consideration for an interoperable health system.

Therefore, while various types of disease surveillance/public health informatics efforts are already used throughout cities in the developing world to help inform appropriate health policies and plans, because they are not integrated into a larger, more systematic enterprise-wide data collection effort, they are limited and suffer from gaps in information. In India, for example, a GIS information system was developed to help urban malaria control in Tamil Nadu (Srivastava and others 2003). This system ensures that if a localized spurt of the disease occurs, it can be rapidly associated with a likely cause, specific vector, and a probable human source. With this information, appropriate preventive action can be taken to address any rising trend. However, each time an analysis needs to be run, the data collection alone takes time and uses already limited resources.

There are also larger, more systematic efforts, ranging from local to national levels in the Global South. In Karachi, Pakistan, for example, the Aga Khan University developed a series of community-based, urban primary health care (PHC) systems to help plan, manage, and evaluate the health of squatter settlements (Husein and others 1993). And in Kenya's Coast Province, the Community Health Department (CHD) of the Aga Khan Health Services, Kenya—with funding from the Rockefeller Foundation—is working on a provincial health information system that could be linked to the province's eight districts (Aga Khan Health Services, Kenya, 2008). This project is expected to enable the aggregation of data at the provincial level to strengthen the entire provincial health system. Both these projects emphasize the value of early community buy-in, particularly since many of the data collectors are local district managers and community practitioners.

Like the earlier versions of e-health systems in the Global North, most of the urban and national systems throughout the developing world are limited by scope (focused on only one disease), institute (only government-administered versus multi-institutional), ineffectual network and community participation, and no clear incentives to comply. These systems also face local-specific challenges, including lower levels of technical managers than in the Global North; data overload without the capacity to develop a clear plan for analysis; lack of a feedback loop for the type and/or quality of data that is collected by stovepiped and siloed Northern-based e-health systems; and the amount of resources it takes to make these systems communicate. There is an opportunity for cities without large stocks of legacy health information technology infrastructure to leapfrog over many of the same hurdles faced in the North. For instance, building standards-compliant systems from the start is much cheaper than retrofitting later and involves less established-stakeholder opposition.

The World Bank reported in 2003 that Tanzanian officials had to compile over two thousand reports every quarter for various donor agencies. Surely the reduction in time required to compile these reports and movement toward standardized reporting of information would do a great deal toward improving the capacity of health systems and health systems managers. One demonstration of this was seen shortly after the implementation of the Mosoriot Medical Record System (MMRS), an electronic medical record (EMR) system, at a health clinic in Western Kenya. Monthly reports for the Kenyan ministry of health, which took two weeks to prepare prior to the installation of MMRS, are now routinely prepared in an hour because of the ability to quickly and accurately retrieve and aggregate data. The ministry of health now ranks the Mosoriot Center first among all Kenyan health centers in terms of speed, accuracy, and completeness of monthly reports.

Through the delivery at the point of care of comprehensive patient information that adheres to standards of health information exchange, e-health systems can also dramatically improve the quality of care. Due to modern technical advances, Web-accessible applications requiring only an Internet connection or cell-phone-based applications requiring minimal investment in hardware can now be easily distributed among a provider community. Through these and other technologies, providers in developing countries may communicate via phone, e-mail, webcast, or videoconference with providers in training and other research institutions to learn about new methods of treatment or disease that would not otherwise be available. E-learning and telehealth are now two very viable means of remotely training and educating health workers at all levels—nurses, physicians, staff, and so on—that require minimal resources and investment on the part of participating institutions. For example, Le Réseau en Afrique Francophone pour la Télémédecine (RAFT), initiated by medical students at the Bamako University School of Medicine in Mali, facilitates continuing medical education, collaboration, and even patient consultations by linking participating institutions in ten African countries and two European countries. Imagine the possibilities of combining all of these e-health technologies not only to efficiently collect and access information but also to present quality standardized information that could be used to guide urban health policy and planning.

The increase in growth of mobile technology projections indicates that the evolution of integrated e-health systems in the Global South has begun. One already existing example of this transformation is seen in the SIGA Saúde integrated e-health system in São Paulo, Brazil.

# A CASE STUDY OF SIGA SAÚDE, SÃO PAULO CITY'S INTEGRATED PUBLIC HEALTH SYSTEM

The history of health information systems in Brazil is characterized by the same system fragmentation experienced in the Global North, with most application systems developed to sort out specific diseases or support specific national programs, such as AIDS, tuberculosis, hypertension, and diabetes. As a result, some reports have counted more than two hundred health information systems of different complexities without any integration (Costa, Leao, and Moura 2007).

In 1999, things began to change with the launching of the National Health Card Project (NHCP), whose main objective was to create a unique health identifier for each individual and to define a core patient dataset for registering the health care outpatient encounter (Cunha 2002). The NHCP project covered 10 million inhabitants in twenty-two towns. Many lessons were learned through this endeavor, such as the importance of keeping the complexity away from the end user and the possibility of deploying person-centered systems in remote regions even without any computer-literate health workers. In August 2000, the national registry of health care providers was launched. Today, the national database contains records for 170 million uniquely identified people, and the national health care providers' database holds 189,564 facilities including medical offices, lab facilities, imaging services, clinics, and hospitals, with a full description of the services, equipment, specialties, and professionals in each one (CNES n.d.). Besides the national unique identifiers and the Family Health Program (FHP), from 2002 the Brazilian minister of health began devising means to optimize the existing health care resources through patient flow management. Essentially, this meant the intelligent scheduling of specialized consultations and exams and of inpatient admissions, including emergencies. "Intelligent scheduling" means that allocating resources to answer to an individual's needs takes into account all relevant factors, such as travel distances, effectiveness, budget, and costs. Although all treatment under Sistema Único de Saúde (SUS), the Brazilian national public health system, are offered free of charge, several procedures have to be authorized beforehand. Therefore, part of the patient flow management function relates to authorizing procedures and inpatient admissions.

São Paulo is the seventh largest city in the world, with 10.3 million people in the city and some 18 million in the metropolitan area. In June 2003, São Paulo Public Health began to operate as a "full managed-care" city, which means resources from the National Health Fund were transferred directly to the São Paulo City Department of Health (SPCDH) on a capitation basis. Soon after, it became clear that it was impossible to deliver proper health services, including FHP, without an integrated e-health information system.

SIGA Saúde is São Paulo City's integrated e-health information system. It has been in operation since 2004, and today it is present in all 703 health facilities, with 14 million people in its database, and it processes 45,000 scheduling requests a day. The system implements all SUS business rules, from family and community care to surveillance and patient flow management. SIGA Saúde is an evolution of the National Health Card Project.

SIGA Saúde has several strong points. The major one is its ability to support SUS policies in an integrated way. Unique national identifiers are provided at the point of care and there is an emphasis on primary care with support to (or from) FHP and the immunization record (routine, campaign, and blockage). Before SIGA Saúde there were long waiting lines for a specialized consultation, such as orthopedics or ophthalmology. Patient flow management offers optimization of resources via intelligent scheduling of specialized consultations and procedures as well as intelligent bed assignment. Patient flow management gives life to the referral and counter-referral model, based on real-time budget allocation and resource availability. SIGA Saúde also provides real-time epidemiological surveillance of all notifiable diseases.

The SIGA Saúde system was developed with methods that incorporate a software development framework and a strong health informatics standards model for interoperability, leading to a robust, scalable system. The system uses a multi-tiered, Java-based platform-independent architecture. In 2005, it received a Duke's Choice Award at the JavaOne conference as the largest Java enterprise project. SIGA Saúde's documentation is one of the most important contributions to the development of integrated e-health architecture to be used in other countries.

São Paulo City gives away the source code free of charge to any other government that wishes to deploy the system, so SIGA Saúde has been deployed in other cities in Brazil. Campinas, a city with 1.6 million people, some 100 kilometers from São Paulo, has recently begun to deploy SIGA Saúde. Camaçdari, a city in the northeast region of Brazil, in the state of Bahia, with 200,000 inhabitants and forty health care providers, has also been running SIGA Saúde for the past two years. This city provides Internet connectivity using WIMAX technology; therefore, neighboring cities can access SIGA Saúde to schedule consultations for their patients.

Similar to other systems in the Global South, SIGA Saúde faces many challenges, including human resources capacity and training issues. However, because of the use of Web machines at the point of care, efforts to collect data have been simplified, which differs from other Brazilian health systems efforts.

One preliminary evaluation of the use of SIGA Saúde showed that it increased access to specialized consultations, such as orthopedics, and specialized exams, such as mammograms, between 20 percent and 30 percent. The information provided by SIGA Saúde has also been shown to improve the work of health care workers. Recently, for example, a pregnant teenager was rushed to the hospital with eclampsia, a life-threatening pregnancy complication. Because she had missed her scheduled prenatal visits, the Family Health Program team decided to visit her at home and found her in critical condition; they rushed her to the hospital, saving her and her child's life. To better capture the impact of the system, São, Paulo City and Health Metrics Network are now working toward a more formal, independent evaluation of SIGA Saúde.

## LESSONS LEARNED FROM E-HEALTH EFFORTS

Much has been learned from the e-health efforts that already exist in both the developed and developing world. Perhaps that is why interest in e-health as a transformative tool to improve the access, affordability, and quality of health has recently increased among donors, governments, industries, researchers, policy makers, and civil societies. Even global institutions such as the United Nations, the World Health Organization (WHO), and the World Bank and groups such as the G8, Asian-Pacific Economic Cooperation (APEC), New Partnership for Africa's Development (NEPAD), the Commission for Africa, the fifty-three-nation Commonwealth Secretariat, and the European and African Unions are examining the possibilities presented by e-health, and they are coming to appreciate its value and potential to support the UN Millennium Development Goals. A Rockefeller Foundation initiative, Making the eHealth Connection: Global Partnership, Local Solutions, is also prominent among current global efforts. This inclusive, action-oriented effort is working on galvanizing all those who are involved in improving health systems, seeking to draw consensus from diverse experts across the world about the way they can successfully operate and sustain e-health technology in low-resource settings. Discussions with stakeholders across borders and health systems, including clinicians and care providers, hospitals, health care information technology suppliers, and donors, echo the efforts presented in and beyond this chapter.

The following list is a summary of the key barriers to information technology adoption that need to be addressed through powerful leadership, policy, and public-private sector cooperation:

- **Lack of standards and interoperable systems.** Interoperable systems and data standards have often been cited as a key to e-health adoption. While some gains could be achieved through the adoption of EHRs and other tools across the health care system, the real value in terms of quality, safety, and efficiency will only be achieved if such systems are interoperable. Health care providers would have key information, such as that related to laboratory tests and prescriptions, when and where it is needed, at the point of care. This was seen in the Indianapolis, New York City, and São Paulo cases.

- **Dearth of upfront funding and poor alignment of incentives.** Hospitals and other health care providers often cite the limited upfront funding and lack of business models to support ongoing usage as key barriers to adoption. Emerging research also indicates a misalignment between those who pay for the implementation and ongoing usage of information technology and those who benefit from its usage. Under most current health system models, benefits related to the gains in quality, safety, and efficiency are spread across all stakeholders while the real costs are borne by only a few. Incentives must be realigned to facilitate the exchange and sharing of data across and between organizations, institutions, providers, and payers. As seen in New York City, encouraging a robust local government role where appropriate should also be a central priority for funding and incentives.
- **Need for leadership.** To drive transformational change, leadership is needed from both the public sector and every segment of the private sector, including clinicians, hospitals, laboratories, payers, employers and other health care purchasers, manufacturers of pharmaceutical and medical devices, public health agencies, and those who build and implement information technology. In the case of Indianapolis, the leader was the Regenstrief Institute, while for New York City and São Paulo, it was each city's health department.
- **Partnerships and community participation.** Ensuring community participation early in the development of an overall integrative strategy is key to the success of an e-health initiative. Especially given the technical nature of health information systems, it is imperative that an urban e-health strategy contain this element. This was particularly important in the Indianapolis model.

In addition to these overarching e-health policy challenges, urban areas also face three hurdles:

- **Policy integration.** Just as global e-health policy collaboration is accelerating, international cooperation on tackling the challenges of urbanization and associated issues (for example, lack of transportation; shortage of basic necessities, such as shelter, clean water, and sanitation; and the threat of climate change) is also increasing. A key question in moving forward is how e-health leaders can coordinate with these urban initiatives and efforts to seek solutions to challenges in transport, population, education, capacity-building, and macro health care policy making. This also highlights the importance of intersectoral models as a new paradigm for the development of urban policy and planning.

- **Capacity challenges.** Health worker shortages are a particularly serious concern. Thousands of people die or are disabled because they cannot get the help and advice that a trained health worker can offer. There is a shortfall of 4.3 million health care workers worldwide. Capacity needs are often felt more acutely in those areas with the greatest health disparities. Not only are health practitioners in high demand but also needed and in short supply are technical practitioners who are able to analyze and manage large amounts of health data that emerge from a health information system. By providing electronic information and training links to underserved areas and by supplying robust clinical data to make informed clinical and managerial decisions, e-health technologies can help bridge many of these capacity gaps. Local leadership, support, and informatics expertise appropriate to the circumstances "on the ground" are vital for the success of an e-health initiative, so e-health and capacity-building policy must be addressed in tandem.

- **Sustainability and replicability.** The ultimate aims of e-health projects are to be person-centered, user-driven, integrated, collaborative, sustainable, scalable, reusable, and demand-driven. Sustainability and replicability are particular challenges in underresourced environments that have natural and monetary resource challenges, political complexities, and unique needs that may limit the applicability of e-health experiments. More demonstration projects must be undertaken in cities around the world to illuminate both challenges and opportunities of an urban e-health environment and to leverage and share these lessons with the broader global e-health community.

# SUMMARY

The purpose of this chapter is to contribute to the thinking on integrated e-health systems, particularly in urban areas in the developing world. One of the key messages interwoven throughout is that if more is not done now, low-resource environments locally, regionally, and nationally could find themselves in ten years with a mishmash of donor-funded health information applications and monitoring systems that cannot interchange information—leaving the Global South with ineffective health systems. While the future for urban integrated e-health systems is bright, many barriers to their adoption remain, including those related to leadership, financing, standards, and the number and types of organizations involved, with the resulting complexity of partnerships and the challenge of community participation.

A 2009 article in *The New Yorker* by Dr. Atul Gawande speaks to the issue of building on what you already have or know, what scientists typically call "path-dependence." Although Gawande specifically addresses the emergence of various national and subnational universal health coverage models, a similar argument can be made about the emergence of integrated e-health systems. That is, building upon the work already being conducted by the public and private sectors in cities throughout the world can serve as the engine for e-health creativity at the national level and lead the way toward development of a larger, perhaps nationally integrated e-health system.

We can even imagine an already existing integrated e-health system such as the Indianapolis, New York City, or São Paulo model serving as a prototype for such a national system. Already, the creators of the São Paulo model are part of a group of international experts working on developing a national framework based on the São Paulo system, to be implemented in various countries in Africa. With an electronic national health information system in place, the possibility for national health reform and universal health coverage may then be one step closer to becoming a reality for many countries.

# REFERENCES

Aga Khan Health Services, Kenya, Community Health Department (CHD). 2008. *Final narrative report: Strengthening health systems in Coast Province, Kenya*, October 1, 2006–September 30, 2008. New York: Rockefeller Foundation.

Cadastro Nacional de Estabelecimentos de Saúde (CNES). n.d. CNESNet. http://www.datasus.gov.br/cnes.

Costa, C.G.A., B. F. Leao, and L. A. Moura. 2007. São Paulo City health information system—A case report. In *Medinfo 2007: Proceedings of the 12th World Congress on Health (Medical) Informatics*, ed. K. A. Kuhn, J. R. Warren, and T-Y. Leong, 377–381. Amsterdam: IOS Press. Also available online at http://search.informit.com.au/documentSummary;dn=784484762660240;res=IELHSS.

Cunha, R. 2002. Cartão Nacional de Saúde—Os desafios da concepção e implantação de um sistema nacional de captura de informações de atendimento em saúde. *Ciência & Saúde* 7(4): Coletiva 7(4):869–878.

Gawande, A. 2009. Getting there from here: How should Obama reform health care? *The New Yorker*, January 26.

Husein, K., O. Adeyi, J. Bryant, and N. B. Cara. 1993. Developing a primary health care management information system that supports the pursuit of equity, effectiveness and affordability. *Social Science & Medicine* 36 (5):585–596.

Matheson, N. W., and J.A.D. Cooper. 1982. Academic information in the health sciences center: Role for the library in information management. *Journal of Medical Education* 57(10 pt. 2):1–93.

McGowan, J. J., and others. 2004. Indianapolis II: The third generation Integrated Advanced Information Management Systems. *Journal of the Medical Library Association* 92(2).

Mostashari, F., M. Tripathi, and M. Kendall. 2009. A tale of two large community electronic health record extension projects. *Health Affairs* 28(2):345–356.

New York City Department of Health and Mental Hygiene. n.d. Primary Care Information Project. http://www.nyc.gov/html/doh/html/pcip/pcip.shtml.

Srivastava, A., B. N. Nagpal, R. Saxena, A. Eapen, K. J. Ravindran, S. K. Subbarao, C. Rajamanikam, M. Palanisamy, N. L. Kalra, N. C. Appavoo. 2003. GIS based malaria information management system for urban malaria scheme in India. *Computer Methods and Programs in Biomedicine* 71(1):63–75.

World Bank. 2003. *World development report 2004: Making services work for poor people*. Washington, DC: World Bank.

//CHAPTER SEVENTEEN

# GOVERNANCE FOR HEALTH IN LONDON: UTILIZING THE HEALTH IMPACT ASSESSMENT

### SUE ATKINSON

---

### LEARNING OBJECTIVES

- Describe the structure and function of the London Regional Office of the Department of Health in relation to the Greater London Authority and the London mayor
- Discuss the role of the London Regional Public Health Group of the Department of Health, in shaping London's health
- Demonstrate the role of *Health Impact Assessment* as a tool to effect change

PUBLIC health entails both improving the health of the population as a whole, as well as reducing the inequalities in health among different sections of the population. It is a wide-ranging discipline that requires a focus on both individual behavior and social determinants, with interventions guided by evidence of what works to improve health.

Public health is both science and art. The science is the epidemiology, statistics, sociology, and evidence of what works while the art is knowing where, when, and how to apply these and how to use the opportunities and systems that are in place to make a difference. The real skill is in the balance of the art and science and putting them together to improve the population's health.

This balance was achieved in London between 1999 and 2006—via the opportunity presented by the establishment of the Greater London Authority (GLA) in 2000, a new form of citywide government. The Greater London Council (GLC), the previous pan-London government body, had been disestablished some eighteen years previously by the Thatcher government. In 1998, the government decided, as part of "regionalism," to establish the GLA with new and different powers and responsibilities.

This chapter provides a case study of using the new city government arrangements and the power of politics in an effort to create a healthier London. In doing so, it recognizes the wider causes (determinants) of health and how work addressing them can best be accomplished within the complex urban health environment.

# LONDON CONTEXT

London is Europe's largest city, with a diverse population of 7.4 million which will increase to 8.1 million by 2016. Nearly half of all UK foreign nationals and two-thirds of recent immigrants live in London, producing a rich diversity of at least ninety-one nationalities speaking three hundred languages. London is economically rich and moderately healthy, but deprivation and affluence are juxtaposed, with 52 percent of children in Inner London living in poverty. Although the main "killers" are cancer and cardiovascular disease, compared with other parts of England, there are higher levels of tuberculosis, childhood obesity, teenage pregnancy, sexually transmitted diseases, drug and alcohol abuse, and poor mental health.

Within London, there are wide inequalities in living, working, and educational conditions and other socioeconomic factors that have an influence on health. These inequalities exist between people living in different parts of London and between different ethnic groups, age groups, and other groups. The inequalities are demonstrated in many of the usual parameters, such as infant mortality and life expectancy across London, with an eight-year gap in life expectancy between the best- and worst-off, in different geographical areas (Barer and others 2002; Findlay and others 2007). People who are less well-off have substantially shorter life expectancies and more illness than the rich. Health is very sensitive to the social circumstances in which people live—the social determinants of health (Wilkinson and Marmot 2003). While those at the bottom of the social ladder run approximately twice the risk of serious illness and early death as those at the top, there is also a clear social gradient. Disadvantage—few assets, poor education, insecure employment, poor housing—all tend to concentrate in particular groups of people and have a cumulative effect.

## SOCIAL DETERMINANTS OF HEALTH

Since the 1970s, there has been increasing knowledge and evidence of the relationship among health, wealth, inequalities, and socioeconomic status. Peter Townsend on poverty (1979), the Black report (Black and others, 1980), the government-commissioned "The Health Divide" (Whitehead 1992), and Acheson (1998) all looked at various aspects of inequalities and demonstrated the relationships between health and socioeconomic status. A treasury-commissioned report by Derek Wanless (2004) identified a need for a much greater focus on prevention and public health issues, encouraging the population in a "fully engaged" scenario, if the National Health Service (NHS) is to be financially viable over the next twenty years. A focus either only on individuals and their lifestyle or only on social determinants will not achieve the "upstream" preventive action shown by Wanless to be needed.

The interrelationship between individual behavior and the various factors that impact on health and well-being is captured in Whitehead and Dahlgren's social model of public health (1991; Figure 17.1).

The concentric semicircles represent the various layers of influence on the individual at the center. The center is the individual whose health is related to individual factors, such as age, sex, ethnicity, and genetics. The inner layer identifies individual lifestyle factors, such as smoking, healthy food, and physical activity. The sequential outer layers include public services and living and working conditions. The outermost layer is the socioeconomic, cultural, and environmental conditions. All layers have influence on the others and determine whether any individual is likely to adopt a healthier lifestyle. Individuals are not in a position to adopt healthier lifestyles unless the outer layers enable relevant choices.

## FIGURE 17.1 Social Model of Public Health

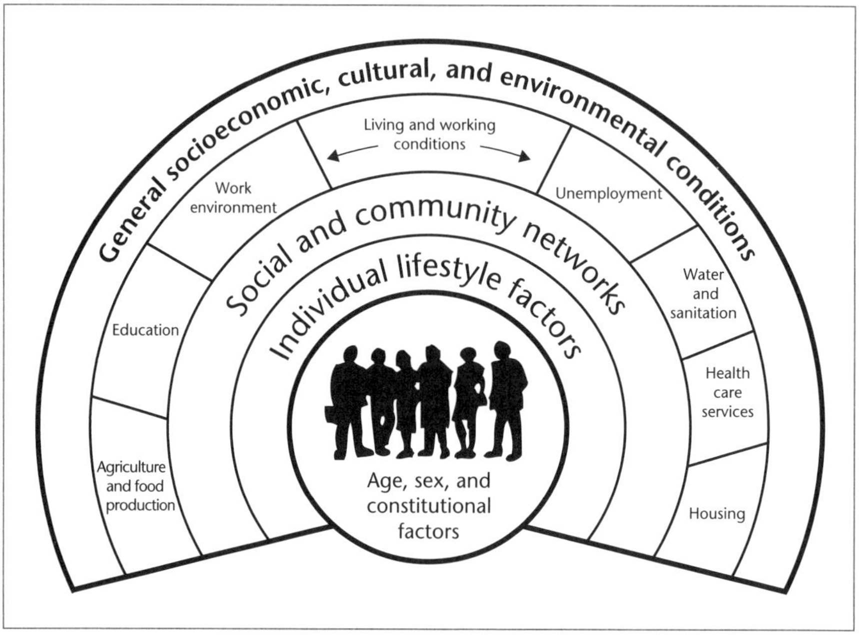

*Source:* G. Dahlgren and M. Whitehead, 1991, *Policies and strategies to promote social equity in health*, Stockholm: Institute of Futures Studies.

Evidence exists and policy implications can be drawn for each individual social determinant: housing, planning, green spaces, transport links, civic amenities, integrated employment, and so on. It is clear what the best outcomes would be, but it may not be known how to bring them about because it may not be apparent how they may interact with each other and what the overall implications may be (Wilkinson and Marmot 2003). The question of how to combine evidence in various research studies from a variety of disciplines to answer the practical questions of how to deliver improved public health also requires development of innovative approaches to both defining the research questions and the methodologies to investigate them. Nevertheless, considerable attempts are being made in the United Kingdom to harness and collate available public health evidence, such as in the National Library for Public Health and in NICE (National Institute for Health and Clinical Excellence) through its public health program.

> **Outcomes of Healthy Urban Development**
>
> - Housing: affordable and health-improving
> - Configuration: social integration and inclusion
> - Transport: integrated, accessible, public, and healthy
> - Social and community infrastructure: schools/libraries/leisure/sports and integrated with health delivery
> - Healthy food: growing, markets, shops, access
> - Lighting: safety and reducing crime
> - Green spaces; access, leisure, exercise
> - Health provision: whole spectrum, modern, integrated with other infrastructure
> - Local employment and skills: in development and longer term, in public and private sector

With these social determinants of health (SDH) in mind and with the formation of the Greater London Authority in 2000, there was an opportunity to address the determinants of health of the population of London via the mayor's strategies.

## A HEALTH STRATEGY FOR LONDON

The Greater London Authority (GLA) was established in 2000 to provide a new form of citywide government. The Greater London Authority Act of 1999 established a directly elected mayor for London and an Assembly of twenty-five members with a scrutiny role. Included in the GLA "family" are four functional bodies—the London Development Agency (LDA), Transport for London, Metropolitan Police Authority, and the London Fire and Emergency Planning Authority, with a specific scope of work as their names imply. The issue of health was raised in drafting the GLA Act of 1999, and Section 30 of the act states that the GLA must exercise its power in a manner calculated "to promote improvements in the health of persons in Greater London." The mayor's responsibilities include developing and implementing eight high-level strategies for Greater London on a range of issues: spatial development (the London Plan), transport, economic development, waste, air quality, ambient noise, biodiversity, and culture. It was also the statutory responsibility of the GLA to "take the health of Londoners into account" and to "promote their health." This resulted in the establishment of the London Health Commission (LHC) as the vehicle that conducted health impact assessments on all of the original mayoral statutory, and some of the non-statutory, strategies.

Established by the mayor in 2000, the LHC is an independent commission whose overall aim is to reduce health inequalities in the capital and to improve the health and well-being of all Londoners by raising awareness of health (not health services) and health inequalities and promoting coordinated action to improve the determinants of health across London, as discussed above. The LHC achieves its goals through influencing key policy makers and practitioners, supporting local action, and driving on specific, priority issues through joint programs. The LHC has a number of forums including SmokeFree London (http://www.smokefreelondon.com) and Urban Development (http://www.londonshealth.gov.uk/urban/tm).

The model of this cross-city partnership has been identified as useful by other cities. Recently, Glasgow set up a "task and finish" Glasgow Health Commission to engage partners and identify the key issues for health in Glasgow (Glasgow Health Commission 2009).

In the eighteen months before the June 2000 mayoral elections, the Department of Health (DH) created, for the first time, a single health body for London, the London Regional Office (LRO) of the DH. Prior to this, regional health authorities and offices had each covered part of London and part of the surrounding counties, for example, the South East Regional Health Authority included the southeast segment of London and Kent. The London Regional Office of the DH enabled a clear focus on London's health and the national health service within London, undiluted by the complexities of differing issues in the counties surrounding London. The Regional Public Health Group, within the LRO, focused on the public health issues in London.

The author was appointed Regional Director of Public Health (RDPH) for London in 1999 and took the opportunity of this new London-only focus to lead a multiagency project to develop the first London Health Strategy. This involved a large steering group (some 30+ people) from a wide range of partner organizations, including health, local government, crime, housing, education, employment and skills, academia, voluntary, and nonprofit sectors. The approach to developing the strategy was managed as a piece of action research with constant feedback from facilitators and participants to shape and modify. Feedback revealed that partner organizations welcomed the approach and considered that it was the first time they really understood the wider health concepts and that they felt involved. The aim was engagement of both of these partner organizations and the wider community. In addition to a number of management techniques, such as a Delphi process on priorities, a major conference formed part of the process, which provided the forum to identify priorities within the strategy. The Coalition for Health was formed.

Four priority areas were identified: inequalities, black and minority ethnic health, regeneration, and transport. Information and evidence and Health Impact Assessment (HIA), a structured method for assessing and improving the health consequences of projects and policies in the nonhealth sector (Lock 2000), were advocated as the foundation for action-underpinning themes. The London Health Strategy (2000) was published and widely distributed. By this time, the mayoral candidates were already identified. Each expressed an interest in the health issues in London and, when the Health Strategy was shared with them, each pledged to pursue it. Several mayoral candidates also included "chief medical officer" for London or "health advisor" as part of their manifesto commitments.

Once Ken Livingston was elected mayor and took office (June 2000), links between the (then) London Regional Office of the DH (which was responsible for the NHS across London) and the Greater London Authority (GLA) started to develop. The Coalition for Health and Regeneration and its Health Strategy were accepted by the mayor, who established the London Health Commission as a successor organization, and the RDPH was appointed as health advisor to the mayor and the Greater London Authority.

## USING HEALTH IMPACT ASSESSMENT AS AN EFFECTIVE TOOL

The mayor agreed that health impact assessment (HIA) provided a tool to "take the health of Londoners into account" in the strategies and that HIA should be undertaken as part of all strategy and policy making to improve the health of Londoners. It was decided to use HIA as a tool at the draft stage of each strategy, when it was with the Assembly and functional bodies for consultation, prior to the draft for public consultation. Although discussed across the United Kingdom, HIA was not widely used at that time, and a rapid method that could be used within a limited timeframe had to be developed. It was also important to explain and demystify HIA for a wider audience, so a brief guide was developed and published jointly by the mayor, the London Assembly, and the RDPH (Cameron and Ison 2000).

The mayoral strategies were developed by teams working within either the Greater London Authority or the appropriate GLA functional body. These teams are specialists in their strategy area, but they do not always understand how their work impacts on health. For example, the London Development Agency was responsible for the writing of the Economic Development Strategy.

During strategy development, they had public health advice from the health team based in the GLA, with the overall guidance of the RDPH (as health advisor) and through her, a wider network of public health expertise, both academic and service-based.

One of the fundamental early stages of the HIAs was a rapid review of the evidence on the topic of strategy and health implications. These were commissioned to inform the HIA but also proved beneficial to strategy writers. While some of the early drafts of strategies encompassed some elements of health, health was not a priority, but by conducting health impact assessments, the GLA ensured that the strategies reflected any relevant health concerns and raised awareness about "health" and its "determinants" within the Greater London Authority and more widely across London organizations. In the later HIAs, it was noticeable that health effects had often already been taken into account in the strategies, at least to some extent, prior to the HIA being undertaken.

Of the first two strategies to be developed, the initial draft Economic Strategy (Mayor of London 2001a) did not overtly reflect health concerns. Some of the recommendations included in the published Economic Strategy after the HIA was conducted were

- Promotion of Londoners' health as a main objective
- Acknowledgment of the links between economic development and health
- Adoption of a broad definition of health in the strategy
- Promotion of social inclusion and renewal among all London's communities included as a revised objective
- Commitment to particular health-enabling projects, such as the London Development Agency, to undertake further work to fund breakfast clubs in schools to promote healthy eating

Likewise, the first-draft Transport Strategy's main health emphasis was on air pollution (Mayor of London 2001b). There was brief mention of modes of transport, such as walking and cycling, but the HIA ensured that these featured more prominently in later drafts (LHC 2001; Mindell and others 2004). The transport strategy after the HIA also included safety and security of public transport and cycling and walking priorities. Key messages from all of the health impact assessments on the strategies were summarized and published (Mountford 2003).

Ensuring that potential health impacts were considered in the development of the mayor's statutory strategies has been a real opportunity to embed health into the work of the Greater London Authority (GLA) and its functional bodies. Along with public health input during strategy development, the HIA process has been an opportunity to create more understanding about the wider determinants of health; how the work of local and regional government impacts on health and health inequalities; and how to incorporate health into all strategies.

## HIA AND EVIDENCE-BASED POLICY CHANGE

London's strategies and the approach is cost-effective. They increased stakeholder awareness of the impact of wider policies on health and encouraged GLA staff to consult public health staff while drafting policies (Opinion Leader Research 2003). This prompted earlier consideration of health in strategy development and contributed to the further development of HIA methods, tools, and the evidence base. The success of the London Health Commission was attributed to political commitment from the mayor, with health as a cross-cutting theme in the GLA Act, and to the Regional Director of Public Health for London being given a joint role as health advisor to the mayor.

Other considerations are related to the nature of public health interventions: evidence from the relevant research may not be able to be implemented at a local level by individual practitioners but require policy changes or strategies in nonhealth sectors and with nonhealth professionals. Obstacles to evidence-based public health policy relate also to the relatively short timeframes that preoccupy politicians. The development and implementation of an effective public health intervention is likely to take longer than one electoral cycle. Beyond the need for quick results, there is also the power of other interests; for example, Nuthall (2006) estimated that the liquor industry had been able to water down the recent EU alcohol plan. Some examples of issues tackled by the Commission are described below.

### Built Environment

The London Plan (GLA 2009) focused on accommodating London's increasing population while promoting a sustainable city and ensuring economic and social inclusion. The Healthy Urban Development Unit (HUDU) was established because of the lack of capacity and knowledge within the health sector on how urban planning works and on how to negotiate with property developers to ensure health is included in the plans (www.healthyurbandevelopment.nhs.uk). Staffed by urban planners, it supported the health service in London in trying to shape local developments to become health promoting and to ensure health services were available to the new communities.

### Healthy Foods

Another issue is tackling obesity. The rates of obesity in London are increasing dramatically, with more than 50 percent of the adult population being classed as overweight or obese, as well an increasing proportion of children. The question is what has influenced this increase and, therefore, what must be done to reverse the trend. It is apparent that to improve the public's health, individuals need to be influenced to change their actions, and wider strategies need to be developed to change the social determinants of people's health. Healthy food is important to the individual, but just disseminating information and imploring people to eat healthily is unlikely to have much impact. London's Food (LDA 2006), the plan, was based on evidence and covered all aspects of food from farm to fork.

### Smoking

Smoking remains an important public health issue. In London, 5,000 cancer deaths annually are related to smoking. It is an important contributor to inequalities, and the risk of making inequalities greater remains, which was seen in smoking policies over the past twenty years. Health promotion messages in the 1970s and 1980s on "stop smoking" were correctly based on the available evidence about the effects of tobacco on health. However, the approach was only one of campaigns and health promotion material to encourage individuals to stop smoking. None of the wider social determinants that influence whether people were able to make the choice to stop smoking were addressed. The outcome was a widening of the inequalities in health as a result of smoking because those in higher socioeconomic groups were able to act on this information, while those in lower socioeconomic groups did not. Smoking in managerial and professional groups now stands at 16 percent compared to 34 percent in routine and manual occupations (ASH 2007).

By contrast, the current smoking policy includes a wider policy to ban smoking in public places within London, and the SmokeFree London forum of the LHC was instrumental in achieving the smoking ban in public places in England. And this smoke-free approach was adopted by other regions, influencing politicians locally and nationally.

## HEALTH INEQUALITIES

Given the wide and widening inequalities in London, addressing inequalities remains a key objective. Three broad policy approaches have been identified to lessen health inequalities: (1) improving the health of disadvantaged groups,

(2) closing the gap between those in the poorest social circumstances and better-off groups, and (3) addressing the entire health gradient, that is, the association between socioeconomic position and health across the whole population. It has been demonstrated by modelling in London that adoption of either of the first two approaches alone at a local level will not achieve the desired targets for reducing inequalities; instead, a comprehensive cross-sector, London-wide approach would be needed. Unfortunately this is counterintuitive to those who are running the thirty-one specific Primary Care Trusts and local authorities who only have a responsibility for their population (Fitzpatrick, Hofman, and Jacobson 2004).

## NEXT STEPS

These various examples illustrate a range of important public health issues and their impact on individuals' lives. They demonstrate how these public health issues were approached and handled in London between 1999 and 2006. They demonstrate that policies and strategies must encourage, enable, and ensure an environment and other factors that are right for individuals to improve their health, and that these are the responsibility of those who have control of policies.

In 2006, when the GLA had been in existence for six years, there was a cross-government review of the powers of the mayor and GLA. The health aspects of the GLA powers formed part of this review. As a result of this and how health issues were already being tackled by the GLA in terms of HIA and wider determinants, the case was made to increase the mayoral health powers to include addressing inequalities in health. The London mayor's health powers were enhanced by the GLA Act of 2007 and now include developing a strategy on health inequalities, in partnership with the Regional Director of Public Health, the NHS, and other relevant partners, and the formalization of the RDPH as health advisor to the mayor and GLA. The London Health Inequalities Strategy has recently been published (GLA 2009).

## SUMMARY

Public health requires a focus on both individual behavior and social determinants, as shown in Dahlgren and Whitehead's social model of public health. In 1998 the Department of Health created a single health body for London, the London Regional Office (LRO), and in 1999 the new Regional Director of Public Health (RDPH) for London led a multiagency project to develop the first London Health Strategy (LHS). The establishment of the Greater London Authority (GLA) in 2000, having a health focus in its statute provided new opportunities to use the power of politics to create a healthier London. The new mayor created the London Health Commission (LHC), which replaced the Coalition for Health and Regeneration, in order to reduce health inequalities and improve the determinants of health across London. His eight strategies for Greater London—on issues from economic development to transport to biodiversity—included the health consequences of the proposed projects and policies identified by health impact assessments.

Tools like the HIA can be powerful in raising awareness of health and health inequalities and in demonstrating the paramount importance of social determinants of health. Central to such efforts is the ability to create partnerships across organizations, within and outside government, both vertically and horizontally. Sharing the process and results of HIA can influence public opinion, which can be a powerful influence for change, not least in terms of influencing politicians. Looking for synergy between improving health and other high-priority actions such as transport, climate change, and reducing inequalities may provide a catalyst for health improvement.

## REFERENCES

Acheson, D. 1998. *Independent inquiry into inequalities in health*. London: HMSO.
ASH. 2007. *Smoking statistics: Who smokes and how much*. London: Action on Smoking and Health.
Barer, R., J. Fitzpatrick, and C. Traoré. 2004. *Health in London report*. London: GLA, London Health Commission and London Health Observatory. http://www.london.gov.uk/lhc/docs/publications/healthinlondon/2004/hilfullreport2004.pdf.
Barer, R., G. Marshall, J. Fitzpatrick, L. Cragg, and B. Jacobson. 2002. *Health in London report*. London: GLA, London Health Commission, and London Health Observatory. http://www.london.gov.uk/lhc/docs/publications/healthinlondon/2002/hinl2002.pdf.
Black, D., J. Morris, C. Smith, and P. Townsend. 1980. *Inequalities in health: Report of a working party*. London: Department of Health and Social Security.
Cameron, M., and E. Ison. 2000. A short guide to Health Impact Assessment: Informing healthy decisions. http://www.london.gov.uk/lhc/docs/publications/hia/strategy/hiaguide.pdf.
Dahlgren, G., and M. Whitehead. 1991. *Policies and strategies to promote social equity in health*. Stockholm: Institute for Futures Studies.
Findlay, G., H. Davies, G. Wilson, and M. Brannan. 2007. *Health in London report*. London: GLA, London Health Commission and London Health Observatory. http://www.london.gov.uk/lhc/docs/publications/healthinlondon/2006/hinl06.pdf.
Fitzpatrick, J., D. Hofman, and B. Jacobson. 2004. *The London health forecast: Can London's health divide be reduced*. London: London Health Observatory.
Foresight Report. 2007. *Tackling Obesities: Future Choices, 2007*. http://www.foresight.gov.uk/OurWork/ActiveProjects/Obesity/Obesity.asp.
Glasgow Health Commission. 2009. Glasgow City Council. http://www.glasgow.gov.uk/en/Residents/HealthCommission.

Graham, H. 2000. The challenge of health inequalities. In *Understanding health inequalities*, ed. H. Graham. Buckingham: Open University Press.
Graham H., ed. 2001. *Understanding health inequalities*. Buckingham: Open University Press.
Greater London Authority (GLA). 2009. Health inequalities strategy. http://www.london.gov.uk/who-runs-london/mayor/publications/health/health-inequalities-strategy.
Lock, K. 2000. Health impact assessment. *BMJ* 320:1395–1398.
London Development Agency. 2006. Healthy and sustainable food for London: The Mayor's Food Strategy. http://www.gos.gov.uk/497417/docs/240251/MayorFoodStrategyMay2006.pdf.
London Health Commission (LHC). 2001. *A report of a health impact assessment of the mayor's draft transport strategy*. London: LHC.
London Health Strategy (LHS). 2000. London's health: Developing a vision together. http://www.londonshealth.gov.uk/strategy.htm.
Marmot, M. G., and S. A. Stansfeld. 2002. *Stress and heart disease*. London: BMJ Books.
Mayor of London. 2001a. Economic development strategy. London: GLA. http://www.london.gov.uk/approot/mayor/strategies/economic_development/success_thru_diversity.jsp.
Mayor of London. 2001b. Transport strategy. London: GLA. http://www.london.gov.uk/approot/mayor/strategies/transport/index.jsp.
Mayor of London. 2004. The London plan. Spatial development strategy. London: GLA. http://www.london.gov.uk/thelondonplan/thelondonplan.jsp.
Mindell, J., J. Fitzpatrick, and F. Seljmani. 2006. *Health inequalities in London: Life expectancy and mortality*. London: London Health Observatory.
Mindell, J., L. Sheridan, M. Joffe, H. Samson-Barry, and S. Atkinson. 2004. Health impact assessment as an agent of policy change: Improving the health impacts of the Mayor of London's draft transport strategy. *Journal of Epidemiology and Community Health* 58:169–174.
Mountford, L. 2003. *Key messages from health impact assessments on the Mayor of London's Draft Strategies*. London: London Health Commission.
Nuthall, K. 2006. Europe waters down alcohol plan. *Environmental Health News*, November: 4.
Opinion Leader Research. 2003. Report on the qualitative evaluation of four Health Impact Assessments on draft Mayoral Strategies for London. London Health Commission. http://www.london.gov.uk/lhc/docs/publications/briefingpapers/hiaeval.pdf.
Ranzetta, L., J. Fitzpatrick, and F. Seljmani. 2003. *Megapoles: Young people and alcohol*. London: GLA.
Tarvol, A, R. 1996. Social determinants of health: The sociobiological translation. In *Health and social organisation: Towards a health policy for the twenty-first century*, ed. D. Blane, E. Brunner, and R. Wilkinson. New York: Routledge.
Townsend, P. 1979. *Poverty in the United Kingdom: A survey of household resources and standards of living*. London: Penguin Books and Allen Lane.
Wanless, D. 2004. *Securing good health for the whole population: Final report*. London: HM Treasury.
Whitehead, M. 1992. The health divide. In *Inequalities in health: The Black Report and health divide*, 2nd ed., ed. P. Townsend, M. Whitehead, and N. Davidson. London: Penguin.
Wilkinson, R., and M. G. Marmot, eds. 2003. *The solid facts*. Copenhagen: World Health Authority.

# CHAPTER EIGHTEEN

# PROVISION OF WATER AND SANITATION SERVICES

### JONATHAN PARKINSON
### MARTIN MULENGA
### GORDON MCGRANAHAN

## LEARNING OBJECTIVES

- Describe how improved water supply and sanitation, combined with improved hygiene behavior, can have synergistic benefits (both direct and indirect) on the livelihoods of communities

- Discuss how the level of service (that is, household, shared, or communal) influences health benefits, particularly as a result of responsibilities for management and maintenance of facilities

- Explain why the socioeconomic dimension of water and sanitation interventions is just as important as knowledge of technical aspects

- Discuss the rationale for engaging public health engineers with health specialists, with more attention on the epidemiological aspects of water and sanitation facilities

- Discuss why water and sanitation facilities may become a health risk if poorly managed or improperly used

- Identify factors that are important determinants of hygienic behavioral change

THE health sector is dominated by medical responses to illness and disease. Interventions are often determined by diseases that are apparent because of their severity. However, a massive urban population suffers from endemic diseases related to poor water supply and inadequate sanitation. The high incidence of diarrhea and other excreta-related diseases is widespread and has become the norm in many communities. Even though there are known to be significant socioeconomic impacts related to loss of work, care of the sick, decrease of learning ability, and so on, improved water and sanitation purely for health reasons is often not considered to be a priority by urban communities. Bearing this is mind, this chapter focuses on the challenges facing the water and sanitation sector in terms of promoting investments to achieve health benefits and promoting a better understanding of the complexities of disease transmission.

## WATER AND SANITATION SERVICES IN LOW-INCOME URBAN SETTLEMENTS

Although governments have made efforts to provide a basic level of service for their constituents, the quality of water and sanitation infrastructure in low-income communities is deplorable throughout much of the developing world. Many communities pay disproportionate amounts compared to their more affluent counterparts for services that are wholly inadequate.

For water supply, the majority of low-income urban communities depend on standpipes or public taps (see Figure 18.1), which are poorly managed and maintained and are prone to service interruptions due to power failures. In many cities, the demand for water totally outstrips the supply, and there is often not enough water to go around.

Water and sanitation facilities can be solely for access and use by private families, but often facilities are shared. In other situations where there are no household latrines, communities use communal facilities. Coverage is consistently lower for sanitation than for water, with contrasts being notably apparent in Africa and South Asia (WHO/UNICEF 2008). McGranahan and Owen (2006) point out that this is a reflection of the simplicity of water distribution and water being generally a more economically saleable and politically negotiable commodity than sanitation.

---

The authors would like to thank Beth Scott from the London School of Hygiene and Tropical Medicine for her comments and advice during the preparation of this chapter.

FIGURE 18.1  Local Residents Waiting for Water from a Tap Stand in an Urban Slum in Freetown, Sierra Leone

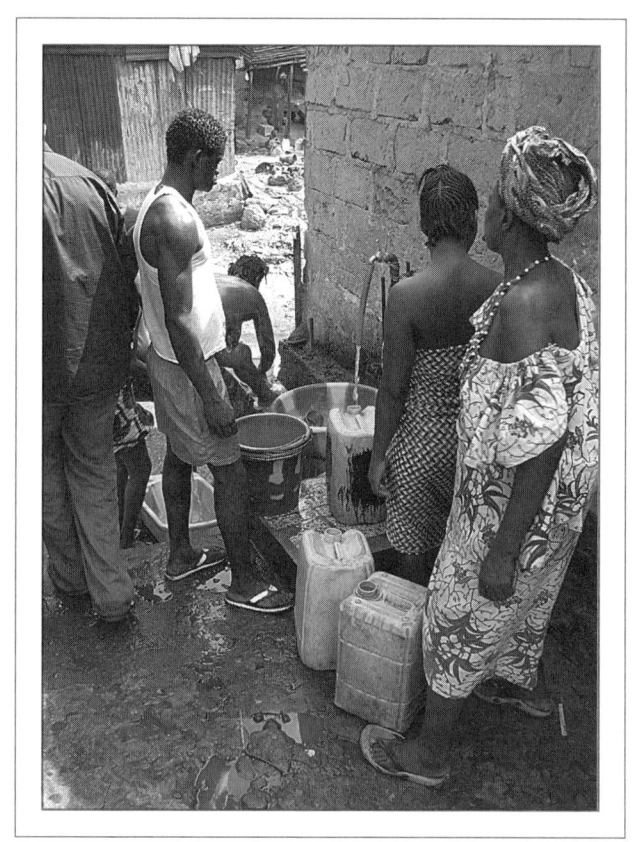

Photo by Jonathan Parkinson.

The vast majority of urban dwellers lack sewer connections and utilize some form of on-site sanitation. Access to individual private household latrines of decent construction is a luxury. Many are shared and overused and rapidly fall into a state of disrepair, and poor hygienic conditions prevail. Inadequate desludging and arrangements for septage disposal mean that many on-site sanitation facilities become unhygienic and become loci for disease transmission.

Communal and public latrines are notoriously bad, and poor maintenance makes them major health concerns (see Figure 18.2). Some communities that lack any form of latrine resort to open defecation, which has significant health risks. Open defecation results in high incidences of diarrheal diseases, often with intermittent outbreaks of cholera. Although cholera epidemics resulting in deaths

FIGURE 18.2 Latrines in an Urban Slum in Freetown, Sierra Leone, Discharging Directly into the Local River System

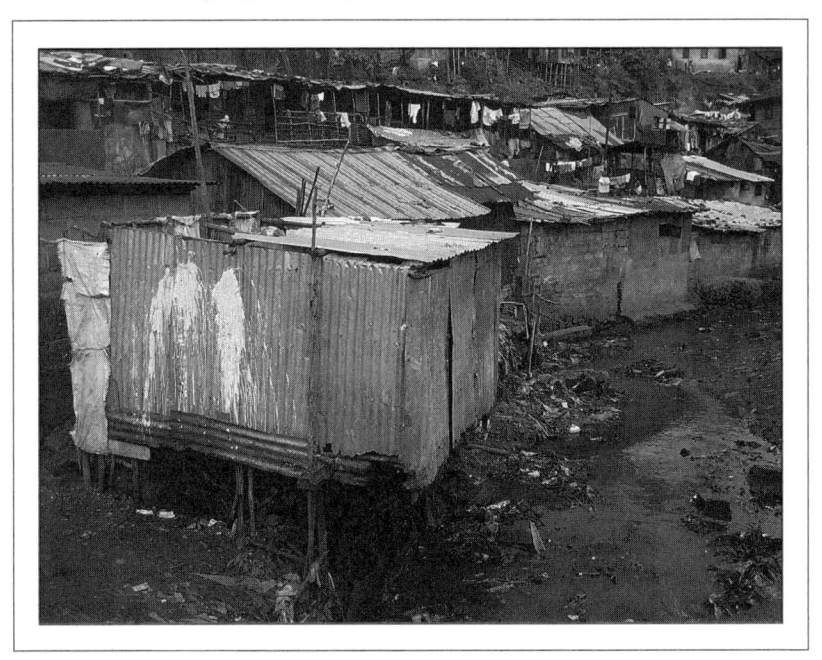

Photo by Jonathan Parkinson.

are reported in the media and become a political concern, endemic diarrheal diseases are a major health concern, especially for those already infected by intestinal worms.

According to the World Health Organization, unsafe water, inadequate sanitation, and insufficient hygiene practices engender at least 9 percent of the global disease burden. However, this may be an underestimate because several significant diseases are unquantifiable (Prüss-Üstün and others 2008). The incidence of diseases related to poor water and sanitation also is likely to be higher in urban areas where fecally contaminated environments pose more immediate threats to health than in rural areas. People living in urban areas face greater health risks because of higher population densities than their rural counterparts even though sanitation coverage is generally higher (Hardoy and Satterthwaite 1989; Mulenga, Manase, and Fawcett 2004).

The resulting combination of environmental hazards creates a *syndemic* situation: multiple diseases and conditions combine synergistically to create an excess burden of disease (Singer and Scott 2003). Prevailing environmental conditions and associated morbidity rates in many low-income neighborhoods in cities throughout the developing world are similar to those in Europe in the nineteenth century (Konteh 2009). The situation is so bad that water and sanitation inadequacies are considered one of the world's most serious environmental health problems (McGranahan, Leitmann, and Surjadi 1997).

## IMPACT OF INADEQUATE WATER AND SANITATION ON LIVELIHOODS

Unsanitary living conditions and environmental health risks related to water and sanitation perpetuate a vicious cycle of poverty because of the increased expenditure on health care and loss of productivity related to illness (Environmental Health Project 2004). Therefore, poverty becomes inseparable from ill health, which is the single most common trigger for the downward slide into poverty (Narayan and others 2000).

Disparities exist within communities, and a greater share of the socioeconomic burden falls on the population without improved sanitation, making inequalities worse (Hutton, Haller, and Bartram 2007) and concentrating economic impacts on poorer communities (Hutton and Haller 2004). A similar picture was seen in Great Britain during the second and third decades of the nineteenth century, when the working population living in urban slums was more severely affected than other elements of society (Rosen, Fee, and Morman 1993).

Diarrheal diseases are more debilitating for the undernourished (Bhandari and others 1989). Diarrhea amplifies malnutrition, which is particularly a problem for those who depend on their physical strength to earn a livelihood. These illnesses therefore have a direct impact on household finances because of loss of working days and because of financial outlay to pay for medicines in severe cases (Pryer 1993). The ill health of one member of the family also has repercussions on the others. In the longer term, illnesses drain household savings, lower learning ability, reduce productivity, and lead to a diminished quality of life.

A disproportionate share of the labor and health burdens related to inadequate water and sanitation services falls upon women. In addition to the higher risk of exposure related to water and sanitation-related diseases, it is often the woman's responsibility to care for people who become sick. To maintain household income, women are likely to replace the labor of those who have fallen ill with their own labor. Women may also suffer from other illnesses as the result of poor sanitation, such as urine retention due to lack of private places for urination and increased vulnerability from harassment (Bapat and Agarwal 2003).

The public health consequences of poor water and sanitation are notably severe for young children (Fry, Cousins, and Olivola 2002), especially infants less than two years old. Repeated diarrhea causes stunting of growth because of malnutrition and, although intestinal worms are unlikely to cause mortality directly, they are responsible for substantial disability. Therefore, chronic infections have long-term impact on future educational performance (Lima and others 2004). Lack of appropriate sanitation facilities in schools also keeps girls out of education with serious adverse consequences on their future opportunities for paid employment (Cairncross 2003; Pearson and McPhedran 2008).

# EPIDEMIOLOGY OF DISEASE TRANSMISSION

Where service provision is poor, water and sanitation problems are interconnected and are also connected with a range of other localized environmental health problems. It is in these situations where infections via fecal-oral routes thrive (McGranahan and others 2001). The linkages between poor environmental health conditions and disease transmission is common knowledge for public health professionals today. But it was only during the 1900s, when a plausible epidemiological theory about disease transmission was identified, that the principles of sanitary reform and community health action developed.

These subsequently formed the basis for action in the industrialized world for the next fifty to sixty years. Mostly, these principles are just as valid today in developing countries as they were when they were first announced, which suggests that sanitary reforms in less-developed countries should still be based upon the principles set forth by Edwin Chadwick more than a hundred years ago (Rosen, Fee, and Morman 1993).

## Factors Affecting Concentrations of Pathogens in the Environment

Although a complex set of factors determines whether a person falls ill, two of the main factors that affect risk of disease transmission in the first place are the level of fecal contamination and the level of exposure. Evidently, the lack of sanitation will result in dangerously high concentration of pathogens in the environment. But when considering health risks, the provision of sanitation facilities cannot be disaggregated from other physical and environment factors, such as those listed in Table 18.1.

Once excreted, pathogens' survival depends on the type of pathogen and on environmental conditions such as light, temperature, and humidity. Survival can also be prolonged by both the type of housing and physical characteristics of the

TABLE 18.1 Physical Factors Influencing Disease Transmission in the Urban Environment

| Topography | Low-lying land | Flooding of latrines results in increased transmission of fecal-oral diseases. Poor drainage creates ponding and damp conditions, which are conducive to microorganism survival and possible regrowth. |
|---|---|---|
| | Steep hillsides | Steep hillsides are often poorly served by water supplies and are hard to reach by vehicles with equipment for desludging pit latrines, which means that they become a health hazard especially during the wet season. |
| Housing | Construction | Poor-quality housing may harbor insects that spread diseases. Dirt floors present a significant health hazard relating to transmission of helminths (hookworm and ascaris). |
| | Overcrowding | Overcrowding creates conditions that are conducive for the spread of communicable/infectious diseases. It also leads to excessive use of water points and latrines. |
| Settlement | High density of unplanned housing | High densities perpetuate overcrowding and problems for installation of infrastructure and access for servicing of facilities. |

settlement itself. Some bacteria can even multiply in the environment in the right conditions, for example, in food kept at ambient temperatures (Curtis, Cairncross, and Yonli 2000).

## Transmission Pathways

Households supplement inadequate supplies of water with unprotected wells and surface waters; many are contaminated by wastewater and other wastes. Low pressures in distribution systems caused by intermittent operation means that supplies are prone to contamination where water supply pipes and the joints are cracked.

Poor access to water facilities, combined with the unreliability of supplies, means that many households have to carry water and store it in the home. Water is often stored in containers in houses where water is not piped directly into the home, and they provide water during times of disruption to the supply. Post-source contamination can occur in storage vessels in homes (Gundry, Wright, and Conroy 2004). Higher levels of microbial contamination are often associated with storage vessels that have wide openings (for example, buckets and pots) because these are vulnerable to the introduction of hands, cups, and dippers that may carry pathogens (WHO 2002).

Water contamination is one way in which diseases are perpetuated, but there has traditionally been a tendency to place too much attention on water quality as a means of disease control. According to Cairncross and Feachem (1993), this may reflect the critical role that inadequate urban water treatment facilities have played in some of the more memorable cholera and typhoid epidemics in European history.

Figure 18.3 shows the routes of transmission of fecal-oral diseases that are most common in the urban environment. Whereas transmission in the public domain can result in a large epidemic, transmission in the domestic domain is less dramatic and often ignored, even though it may account for a substantial number of cases (Cairncross and others 1996).

Contaminated public water supplies tend to be the principal transmission route for the wealthy minority, but for the vast majority of urban dwellers, excreta-related routes predominate. In addition, although polluted water is commonly perceived to be the mechanism for transmission of microbial pathogens, it is direct person-to-person transmission that is more important, especially where fecal contamination of the domestic environment is high (Feachem 1984; Curtis, Cairncross, and Yonli 2000).

## Urban Disparities and Susceptibility to Disease

Figure 18.3 also highlights the important fact that infection may not progress to illness and those carrying pathogens can contribute towards further transmission of disease. Thus, although the species and strain of pathogen influences the infective dose, whether this results in illness is highly dependent on the health and resilience of the individual.

The urban poor are notably more susceptible to illness than their wealthier counterparts due to weakened immune systems caused by fatigue and malnutrition. Other factors that influence whether the host develops symptoms are age and sex. Women, infants, and children typically spend more time in and around the home than adult men do, so they are more likely to be exposed to household and neighborhood environmental hazards (Songsore and McGranahan 1998).

Women's lives differ from those of men, and their daily activities expose them to different environmental hazards (Kettel 1996). In many situations, women are prone to greater exposure and risk, as they are generally responsible for water, waste disposal, and maintenance of latrines. As they also tend to be responsible for cooking, child care, and care of the sick, they are the most important proponents of household facilities.

### FIGURE 18.3 Fecal-Oral Pathogen Transmission Routes in the Urban Environment

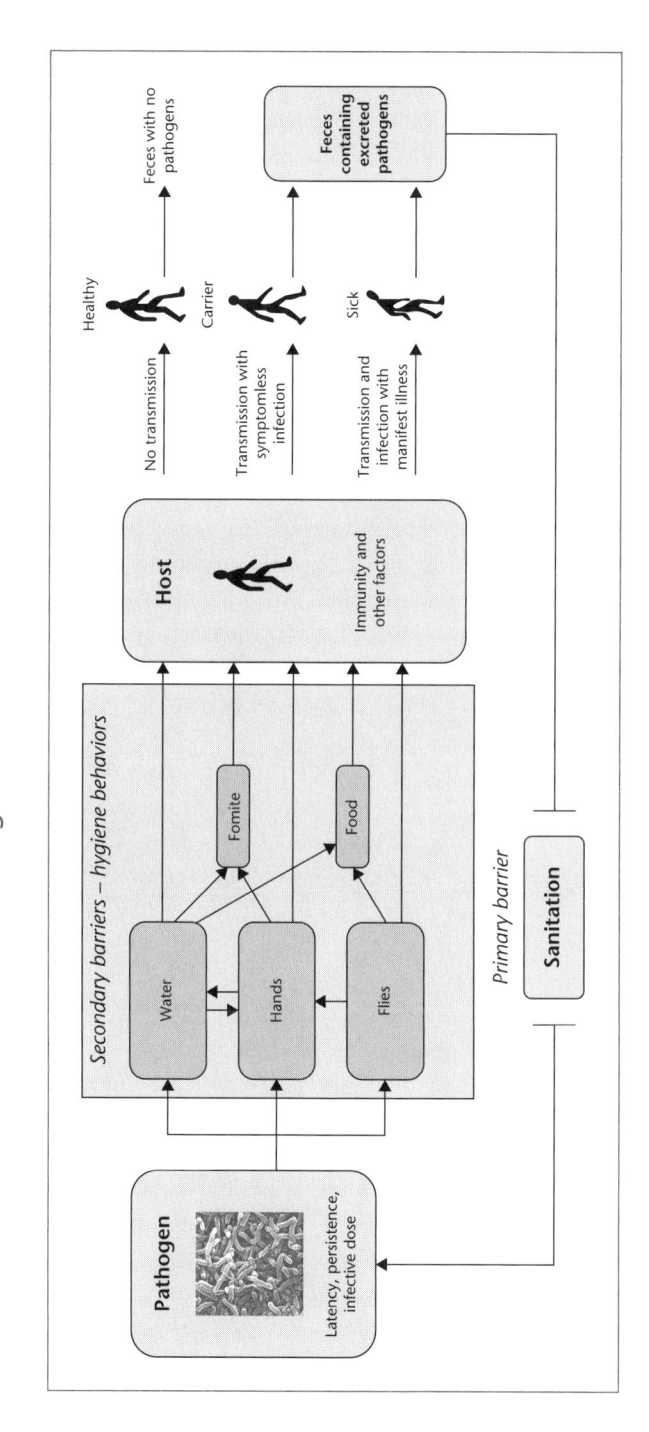

*Source:* Adapted from R. Carr, 2001, Excreta-related infections and the role of sanitation in the control of transmission. In *Water quality: Guidelines, standards and health,* ed. L. Fewtrell and J. Bartram. London: IWA/WHO.

There may be few benefits from improved sanitation for children even if they use a latrine if they continue to play in a contaminated environment (Bartlett 2003). The health risks for children are also exacerbated because children's feces contain higher concentrations of pathogens (Cairncross and Feachem 1993). As a result, designing sanitation facilities without children in mind can undermine the best intentions of public health engineers, who often focus on the larger-scale downstream infrastructure rather than the more important household environment.

# PERCEPTIONS OF Ill HEALTH AND DEMANDS FOR IMPROVEMENT

Residents from deprived neighborhoods frequently rank ill health as one of the key dimensions of poverty and describe a strong link between illnesses and livelihood impacts, such as cost of health care and subsequent indebtedness (Cities Network 2003). However, demands for improved access to better water and sanitation facilities are rarely driven by health benefits. Among the range of urban services, water supply is usually the priority of local residents (Mulenga, Manase, and Fawcett 2004), even though this may have the least benefit in health terms.

Urban dwellers living in deprived neighborhoods often set water and sanitation improvements as priorities (Mulenga, Manase, and Fawcett 2004). It is more common for poor people to talk about the devastating consequences of ill health than to make specific reference to particular illnesses or their causes. Of particular importance for them is addressing acute health concerns that cause immediate suffering as opposed to reducing the risks of excreta-related diseases, which are not usually as severe as other diseases (Narayan and others 2000).

While health may rarely be the specific reason for the demand for improved services, or indeed why people change their behavior, they do generally want better health for themselves, their families, and their communities (McGranahan 2007). An increased awareness of health risks is therefore potentially an important motivating factor for both investments in facilities and infrastructure as well as changes in behavior. Table 18.2 summarizes the expected health improvements associated with different components of water and sanitation infrastructure and the reasons commonly expressed by residents for improvements.

Deficiencies of service provision are particularly apparent in the sectors of water and sanitation, but particularly so in the case of sanitation due to its low political priority and institutional neglect. In Great Britain in the nineteenth century, recognition of the social and economic costs of preventable disease provided

TABLE 18.2   Components of Environmental Health Infrastructure: Reasons for Prioritization and Health Improvements

| Component | Public's Reason for Prioritization | Related Health Improvements |
| --- | --- | --- |
| Water supply | Water is required for cooking, cleaning, washing. Carrying water is very onerous, especially when the sources are far. Water quality matters depending on the use. | Potable water, water for cleanliness and washing (especially hand washing). |
| Drainage of wastewater and storm water runoff | Ponded water is an inconvenience, flooding causes disruption and damage. | Drained water removes habitats for insect (flies and mosquitoes) breeding, and better drainage can stop latrines from flooding. |
| Latrines and pit desludging | Convenient access to a safe and private place for excretion is a prime concern. Improved servicing of on-site sanitation is frequently a priority as pits rapidly become unusable when full. | Access to well-maintained latrines that are affordable and can be accessed easily is a necessary prerequisite of improved health. |
| Solid waste collection | Uncollected waste is an inconvenience, looks unsightly, blocks drains, and can be dangerous for children. | Reduced insects and rats. |

additional stimulus for action to improve public health. Although there also was evidently a political concern for the well-being of the lower classes, the wealthy groups also felt threatened by disease epidemics, and this fear contributed to sanitary reforms and major investments in sanitation in the form of sewerage (Rosen, Fee, and Morman 1993).

Unfortunately, few governments in the developing world can demonstrate a similar level of political commitment to improve public health. In addition to the lack of recognition of the true cost to the economy caused by endemic diarrheal diseases, there are major financial deficits to contend with, compounded by a complex set of institutional and legal constraints.

A particular problem is that utilities are often not allowed to provide services to households in informal settlements due to lack of legal tenure. Therefore, for political and financial reasons, urban authorities and utilities usually set as a priority more affluent residential areas where there is a perception of a greater capacity to pay, and residents are in a stronger position to lobby for better services.

## HEALTH BENEFITS OF WATER AND SANITATION INTERVENTIONS

Even where political will and resources are made available to invest in improved water and sanitation, increased coverage may not translate into health benefits. This is because there are no guarantees that facilities will be properly used or adequately maintained.

Provision of facilities (known as "hardware") has traditionally been the main focus of interventions to decrease the incidence of water- and excreta-related disease in low-income settlements. All types of hardware inherently have a software aspect and, as small design features can be critical for the successful use of facilities, the ergonomics of water and sanitation are critical for disease control.

Other types of "hardware" may include household water treatment systems, containers for washing hands with soap, and potties for small children (EHP 2004). Improved facilities can greatly reduce the incidence of diarrheal disease, but to be effective, they need to be implemented in tandem with campaigns to promote better hygiene behavior.

There have been a number of studies (originally Esrey and others 1990, but more recently Fewtrell and others 2005 and Cairncross and Valdmanis 2006), that have carried out meta-analyses to compare the effectiveness of different types of intervention. The results highlight the importance of hygiene promotion and indicate that public water supply connections may not result in significant health benefits compared with house connections. But attributing health benefits to one particular type of intervention is problematic because the boundaries between water, sanitation, food contamination, insects, and solid waste problems are blurred (McGranahan, Leitmann, and Surjadi 1997).

### Water

There is a common perception that water quality is the main factor that affects health, and therefore provision of potable water is the only concern for achieving health benefits. Water quality is obviously important, but it is necessary to consider that water is often contaminated between the source and the point of consumption (Wright, Gundry, and Conroy 2004). Therefore, there may be a need for additional treatment by filtration in the home prior to consumption.

It is not only necessary to provide communities with sufficient water of good quality for drinking. There is also a need to provide water for a range of other domestic purposes. Water supplies are particularly important for maintaining good hygiene. Washing, even with water that might not be good to drink, can help curb fecal-oral diseases (Cairncross 1987) as well as a variety of other health problems ranging from scabies to louse-borne typhus. Thus, increasing the quantity of water that is available may be just as important for curbing diarrhea as improving water quality.

## Sanitation

When it comes to endemic diarrhea, there is a strong argument to set as a priority disposal of feces to prevent pathogens from entering the home environment (Curtis, Cairncross, and Yonli 2000). So sanitation interventions are those that are aimed at the disposal of human excreta in a manner designed to reduce direct or indirect human contact.

Given the obvious importance of sanitation as a primary barrier to excreta-related diseases (see Figure 18.3), the results from the meta-analyses are somewhat disappointing. However, the relative low effectiveness may be explained by the fact that effectiveness is just as much about the quality of the service as the existence of facilities in the first place (coverage).

A key consideration is the level of service, as mentioned above. Communal and shared latrines, which are ubiquitous in low-income cities in the developing world, are beset with problems of ownership, management responsibility, and poor maintenance. However, where the responsibility is divulged, there are much greater opportunities to promote local management of facilities by people who are better equipped to ensure sustained operation and cost recovery; this is the case in some of Mumbai's urban slums (Nitti and Sarkar 2003).

## Hygiene Promotion

The results from the meta-analyses indicate that hygiene promotion is the most effective intervention for controlling endemic diarrhea. From a health perspective, washing hands at critical times, such as after defecation or the handling of children's feces, is seen to be a priority over water supply (Curtis, Cairncross, and Yonli 2000).

The evidence is backed up by a consideration of the transmission routes. Many infections are transmitted by direct hand-to-hand contact—either directly or indirectly by use of objects capable of carrying infectious organisms and transferring them from one individual to another (fomites). Hand washing is therefore the most important hygiene behavior. A review of epidemiological studies of the impact of hand washing on diarrhea found that on current evidence washing hands with soap can reduce the risk of diarrheal diseases by 42–47 percent (Curtis and Cairncross 2003).

## SUMMARY

Promoting improvements in health via water and sanitation requires an understanding of the disease transmission pathways and the role of different technologies and service levels on resultant health outcomes. Also, those responsible for sanitation improvements need to take on board the critical importance of hygiene behavior related to the use of water and sanitation facilities, which may either undermine or enhance health outcomes.

Health benefits of improved water and sanitation are not always directly perceived at the community level, but more general health concerns linked to inadequate provision of water and sanitation facilities are frequently raised by residents from underserved areas. Thus, improved sanitation is a key concern from a public health benefit perspective, manifesting in improved livelihood and economic benefits for the community. These benefits perceived by the community may be important motivating factors for investments in improved household facilities and hygiene behavioral change.

Health benefits can never be achieved without the foundation of affordable services that meet the needs of the populations that they are designed to serve. Bearing this in mind, an understanding of the broader poverty aspects and multiple priorities for development is required to ensure that initiatives to improve water and sanitation result in sustainable service delivery and consequently in sustained health improvements.

## REFERENCES

Bapat, M., and I. Agarwal. 2003. Our needs, our priorities: Women and men from the slums in Mumbai and Pune talk about their needs for water and sanitation. *Environment and Urbanization* 15(2):71–86.

Bartlett, S. 2003. Water, sanitation and urban children: The need to go beyond improved provision. *Environment and Urbanization* 15:57–70.

Bhandari, N., M. K. Bhan, S. Sazawal, J. D. Clemens, S. Bhatnagar, and V. Khoshoo. 1989. Association of antecedent malnutrition with persistent diarrhea: A case-control study. *British Medical Journal* 298(6683):1284–1287.

Cairncross, S. 1987. The benefits of water supply. In *Developing world water* II, ed. J. Pickford. London: Grosvenor Press.

Cairncross, S. 2003. Sanitation in the developing world: Current status and future solutions. *International Journal of Environmental Health Research*, 13(1):S123-S131(1).

Cairncross, S., U. Blumenthal, P. Kolsky, L. Moraes, and A. Tayeh. 1996. The public and domestic domains in the transmission of disease. *Tropical Medicine & International Health* 1(1):27–34.
Cairncross, S., and R. Feachem. 1993. *Environmental health engineering in the tropics*, 2nd ed. Chichester, UK: Wiley.
Cairncross S., and V. Valdmanis. 2006. Water supply, sanitation, and hygiene promotion. In *Disease control priorities in developing countries*, 2nd ed., 771–792. New York: Oxford University Press.
Carr, R. 2001. Excreta-related infections and the role of sanitation in the control of transmission. In *Water quality: Guidelines, standards and health*, ed. L. Fewtrell and J. Bartram. London: IWA/WHO.
Cities Network. 2003. *A South African urban renewal overview*. Johannesburg: South African Cities Network.
Curtis, V., and S. Cairncross. 2003. Effect of washing hands with soap on diarrhea risk in the community: A systematic review. *Lancet Infectious Diseases* 3(5):275–281.
Curtis, V., S. Cairncross, and R. Yonli. 2000. Review: Domestic hygiene and diarrhea: Pinpointing the problem. *Tropical Medicine and International Health* 5(1):22–32.
Environmental Health Project (EHP). 2004. *Improving the health of the urban poor: Learning from USAID experience*, EHP Strategic Report 12 (August 2004). Washington, DC: Environmental Health Project, U.S. Agency for International Development.
Esrey, S. A., L. Roberts, J. B. Potach, and C. Shiff. 1990. Health benefits from improvements in water supply and sanitation: Survey and analysis of the literature on selected diseases. *WASH Technical Report* 66.
Feachem, R. 1984. Interventions for the control of diarrhoeal diseases among young children: Promotion of personal and domestic hygiene. *Bulletin of the World Health Organization* 62(3):467–476.
Fewtrell, L., R. B. Kaufmann, D. Kay, W. Enanoria, L. Haller, and J. M. Colford, Jr. 2005. Water, sanitation, and hygiene interventions to reduce diarrhea in less developed countries: A systematic review and meta-analysis. *Lancet Infectious Diseases* 5(1):42–52.
Fry S., B. Cousins, and K. Olivola. 2002. Health of children living in urban slums in Asia and the near east: Review of existing literature and data. *An urban environmental health initiative in Egypt*, EHP Activity Report 109. Washington, DC: Environmental Health Project, U.S. Agency for International Development.
Gundry, S., J. Wright, and R. Conroy. 2004. A systematic review of the health outcomes related to household water quality in developing countries. *Journal of Water & Health* 2(1):1–13.
Hardoy, J. E., and D. Satterthwaite. 1989. *Squatter citizen: Life in the urban Third World*. London: Earthscan.
Hutton, G., and L. Haller. 2004. Evaluation of the costs and benefits of water and sanitation improvements at the global level, Report No. WHO/SDE/WSH/04.04. Geneva: World Health Organization. http://www.who.int/water_sanitation_health/wsh0404.pdf.
Hutton, G., L. Haller, and J. Bartram. 2007. Economic and health effects of increasing coverage of low cost household drinking water supply and sanitation interventions. Background document to *Human Development Report 2006*, United Nations Development Programme. Geneva: World Health Organization.
Kettel, B. 1996. Women, health and the environment. *Social Science and Medicine*, 42(10):1367–1379.
Konteh, F. H. 2009. Urban sanitation and health in the developing world: Reminiscing the nineteenth century industrial nations. *Health and Place*,15:69–78.

Lima, M.D.C., M.E.F.A. Motta, E. C. Santos, and G.A.P.D. Silva. 2004. Determinants of impaired growth among hospitalised children: A case study. *Sao Paulo Medical Journal* 122:117–123.

McGranahan. G. 2007. Evolving urban health risks in low- and middle-income countries: From housing, water and sanitation to cities and climate change. Improving Urban Population Health Systems. Center for Sustainable Urban Development. Background paper prepared for Global Urban Summit, Bellagio, Italy, July 15–20, 2007.

McGranahan, G., P. Jacobi, J. Songsore, C. Surjadi, and M. Kjellen. 2001. *The citizens at risk: From urban sanitation to sustainable cities*. London: Earthscan.

McGranahan, G., J. Leitmann, and C. Surjadi. 1997. Understanding environmental problems in disadvantaged neighborhoods: Broad spectrum surveys, participatory appraisal and contingent valuation. *Urban Management and The Environment*. UNDP/UNCHS (Habitat), World Bank, SEI (Stockholm Environment Institute).

McGranahan, G., and D. L. Owen. 2006. Local water and sanitation companies and the urban poor. London. International Institute for Environment and Development.

Mulenga, M., G. Manase, and B. Fawcett. 2004. Building links for improved sanitation in poor urban settlements: Recommendations from research in Southern Africa. University of Southampton, UK.

Narayan, D., R. Chambers, M. Kaul Shah, and P. Petesch. 2000. *Voices of the poor: Crying out for change*. New York: Oxford University Press (for World Bank).

Nitti, R., and S. Sarkar. 2003. The slum sanitation program in Mumbai. *Urban Notes* (Thematic Group on Services to the Urban Poor), No. 7. Washington, DC: World Bank.

Pearson, J., and K. McPhedran. 2008. A literature review of the non-health impacts of sanitation. *Waterlines* 27(1):48–61.

Prüss-Üstün A., R. Bos, F. Gore, and J. Bartram. 2008. *Safer water, better health: Costs, benefits and sustainability of interventions to protect and promote health*. Geneva: World Health Organization.

Pryer, J. 1993. The impact of adult ill-health on household income and nutrition in Khulna, Bangladesh. *Environment and Urbanization* 5(2): 35–49.

Rosen, G., E. Fee, and E. T. Morman. 1993. *A history of public health*, expanded ed. Baltimore: John Hopkins University Press.

Singer, M., and C. Scott. 2003. Syndemics and public health: Reconceptualizing disease in bio-social context. *Medical Anthropology Quarterly* 17(4):423–441.

Songsore, J., and G. McGranahan. 1998. The political economy of household environmental management: Gender, environment and epidemiology in the greater Accra metropolitan area. *World Development* 26(3):395–412.

Wagner, E. G., and J. N. Lanoix. 1958. *Excreta disposal for rural areas and small communities*, WHO Monograph Series no 39. Geneva: WHO.

World Health Organization (WHO). 2002. *Managing water in the home: Accelerated health gains from improved water supply*. Geneva: WHO.

WHO/UNICEF Joint Monitoring Programme for Water Supply and Sanitation. 2008. A snapshot of sanitation in Africa. Geneva: World Health Organization.

Wright, J., S. Gundry, and R. Conroy. 2004 Household drinking water in developing countries: A systematic review of microbiological contamination between source and point-of-use. *Tropical Medicine and International Health*, 9:106–117.

# CHAPTER NINETEEN

# URBAN TRANSPORTATION

## RAE ZIMMERMAN
## CARLOS E. RESTREPO

### LEARNING OBJECTIVES

- Describe indicators that characterize transportation systems and how they change over time
- Identify important trends and patterns in transportation and their impact on public health
- Discuss how transportation affects climate change
- Identify new technologies and programs aimed at reducing the impacts of transportation on health

**URBAN** transportation comprises diverse services that are provided and used in different ways. This diversity has considerable implications for the health of transportation users and people living in cities. This chapter presents a foundation for understanding some of the relationships between health and transportation and an overview of options emerging to improve transportation systems and reduce adverse health impacts. The focus is primarily on land-based transport in urban areas, for example, automobile travel, bicycling, walking, and rail and bus transit for passengers, and truck and rail transport for freight.

First, some broad transportation trends and patterns, primarily in the United States, are presented to set the stage for an urban focus. Significant health and safety effects associated with characteristics of road transportation and transit are identified. Then two major public issues—climate change and security—are addressed as they bear upon human health. Second, new, innovative ways of improving transportation while directly and indirectly reducing the sector's impact on human health are discussed. Cities in developing countries are experiencing very rapid rates of urban population growth and consequently, these cities are facing important transportation and health challenges. These challenges have in turn resulted in innovative transportation solutions, such as Curitiba's Bus Rapid Transit (BRT) system, which are being emulated in diverse settings around the world.

# TRANSPORTATION CHARACTERISTICS AND HEALTH ISSUES

## How We Travel, How Much, and Who Travels

Transportation infrastructure is a critical element of urban society and has reached unprecedented levels of complexity and size. The transportation system is generally categorized by mode of travel: highways, pipelines, rail, transit, air, and water. Within those categories, transport is typically divided into the movement of passengers, freight or goods, and information. As Table 19.1 shows, transportation in the United States comprises a myriad of networks, nodes, and vehicles.

---

This research was supported in part by the United States Department of Homeland Security through the Center for Catastrophe Preparedness and Response at New York University (grant number 2004-GTTX-0001, for the project Public Infrastructure Support for Protective Emergency Services) and by the United States Department of Homeland Security through the Center for Risk and Economic Analysis of Terrorism Events (CREATE; grant number 2007-ST-061-000001). However, any opinions, findings, and conclusions or recommendations in this document are those of the authors and do not necessarily reflect views of the United States Department of Homeland Security.

TABLE 19.1    Characteristics of U.S. Transportation Infrastructure

**Air**
Public use airports: 5,233
Private use airports: 14,757
Certified air carrier aircraft: 8,024
Airplane-miles traveled: 6.6 billion
Passenger-miles traveled (air): 592.4 billion

**Highways**
Paved roads: 2,601,490 miles
Unpaved roads: 1,408,757 miles
Highway bridges: 599,893
Passenger cars: 136,568,083
   Vehicle-miles traveled (passenger cars): 1,689,965 million
Light trucks: 95,336,839
   Vehicle-miles traveled (light trucks): 1,059,590 million
Motorcycles: 6,227,146
   Vehicle-miles traveled (motorcycles): 10,770 million
Heavy trucks: 8,481,999
   Vehicle-miles traveled (heavy trucks): 222,836 million

**Pipelines**
Hazardous liquid pipeline: 159,512 miles
Natural gas gathering and transmission pipeline: 296,400 miles
Natural gas distribution pipeline: 1,117,800 miles

**Rail**
Rail (Class I, regional, local, and Amtrak-operated railroads): 162,442 miles
Class I freight cars: 474,839 thousand
Amtrak-owned passenger cars in service: 1,186

**Transit**
Buses: 82,000
  Directional route-miles of bus: 165,854
  Bus passenger-miles: 21,825 million
  Unlinked bus trips: 5,855 million
Heavy rail cars: 11,000
  Directional route-miles of heavy rail: 1,622
  Heavy rail car passenger-miles: 14,418 million
  Unlinked heavy rail car trips: 2,808 million
Commuter rail cars and locomotives: 6,000
  Directional route-miles of commuter rail: 8,076
  Passenger-miles (commuter rail cars and locomotives): 9,473 million
  Unlinked trips (commuter rail cars and locomotives): 423 million

*(Continued)*

## TABLE 19.1 (Continued)

Light rail cars: 1,400
 Directional route-miles of light rail: 1,188
 Passenger-miles (light rail cars): 1,700 million
 Unlinked light rail car trips: 381 million

**Water-Related Transportation**
Navigable waterways: 26,000 miles
Non-self-propelled vessels: 32,052
Self-propelled vessels: 8,976
Oceangoing steam and motor ships in the U.S.-flag domestic fleet: 357

*Source:* Adapted from U.S. DOT, BTS, 2007, *Transportation Statistics Annual Report 2007*, pp. 6–8.

### Trends in Road Transportation of Passengers

Trends in transportation use are influenced by many factors, and one strong influence is the price of fuels. Roadway travel experienced declines in 2008 as gasoline prices were increasing (U.S. DOT, FHA 2009). In contrast, in urban areas throughout the United States, transit ridership reached record levels. The American Public Transportation Association (APTA) reported in March 2009 that "Americans took 10.7 billion trips on public transportation in 2008, the highest level of ridership in 52 years."

Longer-term trends for transportation show significant increases in roadway ridership expressed as vehicle miles of travel (VMT) over the last few decades. VMT is a major indicator of roadway transportation activity. In the United States, this figure doubled between 1980 and 2007, increasing from about 1.5 trillion to 3 trillion (U.S. DOT, FHA 2008b). Considerably greater increases occurred in urban areas than in rural areas (U.S. DOT, BTS 2007).

Motor vehicle registrations reflect the population of vehicles in use. In the United States, the number of registered vehicles increased dramatically between 1950 and 2006; the rate of growth was greatest for trucks and lowest for buses. The number of automobiles registered (publicly and privately owned) is still significantly greater than the other two vehicle types (U.S. DOT, FHA 2003).

The U.S. Department of Transportation (DOT) provides the main transportation variables to assess sector time trends. Figure 19.1 shows several trends indexed to 1987. As shown, vehicle miles traveled, vehicle registrations, and motor fuel consumption all increased rapidly between 1960 and 2006. The only indicator that stabilized in the late 1970s/early 1980s is motor fuel consumption in gallons per vehicle (U.S. DOT, FHA 2008a), reflecting improvements in U.S. average vehicle fuel efficiency as a result of the Corporate Average Fuel Economy (CAFE) standards.

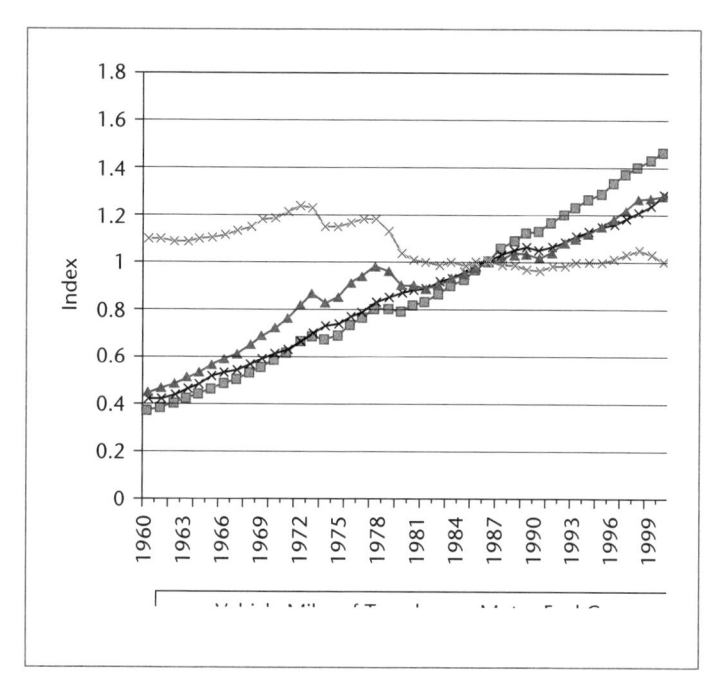

**FIGURE 19.1** Aggregate Transportation Trends in the United States, 1960–2006, Indexed to 1987

*Source:* Graphed using data from U.S. DOT, Federal Highway Administration, *Highway Statistics 2006*.

In 2005, the CAFE standards were 27.1 miles per gallon for a passenger vehicle and 21.6 miles per gallon for light trucks. The average passenger car fuel efficiency in the same year was 22.9 miles per gallon for passenger cars and 16.9 miles per gallon for other two-axle, four-tire vehicles (U.S. DOT, BTS 2007, 93). Improvements in fuel efficiency have had a positive impact on air quality. Between 1995 and 2005 transportation-related emissions of carbon monoxide (CO) in the United States decreased from about 84 to about 54 million short tons, and transportation-related emissions of nitrogen oxides decreased from about 8.9 to about 6.6 million short tons (U.S. DOT, BTS 2007, 94).

Trends in increased vehicle travel translate into considerable roadway congestion and travel delay in urban areas. Schrank and Lomax (2009) noted a steady increase over time in annual delay per peak traveler, wasted fuel, and congestion cost in 439 U.S. urban areas, with more dramatic levels in large metropolitan areas. In terms of annual delay (in hours) per traveler, in 2007 seven very large cities out of fourteen exceeded the very-large-city average of 51 hours, and sixteen large cities out of twenty-nine exceeded their average of 35 hours. For example, very large cities exceeding the 51-hour average were the Los Angeles metro area; Washington, DC; Atlanta, GA; Houston, TX; San Francisco; and the Dallas metro area (Schrank and Lomax 2009, 22).

With congestion becoming an increasing problem, some cities around the world are implementing economic incentives to manage congestion and reduce peak air pollution emissions. As discussed in Chapter 20, Urban Air Quality, London has successfully implemented a congestion-charging scheme.

## Global Trends in Vehicle Ownership

The increasing trends in transportation infrastructure and use over time in the United States are being observed around the world. Vehicle ownership, like vehicle registration, is one way to capture this trend. As shown in Table 19.2, vehicle ownership

TABLE 19.2  Projected Vehicle Ownership, 2002–2030, Millions of Vehicles

|  | 2002 | 2010 | 2020 | 2030 |
|---|---|---|---|---|
| **World** | 751 | 939 | 1,255 | 1,660 |
| **OECD** | 625 | 720 | 827 | 920 |
| United States | 234 | 260 | 288 | 312 |
| Germany | 48 | 54 | 60 | 63 |
| France | 35 | 40 | 46 | 50 |
| Italy | 37 | 39 | 41 | 41 |
| United Kingdom | 31 | 37 | 44 | 50 |
| Japan | 76 | 87 | 95 | 96 |
| Korea | 14 | 22 | 31 | 36 |
| Australia | 12 | 15 | 18 | 19 |
| Other OECD | 137 | 164 | 205 | 252 |
| **Non-OECD** | 126 | 219 | 429 | 741 |
| Africa | 11 | 15 | 23 | 33 |
| Brazil | 21 | 27 | 42 | 71 |
| Other Latin America | 12 | 19 | 33 | 54 |
| China | 21 | 80 | 209 | 387 |
| Other Asia | 58 | 72 | 113 | 184 |
| **Rest of world** | 4 | 6 | 8 | 11 |

*Source:* M. Sommer, 2005, Will the oil market continue to be tight? *World economic outlook, globalization and external imbalances*, Ch. 4, Washington, DC: International Monetary Fund.

rates are increasing worldwide. These rates are expected to increase fastest in rapidly growing developing countries such as China and India. Table 19.2 shows vehicle ownership projections estimated by the International Monetary Fund (IMF). As the table shows, vehicle ownership in China is expected to increase from about 21 million in 2002 to 387 million by 2030. Those figures suggest that by 2030, China may have more vehicles than the United States, where the number of vehicles is expected to increase from 234 million in 2002 to 312 million in 2030. Given population trends, in 2030 the United States is still expected to have the highest number of vehicles per capita in the world (Sommer 2005, 182).

## Trends in Road Transportation of Freight

Freight transportation is critical to the movement of goods and services that our economies rely on. Like passenger travel, freight movement indicators in the United States show significant increases over time. The four main modes of freight transport in the United States are rail, truck, waterborne, and air freight. In the period 1990–2001 rail and truck movement, the first and second largest modes of freight travel, respectively, increased in terms of ton-miles while waterborne freight decreased. Air freight also increased, but it is relatively small compared to the other modes (U.S. DOT, FHA 2005).

## Trends in Transit

There are various modes of transit. First is rail transit, classified as heavy rail, light rail, and commuter rail. Second are modes of transit that primarily use streets or tracks over streets—buses, trolleys, and various forms of paratransit. APTA (2009) reports historical figures for both passenger trips and miles of travel in the United States consistently from 1977 through 2006. Rates of change based on APTA figures show that during that time period, passenger trips for all transit increased 37.8 percent, while rail increased by 67.6 percent. Passenger miles traveled increased more dramatically for rail relative to all transit. For all transit, passenger miles increased by 73.7 percent, while rail increased 167.6 percent.

Transit is primarily concentrated in urban areas. Sixty-two urban area rail transit systems were listed in the National Transit Database for 2007 in the United States. This concentration is largely a function of population. For example, the rail transit systems that service the New York–New Jersey metropolitan area account for the largest share of U.S. rail transit trips. The dominance of other world cities in terms of mass transit is reflected in the fact that although New York City ranks fourth in the world in transit ridership (not including PATH or the Staten Island Railway), the second largest U.S. system, Washington DC, ranks thirtieth, and the third largest, Chicago, ranks forty-second among world cities. The metro systems with the highest passenger rides per year outside the United States are in the following cities: Tokyo, Moscow, Seoul, Mexico City, Paris, Hong Kong, Beijing, London, Shanghai, and São Paulo (Wikipedia n.d.).

# HEALTH AND SAFETY RISKS ASSOCIATED WITH TRANSPORTATION

## Quantity of Fuel Used

In the United States, transportation is a large contributor of air pollutant emissions primarily through fuel combustion. In spite of fuel economies, the consumption of fuel continues to grow, as indicated earlier.

In Delhi, India, emissions from vehicles are estimated to account for about 67 percent of air pollution levels (Ministry of Environment and Forests 2009). With a population of 16 million, Delhi is the second largest urban area in India after Mumbai. After years of economic growth, and increasing rates of car ownership, Delhi has some of the worst air pollution levels in the world. As a result, the population of Delhi is constantly exposed to environmental health risks associated with high levels of air pollution, such as respiratory and cardiovascular disease, asthma, and other ailments. According to recent estimates, over 900 new private vehicles are registered in Delhi every day, and this figure is expected to rise in the future (Gentleman 2007). Studies of the association between air pollution and human health show clear and positive relationships between increasing air pollution levels and mortality in Delhi. A 100-microgram increase in total suspended particles has been associated with a 2.3 percent increase in deaths. Moreover, the number of life years that could be saved per avoided death by improving air quality are expected to be greater for an urban area like Delhi, where the population is relatively young, than for cities in the United States (Cropper and others 1997).

## Fuel Types

Diesel fuel is one example of a fuel type used by a large number of public and private vehicles which has emissions containing chemicals with adverse consequences for human health. U.S. Environmental Protection Agency (EPA 2002) studies summarized by Zimmerman (2004, 194) indicate that diesel emissions account for a large portion of nitrogen oxide emissions in the United States. Approaches to reducing this risk include substituting clean diesel, which attempts to address nitrogen oxides, particulate matter, and sulfur dioxides (Zimmerman 2004, 197).

### Fuel Additives

Fuel additives are major contributors to human health. As summarized by Zimmerman (2004), additives have been a basic part of gasoline, since the automobile was introduced, serving a variety of functions. One is "anti-knock," that is, preventing premature combustion of the fuel that produces knocking in the engines. Another function is to meet oxygenated fuel requirements under the Clean Air Act. A number of additives have had unanticipated health side effects. Tetraethyl lead was originally an anti-knock additive until 1978 when it was withdrawn. It was withdrawn because it interfered with catalytic converters that cleaned car exhausts, yet it had a dramatic effect on human health, measured in terms of blood lead levels. Tetraethyl lead was replaced by methyl tertiary butyl ether (MTBE), which was also withdrawn since it contaminated water supplies.

### Hazardous Material Spills

Spills from truck transport of petroleum and chemical products pose health and safety problems. In 2002, the U.S. DOT reported 2.2 billion tons of hazardous materials shipments. Materials representing the largest number of miles in transit in 2002 were explosives, toxics (poison), and oxidizers and organic peroxides (U.S. DOT, BTS, and U.S. Bureau of the Census 2004b).

By mode, hazardous materials are reported to move by truck, rail, air, pipeline, water, and parcel (U.S. Postal Service). Trucks predominate, accounting in 2002 for 53 percent of all hazardous materials transport modes, based on tonnage transported (U.S. DOT, BTS, and U.S. Bureau of the Census 2004a). For pipelines, an analysis of Office of Pipeline Safety data and U.S. Government Accountability Office (GAO) findings from 1989 to 1998 revealed an average of about 22 deaths per year from hazardous liquid accidents (Restrepo, Simonoff, and Zimmerman 2009).

### Other Health Risks Associated with Transit

Risk factors for human health associated with transit, other than those related to types of fuel used, are very varied and include steel dust released from steel wheels and rails, noise, track fires from debris, electric problems, and electro-magnetic fields (Zimmerman 2005).

### Climate Change and Associated Health Impacts

The link between climate change, transportation, and human health and safety is twofold. First, transportation contributes to about a third of greenhouse gas

(GHG) emissions. Between 1995 and 2005, U.S. passenger cars and light-duty trucks accounted for about 61 percent of all transportation-related carbon dioxide ($CO_2$) emissions. Second, the link to health and safety is that the consequences of climate change can contribute to deaths and injuries through sea level rise, extreme weather, and heat, and these are increasing. The New York City Panel on Climate Change (NPCC 2009, 3–4), for example, showed that by the 2080s, temperature is estimated to rise by 4–7.5 degrees F, precipitation by 5–10 percent, sea levels by 12–23 inches, with extreme events increasing in frequency and severity.

The U.S. Department of Energy (DOE 2007, 15, Figure 9) has summarized $CO_2$ emissions from energy use by transportation (including gasoline and diesel fuel use): transportation emissions of $CO_2$ from energy from 1990 to 2006 increased 25.6 percent (407.5 million metric tons) and represented 46.4 percent of the increase in total $CO_2$ from all sectors; in 2005 and 2006 (estimated), petroleum accounted for 98 percent of the $CO_2$ emissions from transportation-sector energy consumption. Moreover, the U.S. EPA (2008, ES-8) noted that transportation accounts for about one-third of the fossil-fuel-combustion $CO_2$ emissions. Passenger cars contribute the most carbon dioxide, and trucks are second.

Growing congestion in urban areas increases fuel use and air pollution emissions, including $CO_2$ (Frank and Engelke 2005). According to the Texas Transportation Institute, total fuel wasted from congestion increased from 0.5 billion gallons to 2.9 billion gallons between 1982 and 2005 (Schrank and Lomax 2009, 3).

## Safety

Modes of travel vary dramatically in terms of safety. Basic accident statistics by mode from the U.S. DOT (DOT, BTS 2007, 40, Table B-1) show that in 2006, highway travel led all modes in terms of fatalities, accounting for 42,642 fatalities, or 95 percent of the total, and was the sector in which fatalities increased over time. Within that category, passenger car occupants accounted for the largest number of fatalities (42 percent), followed by light truck occupants (30 percent). Railroad, waterborne (primarily recreational boating), air, and transit ranked next in that order in fatalities in 2006. Injuries showed a somewhat similar pattern, with highway travel accounting for by far the largest number of injuries, followed by railroad, transit, waterborne, and air travel (U.S. DOT, BTS 2007, 43, Table B-4).

Road traffic deaths and injuries are a major public health concern worldwide. Over one million people are killed in road accidents every year. In 2002, this was the eleventh leading cause of death in the world and one of the top causes of deaths among people aged 10–24 years. Moreover, between 30 and 50 million people are injured in road traffic accidents every year. Injuries and fatalities associated with transportation around the world are expected to rise in the future, as car ownership is increasing rapidly in many countries (see Table 19.2). In 2000, the fatality rate for the world was estimated as 13 deaths per 100,000 people. Among regions, Latin America and the Caribbean recorded the highest figure: 26 deaths per 100,000 people. In addition, the cost of road accidents is estimated to exceed $500 billion around the world (WHO 2004).

## Transportation and Security

Transportation systems, with long stretches of unprotected areas, are vulnerable to intentional attacks due to vandalism, sabotage, and terrorism. Points where vehicles and stations concentrate are also vulnerable. Transportation security in general in the United States is governed by the National Infrastructure Protection Plan (NIPP) and the Sector Specific Plan for transportation.

For transit, the Mineta Institute found 631 attacks from 1920–1997 worldwide; these were primarily outside the United States, led by India and Pakistan (Mineta International Institute 1997; Zimmerman 2005, 25). The 1995 sarin attack on Tokyo subways was a chemical attack, but most transit attacks are bombings. The larger attacks in London and Madrid from bombing have underscored the vulnerability of transit systems and increased human exposure. Public transportation terrorism-prevention legislation and funding in the United States has included transit security, and vulnerability assessments are an important part of the process of maintaining security (Zimmerman 2005, 25). Transit systems can recover relatively quickly (Zimmerman and Simonoff 2009).

Roadway attacks in the form of sniper attacks in the United States instill fear as well as take lives. According to the U.S. GAO (2009), critical highway segments were identified in 2007, and vulnerability assessments have been completed for them.

# IMPROVING THE SYSTEM

Many options exist to lower the health impacts of urban transportation. These include changing travel behavior in a way that reduces travel and fuel use, using alternative fuels, changing modes of travel to those that reduce exposure to emissions and promote exercise, and adopting new vehicle technologies and alternative fuels that lower emissions.

## Reduction in Fuel Use

The federal government has had a targeted program to increase fuel efficiency by reducing emissions per mile traveled. In spite of reductions in fuel economy fostered by the CAFE standards of Title V of the Energy Policy Conservation Act of 1975 (described previously), increases in VMT have overshadowed the savings.

## Alternative Fuels

New fuels are being developed—including biofuels, hydrogen, clean diesel, and compressed natural gas—that potentially reduce GHG and other polluting emissions from their use in transportation. The use of hydrogen as a potential fuel has been debated on a number of grounds, including the need for fuel cells for storage. Fuel cell technology is still in development and encompasses a very wide variety of technologies. According to the U.S. EPA (2007), fuel cells "convert chemical energy to electrical energy by combining hydrogen from fuel with oxygen from the air."

Because of the poor air quality in Delhi, as seen in the example above, the Centre for Science and Environment, a nongovernmental organization, sued the authorities to improve air quality. The Supreme Court of India mandated a program to end the use of diesel-powered buses in Delhi and the use of compressed natural gas (CNG) was mandated for the public transport system. The Delhi Transport Corporation now operates the world's largest fleet of CNG buses, and by December 2002, all diesel buses had been taken off the street. There are about 10,000 taxis, 12,000 buses and 80,000 rickshaws powered by CNG (Clean Air Initiative in Latin American Cities 2009; Centre for Science and Environment 2009). Despite these transportation improvements, the air pollution benefits of this program have not stopped the deterioration of air quality in Delhi as economic growth and car ownership continue to increase.

## Green Auto Technologies

In the automobile industry, many new technologies for vehicle design, fuel use, and fuel type have moved to the forefront of the public's attention. These include electric vehicles, such as hybrid electric vehicles, plug-in hybrid electric vehicles, battery electric vehicles, and zero-emission vehicles. Limiting factors are their reliance on batteries, which have limited storage capacity, and reliance on chemicals that are rare and often not found in the United States.

## Fuel-Efficient Modes: Promoting Walking

After decades of promoting the use of private vehicles and the construction of roads and highways, many urban areas are now actively promoting walking as an alternative transportation mode. It is both environmentally friendly and promotes physical exercise and a healthy lifestyle. Interest in promoting walking has been sparked by increasing trends in obesity. In 2007, thirty states in the United States had a prevalence of obesity of 25 percent of the population or greater (Centers for Disease Control [CDC] 2009a). Perhaps of greatest concern are the increases in childhood obesity rates. For children aged 6 to 11 years, prevalence increased from 6.5 percent to 17.0 percent. Similarly, for children aged 12–19 years, prevalence increased from 5.0 percent to 17.6 percent (CDC 2009b).

In response to these trends, a number of programs are being implemented in urban areas around the world to promote walking. One simple and effective example is the use of "walking school buses," which allow children to walk to school while supervised by adults. The more complex walking school buses include structured routes with meeting points, a timetable, and a set of adult volunteers. Given safety and liability concerns, most structured walking school buses may also require cooperation of security authorities and others (Pedestrian and Bicycle Information Center 2009). The CDC has developed a program called KidsWalk-to-School as part of its efforts to better health through physical activity (CDC 2007).

Sometimes promoting walking and physical activity can be accomplished by providing the general public and public transit users with adequate information. Besides promoting physical activity and a healthy lifestyle, walking can sometimes be an optimal transportation mode, saving time and reducing congested public transportation systems and the use of vehicles. In London, for example, walklines are being added to maps of the London Underground to inform users about distances and expected times to popular destinations where walking can save time by avoiding changing metro lines and travel through various stations (Rodcorp 2009).

Promoting health through physical activity and walking is also being done through more comprehensive urban planning programs that encourage walking and bicycling. One example is the Greenway Project in the South Bronx, New York City, initiated by two local groups—Sustainable South Bronx and the Point Community Development Corporation. The centerpiece of this project is a continuous bicycle and pedestrian trail along the Hunts Point waterfront to provide local communities with access to the waterfront and increased opportunities for physical exercise in an area that has traditionally had high densities of diesel-truck traffic associated with industrial and manufacturing activities such as waste transfer stations, food markets, and others (Mathews Nielsen Landscape Architects, PC 2006).

## Fuel-Efficient Modes: Promoting Bicycling

Many cities around the world are also promoting bicycling to increase the diversity of transportation modes, provide alternatives to more conventional modes of transportation, encourage environmentally friendly transportation, and to provide opportunities for increased physical exercise. Programs to promote bicycling are gaining popularity as cities attempt to reduce their carbon footprints and reduce obesity rates.

Self-service bike transit systems are among the most popular, consisting of stations where people can pick up and drop off bicycles by using a technology similar to that used for shopping carts in shopping centers and supermarkets. Users can pick up a bicycle at a station and drop it off at any other station, depending on their destination by simply unlocking and locking the bicycles at the terminals. A bank or credit card or a prepaid user card is usually used for this purpose. The bicycle terminals are generally close to other modes of transportation, such as metro stops, do not require any staff, and are always available. Most programs give users an initial free period to use the bicycles, for example, thirty minutes or one hour, charging a fee per hour thereafter. In Europe, these programs are in use in Paris, Lyon, and Vienna. London, Montréal, San Francisco, and New York City are at various stages of considering or implementing similar programs.

Vienna started a bike transit program called Citybike Wien in 2003. It now has 60 terminals around the city, most close to a metro station. Due to high levels of vandalism in a previous program, users are now required to pay 1 Euro to register in the program with a bank or credit card. Figure 19.2 shows a bicycle terminal. The Citybike Wien program allows users to use a bicycle for free for one hour and charges a fee of 1 Euro for the second hour, 2 Euros for the third hour, and 4 Euros for each additional hour (Citybike Wien 2009).

## Fuel-Efficient Modes: Promoting Transit

The environmental economies achieved by rail and bus transit, the two major transit modes, depend on vehicle use relative to capacity (since an "empty seat" uses energy but does not increase transit use) and the use of green technologies aimed at transit, for example, in the area of fuel use and fuel efficiency.

**Bus Rapid Transit Systems**  Public transportation is a critical component of people's mobility alternatives in urban areas around the world, especially bus transport. The city of Curitiba in the state of Paraná in the south of Brazil has one of the most famous public transportation systems in the world. It evolved

FIGURE 19.2  Citybike Wien Self-Service Bike Transit System

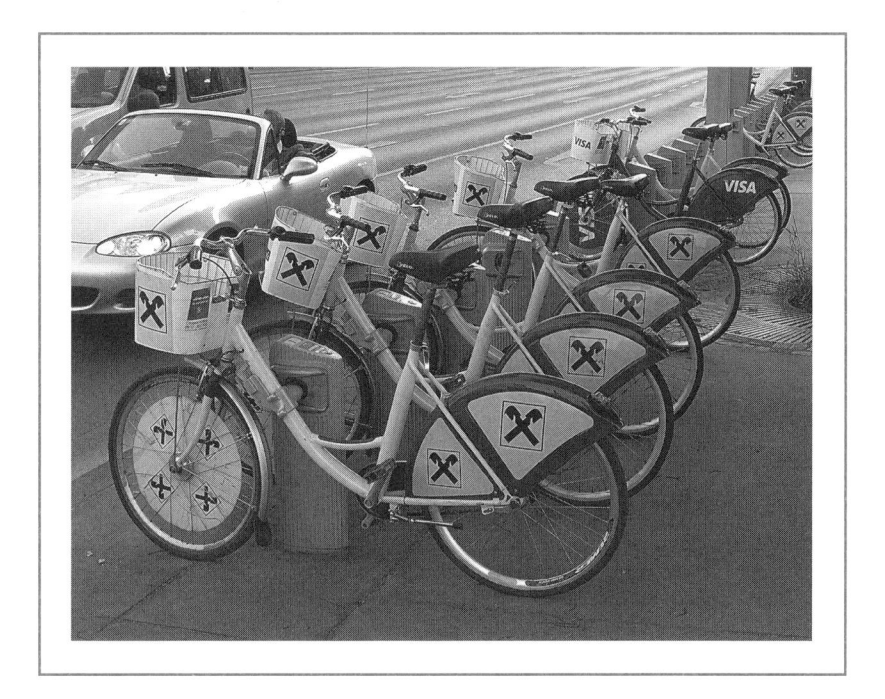

Photo by Carlos E. Restrepo.

under the leadership of Mayor Jaime Lerner in the early 1970s as part of a broad array of innovative urban planning initiatives. Curitiba, like many cities in the developing world, experienced a very rapid rate of population growth in the second half of the twentieth century, growing from about 300,000 people in 1950 to over 2.1 million in the 1990s. This rising population and a rising rate of car ownership were also causing high levels of air pollution (Rabinovitch and Leitman 1996).

To address these issues, zoning for growth and transportation were gradually oriented along five transportation axes over this period. Express bus lanes were included in the middle lanes, which greatly enhanced access to public transportation and efficiency. These were also connected to feeder buses. The centerpiece of Curitiba's transportation system is a Bus Rapid Transit (BRT) system that uses double- and triple-length articulated buses that can carry up to 270 passengers on express lanes.

Tube stations made of glass and steel allow passengers to pay the fare at a turnstile when they enter the stations and before boarding the buses. These stations work like subway stations and make boarding and exiting the buses much

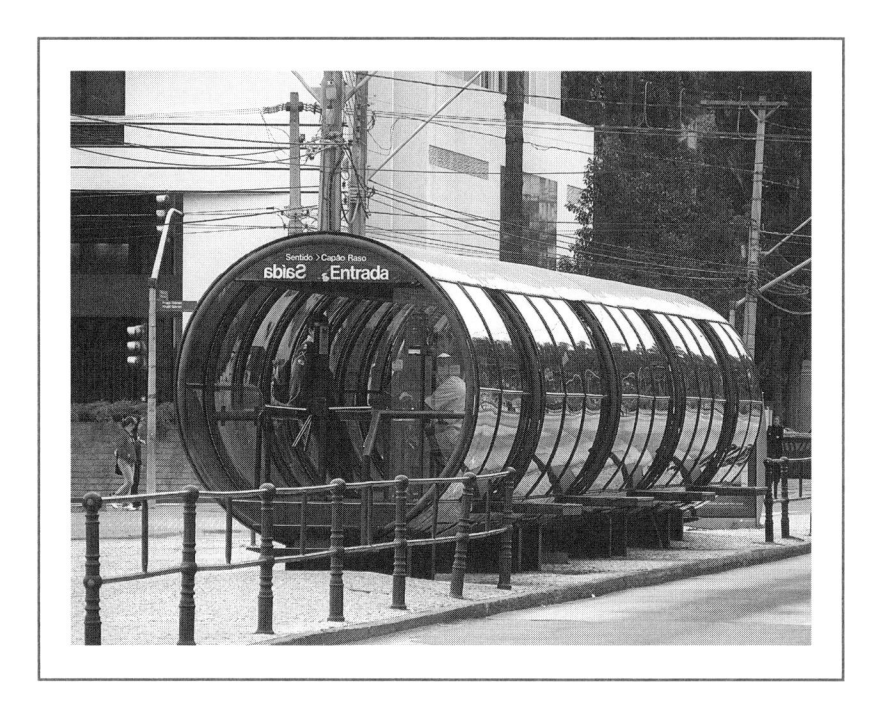

## FIGURE 19.3  A Tube Bus Station in Curitiba, Brazil

Photo by Carlos E. Restrepo.

quicker. According to some estimates, having such bus stations has reduced total travel time by one-third. They also allow the passengers to wait for the buses in an "indoors" environment. Some stations also allow passengers to transfer to other routes and change the direction of their travel while paying a single fare (Rabinovitch and Leitman 1996). Figures 19.3 and 19.4 show the tube bus stations in Curitiba, Brazil.

The BRT system in Curitiba evolved from a need to improve public transportation with limited financial resources. Constructing a subway system would have cost about $60–70 million per kilometer in Curitiba. But the BRT system cost approximately $200,000 per kilometer, including the tube stations (Rabinovitch and Leitman 1996). About 70 percent of commuters in this city use the BRT system and as a result, the per capita use of fuel and air pollution emissions are lower than other cities of comparable size in Brazil (Goodman, Laube, and Schwenk 2005). The system is also highly regarded for its accessibility to disabled people (Lima Camisão Costa 2001). The success of this system has been adapted by many

FIGURE 19.4  A Tube Bus Station and Articulated Bus in Curitiba, Brazil

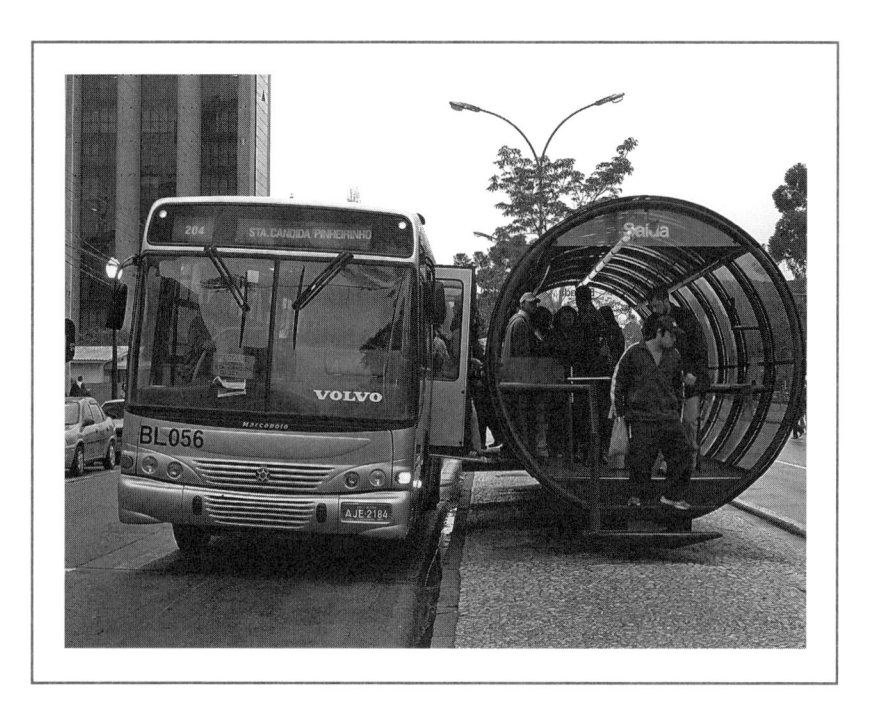

Photo by Carlos E. Restrepo.

other cities around the world, where transportation access, time travel reductions, and environmental benefits are often cited as important considerations.

The city of Bogotá has also implemented a successful BRT system called Transmilenio (DANE 2005). Similarly, México City has adopted a BRT system named Metrobús as part of a broad plan to improve air quality and transportation access and efficiency (City Mayors Statistics 2006).

**Rail Transit**  Rail transit systems are characterized by fuel efficiency and generally lower air emissions per unit of travel (ridership, miles of travel) relative to travel by buses and personal vehicles. However, rail does use electric power, which may be associated with air pollution and greenhouse gas emissions if it is generated using coal or fossil fuels. Rail transit usage in major systems throughout the world has in general been on the rise. The Phoenix, Arizona, metro area is one recent example, which began operating a light rail system in December

2008 that covers a distance of 20 miles and includes twenty-eight stations. The light rail system services customers in the cities of Phoenix, Tempe, and Mesa. In April 2009, the system had over one million total boardings, and there are plans to extend the system (Valley Metro 2008). Wide use of such rail transit systems in urban areas can result in reduced fuel use per capita, reduced air pollution emissions per capita, and reduced environmental health risks associated with air pollution.

## Promoting Transportation Access and Economic Development: Medellín's Metrocable

The world's population is growing predominantly in urban areas in developing countries. According to United Nations estimates in 2008, over half of the world's population was living in urban areas. Unfortunately, a large part of this growth is taking place in poorly planned areas characterized by minimal or nonexistent basic infrastructure services, including water, sanitation, and transportation, and by nondurable housing. About one-third of the world's population is living in slums, with about 60 percent of all slum dwellers living in Asia, 20 percent in Africa, and 14 percent in Latin America and the Caribbean. In some urban areas of Africa, over 90 percent of the population lives in slums (United Nations Human Settlements Programme 2003). In terms of transportation, these areas often lack access to public transportation, which limits the ability of residents to obtain employment, and often they are very close to rail lines and highways, adding to the environmental health risks faced by these communities.

An innovative transportation project in the metropolitan area of Medellín, Colombia's second largest urban area, shows that improving access to transportation in poor neighborhoods and promoting economic development can go hand in hand. A cable-car system named Metrocable was developed to connect Santo Domingo Savio, a densely populated poor suburb of Medellín, located on a mountainside, with the main metro line that provides access to the downtown area. The location of Santo Domingo Savio made transportation access there difficult, and the aerial cable car has solved this problem while providing opportunities for economic development and tourism in an area that has traditionally been considered low-income and plagued by crime and violence.

As a result of this innovative transportation project, Santo Domingo Savio is changing. Nearly 45,000 passengers ride Metrocable every day. The length of the route is 2,072 meters, and the elevation is 399 meters. A projected extension to the line will allow passengers to access an ecotourism park. Besides the transportation and economic benefits, this transit system is considered environmentally friendly because it is run by electricity from hydro resources, so there are virtually zero emissions of greenhouse gases. At night, each cable car uses a light powered with energy stored in batteries and produced from photovoltaic cells mounted on its roof (MedellinInfo 2009).

## SUMMARY

Urban transportation affects public health directly for passengers and indirectly for bystanders and community residents. The human health effects range from the impact of vehicle emissions on cardiopulmonary and other diseases to health problems related to lack of physical activity. The latter is reflected in high and rising obesity rates in many countries around the world, which result from transportation systems that have traditionally discouraged walking and other forms of exercise. The amount of travel reflected in VMT and the way travel is accomplished, as indicated by congestion and choice of mode, are also key factors influencing health.

Transportation-related accidents, and road traffic in particular, are a leading and rising cause of injuries and fatalities around the world. New technologies and modifications to existing transport practices through fuel economy and improvements, as well as the public and political will to implement these approaches, are now moving toward ways of transcending these problems that should benefit health. A number of innovative improvements to transportation systems aim to reduce dangerous air pollution emissions, change to more environmentally friendly fuel sources, and promote greater physical activity such as walking and bicycling.

## REFERENCES

American Public Transportation Association (APTA). 2009. *Public transportation fact book*, Appendix A: Historical tables. Washington, DC: APTA. http://www.apta.com/research/stats/factbook/documents09/2009_fact_book_final_part_2.pdf.

Centers for Disease Control and Prevention (CDC). 1982. Current trends blood-lead levels in U.S. population. *MMWR Weekly* 31(10):132–134.

Centers for Disease Control and Prevention (CDC). 2007. *KidsWalk-to-School*. http://www.cdc.gov/nccdphp/dnpa/kidswalk/index.htm.

Centers for Disease Control and Prevention (CDC). 2009a. U.S. obesity trends 1985–2007. *Overweight and obesity*. http://www.cdc.gov/nccdphp/dnpa/obesity/trend/maps/.

Centers for Disease Control and Prevention (CDC). 2009b. Childhood obesity. *Healthy youth*. http://www.cdc.gov/healthyyouth/obesity/.

Centre for Science and Environment. 2009. *Air pollution*. http://www.cseindia.org/.

Citybike Wien. 2009. Citybike Wien—The free city bike in Vienna. http://www.citybikewien.at/.

City Mayors Statistics. 2006. The world's largest cities and urban areas in 2006. http://www.citymayors.com/statistics/urban_2006_1.html.
Clean Air Initiative in Latin American Cities. 2009. CNG buses in Delhi. *Infopool*. http://www.cleanairnet.org/infopool/1411/propertyvalue-19513.html.
Cropper, M. L., N. B. Simon, A. Alberini, and P. K. Sharma. 1997. The health effects of particulate air pollution in Delhi, India. Policy Research Working Paper 1861, World Bank.
Departamento Administrativo Nacional de Estadisticas (DANE). 2005. Censo general 2005 (Colombia). http://www.dane.gov.co/files/censo2005/resultados_am_municipios.pdf.
Frank, L. D., and P. Engelke. 2005. Multiple impacts of the built environment on public health: Walkable places and the exposure to air pollution. *International Regional Science Review* 28(2):193–216.
Gentleman, A. 2007. Study finds air quality in Delhi has worsened dramatically. *International Herald Tribune*, November 6. http://www.iht.com/articles/2007/11/06/asia/delhi.php.
Goodman, J., M. Laube, and J. Schwenk. 2005. Curitiba's bus system is model for rapid transit. *Race, Poverty and the Environment*, Winter 2005/2006. Oakland, CA: Urban Habitat.
Lima Camisão Costa, V. 2001. The Curitiba transport system in Brazil: An example of universal design within developing economies. *Disability World*, January–February, n.p. http://www.disabilityworld.org/01-02_01/access/curitiba.htm.
Mathews Nielsen Landscape Architects, PC. 2006. South Bronx Greenway Executive Summary. http://www.ssbx.org/documents/SouthBronxGreenwayExecSummarySection1.pdf.
MedellinInfo. n.d. Metrocable. http://www.medellininfo.com/metro/metrocable.html].
Mineta International Institute for Surface Transportation Policy Studies. 1997. *Protecting surface transportation systems and patrons from terrorist activities*. Washington, DC: The Institute.
Ministry of Environment and Forests, Government of India. 2009. White paper on pollution in Delhi with an action plan. http://envfor.nic.in/divisions/cpoll/delpolln.html.
National Transit Database. 2007. Annual databases: RY 2007 data tables. http://www.ntdprogram.gov/ntdprogram/data.htm.
New York City Panel on Climate Change (NPCC). 2009. Climate risk information. http://www.nyc.gov/html/planyc2030/downloads/pdf/nyc_climate_change_report.pdf.
Pedestrian and Bicycle Information Center for the Partnership for a Walkable America. 2009. Starting a walking school bus. http://www.walkingschoolbus.org/.
Rabinovitch, J., and J. Leitman. 1996. Urban planning in Curitiba. *Scientific American* March: 46–53.
Restrepo, C. E., J. S. Simonoff, and R. Zimmerman. 2009. Causes, cost consequences, and risk implications of accidents in U.S. hazardous liquid pipeline infrastructure. *International Journal of Critical Infrastructure Protection* 2(1+2):38–50.
Rodcorp. 2003. London Tube Map with Walklines: Sometimes it's quicker to walk. http://rodcorp.typepad.com/rodcorp/2003/10/london_tube_map.html.
Schrank, D., and T. Lomax. 2009. *Urban mobility report 2009*. College Station, TX: Texas Transportation Institute, Texas A&M University. http://tti.tamu.edu/documents/mobility_report_2009_wappx.pdf
Sommer, M. 2005. Will the oil market continue to be tight? In *World economic outlook, globalization and external imbalances*, Ch. 4. Washington, DC: IMF. http://www.imf.org/external/pubs/ft/weo/2005/01/pdf/chapter4.pdf.

United Nations Human Settlements Programme. 2003. *The challenge of slums: Global report on human settlements.* London: Earthscan.

U.S. Department of Energy (DOE). 2007. *Greenhouse gas emissions in the U.S. 2006.* Washington, DC: Energy Information Administration, Office of Integrated Analysis and Forecasting. ftp://ftp.eia.doe.gov/pub/oiaf/1605/cdrom/pdf/ggrpt/057306.pdf.

U.S. Department of Transportation (DOT), Bureau of Transportation Statistics (BTS). 2007. *Transportation statistics annual report 2007.* Washington, DC: U.S. DOT. Also available online at http://www.bts.gov/publications/transportation_statistics_annual_report/2007/pdf/entire.pdf.

U.S. Department of Transportation (DOT), Bureau of Transportation Statistics (BTS). 2009. National transportation statistics, Table 1-1: System mileage within the United States (statute miles). http://www.bts.gov/publications/national_transportation_statistics.

U.S. Department of Transportation (DOT), Bureau of Transportation Statistics (BTS), and U.S. Bureau of the Census. 2004a. *Hazardous Materials, 2002 Economic Census, Transportation, 2002 Commodity Flow Survey*, Table 1a. Also available online as Table 1–56: U.S. Hazardous Materials Shipments by Transportation Mode, 1997. http://www.bts.gov/publications/national_transportation_statistics/2004/html/table_01_56.html.

U.S. Department of Transportation (DOT), Bureau of Transportation Statistics (BTS), and U.S. Bureau of the Census. 2004b. *Hazardous Materials, 2002 Economic Census, Transportation, 2002 Commodity Flow Survey*, Table 2a. Also available online as Table 1–57: U.S. Hazardous Materials Shipments by Hazard Class, 1997. http://www.bts.gov/publications/national_transportation_statistics/2004/html/table_01_57.html.

U.S. Department of Transportation (DOT), Federal Highway Administration (FHA). 2003. Highway statistics summary to 1995: Motor vehicles. http://www.fhwa.dot.gov/ohim/summary95/section2.html.

U.S. Department of Transportation (DOT), Federal Highway Administration (FHA). 2005. *Assessing the effects of freight movement on air quality at the national and regional level, final report*, Chapter 2. http://www.fhwa.dot.gov/environment/freightaq/chapter2.htm#fig2_4.

U.S. Department of Transportation (DOT), Federal Highway Administration (FHA). 2008a. *Highway statistics 2006*, Vehicle registrations, fuel consumption, and vehicle miles of travel as indices: Table MVFVM. http://www.fhwa.dot.gov/policy/ohim/hs06/htm/mvfvm.htm.

U.S. Department of Transportation (DOT), Federal Highway Administration (FHA). 2008b. *Highway statistics 2007*, Annual vehicle distance traveled in miles and related data: Table VM-1. http://www.fhwa.dot.gov/policyinformation/statistics/2007/vm1.cfm.

U.S. Department of Transportation (DOT), Federal Highway Administration (FHA). 2009. December 2008 traffic volume trends. http://www.fhwa.dot.gov/ohim/tvtw/08dectvt/index.cfm.

U.S. Department of Transportation (DOT), Federal Transit Administration (FTA). 2008. National transit database (Annual Issues), Table 21. http://www.ntdprogram.gov/ntdprogram/pubs/dt/2008/2008_Data_Tables.htm#57.

U.S. Environmental Protection Agency (EPA). 2002. *Health assessment document for diesel engine exhaust.* Washington, DC: U.S. Government Printing Office.

U.S. Environmental Protection Agency (EPA). 2007. Basic information. *Fuel cells and vehicles*. http://www.epa.gov/fuelcell/basicinfo.htm.

U.S. Environmental Protection Agency (EPA). 2008. *Inventory of U.S. greenhouse gas emissions and sinks: 1990–2006*. Washington, DC: U.S. EPA. Also available online at http://www.epa.gov/climatechange/emissions/downloads/08_CR.pdf.

U.S. Government Accountability Office (GAO). 2009. *Federal efforts to strengthen security should be better coordinated and targeted on the nation's most critical highway infrastructure*. Washington, DC: U.S. GAO.

Valley Metro. n.d. News and Media Center. http://www.valleymetro.org/valley_metro/pressroom/.

Wikipedia. n.d. Metro systems by annual passenger rides. http://en.wikipedia.org/wiki/Metro_systems_by_annual_passenger_rides (accessed September 26, 2009).

World Health Organization (WHO). 2004. *World report on road traffic injury prevention*. Geneva: WHO.

Zimmerman, R. 2004. Social and environmental dimensions of cutting-edge infrastructures. In *Moving people, goods and information in the 21st century*, ed. R. E. Hanley, 189–210. London: Routledge.

Zimmerman, R. 2005. Mass transit infrastructure and urban health. *Journal of Urban Health* 82(1):21–32.

Zimmerman, R., and J. S. Simonoff. 2009. Transportation density and opportunities for expediting recovery to promote security. *Journal of Applied Security Research* 4:48–59.

# CHAPTER TWENTY

# INFORMAL SETTLEMENTS: IN SEARCH OF A HOME IN THE CITY

**VANESSA WATSON**

## LEARNING OBJECTIVES

- Review current debates and issues regarding informal settlements
- Identify reasons informal settlements develop and persist
- Discuss the advantages and disadvantages to poor households of living in informal settlements
- Determine the serious problems which the scale and rate of growth of informal settlements is likely to present in poorer cities
- Review the range of strategies which have been used in the past to address the growth of informal settlements and those which at the present time appear to have greater potential
- Discuss the role that community-based and "bottom-up" strategies play in generating meaningful policies and actions in informal settlements

IN many cities and towns, particularly in poorer countries, large numbers of people live in informal settlements. Very often, the majority of these urban populations lives in informal environments, and in many urban areas this form of shelter can now be considered the norm rather than the exception. This chapter will define and characterize informal settlements, give an idea of their extent and location, review the reasons why they emerge and persist, and counter some of the myths that surround them. These settlements present a range of problems, both to the people who have to live in them and to urban managers and administrators. That living in such settlements may not be conducive to health is self-evident, and this chapter will not dwell on the links between informality and health. Some of the approaches that have been taken to address the issue of informal settlements will be discussed, highlighting those ideas that appear to have the potential to improve living conditions.

Informal settlements cannot be viewed in isolation from the wider range of socioeconomic, political, spatial, and institutional aspects of urban areas. Current thinking on informal settlements has moved away from a narrow sectoral perspective on housing alone. Now, informal settlements are understood as the product of poverty and inequality, social and spatial exclusion, and inappropriate urban planning that fails to deliver well-located serviced land and that enforces a regulatory framework which requires people to step outside of the law to survive in urban areas. The clear implication of this is that urban strategies to address informal settlements need to go well beyond the physical planning and upgrade of infrastructure and buildings, which still tends to be the policy focus in many parts of the world.

## DEFINITIONS OF INFORMAL SETTLEMENT

In 1999, the United Nations launched its "cities without slums" initiative, and since that time, numerous international development agencies and publications have used the term *slums* to refer to areas of inadequate shelter. Particularly prominent was the 2003 UN-Habitat Global Report entitled *The Challenge of Slums*. In these reports, the word *slums* is used to describe all kinds of inadequate shelter: informal settlements, inner-city older tenement blocks, and working-class housing areas that have become overcrowded and run-down. This chapter avoids the use of the word *slums*, both because it confuses many different types of inadequate living environments and because it can be used to homogenize both the occupants of these areas and the strategies needed to improve them.

To complicate matters further, different parts of the world use different terms to refer to informal settlements. In some parts of the world, the term *squatter settlements* is used; in Brazil, *favelas* are settlements founded through land invasions and established through processes of self-help; in Argentina, *villa miseria* describes invaded settlements; in Chile, *callampa* refers to settlements that have mushroomed overnight (Gilbert 2007). Some terms refer to the process that established the settlement, some refer to the nature of land tenure and occupation, and some refer to the materials from which houses are made. In most cases, the implication is that the settlements are in some way illegal, but this does not automatically imply that they will be subject to legal action.

More problematically, the terms referring to informal settlements are often understood to characterize the people living within them. It is often assumed that inhabitants are poor, unemployed, uneducated, disorganized, apathetic, unhealthy, criminal, rurally oriented, and unwilling to meet their responsibilities as urban citizens. While this may be true of some people in informal settlements, it can also be true of people living in other types of accommodation or areas, and it is usually not true for all people living in an informal settlement. Populations of informal settlements are complex and heterogeneous. The problem with assumptions of demographic homogeneity is that they can lead to the belief that a single type of approach to improvement and upgrade can be used, regardless of location and context; in reality, careful contextual research and community engagement needs to be undertaken to understand the precise nature of informal settlements and the processes which underlie them, before improvement programs can be initiated. For the purposes of this chapter, informal settlements will be regarded as those areas that have been developed largely through community or individual effort and outside of formal institutional processes and regulations; aspects of the settlement (infrastructure, services, shelters, tenure) may not conform to formal legal requirements and may be deficient in ways that are detrimental to health and well-being.

# SCALE, LOCATION, AND TRENDS OF INFORMAL SETTLEMENTS

Informal settlements are widespread in cities and towns of the Global South (or developing countries), but they are also common in cities of transitional countries (Eastern European countries once part of the Soviet Union) and are not unknown in cities of the Global North (developed countries). Rapid urbanization, increasing poverty, and governments lacking the resources, capacity, or political will to increase supplies of serviced urban land have meant that increasing numbers of people have been unable to access formal shelter and serviced urban land, so informal settlements have grown rapidly over the past decades. It is estimated that the most rapid rates of urbanization will, in future years, occur in Africa and Asia. The "demographic transition" in these continents is yet to come and will occur (certainly in the context of Africa) under conditions of low economic growth (UN-Habitat 2008). It can therefore be expected that informal settlements will continue to proliferate.

The largest number of "slum dwellers" (which includes informal settlements) is found in Asia (particularly China and India), followed by sub-Saharan Africa and then Latin America (UN Millennium Project 2005). In many cities in these regions, the majority of urban populations live in informal settlements: in Brazil in the second half of the 1990s, 84 percent of all new housing units were built informally, mostly by low-income groups with no access to formal finance (Mitlin and Satterthwaite 2004); in sub-Saharan Africa, one-half to three-quarters of the populations of most cities live in informal settlements, and the bulk of new housing is provided this way (UN-Habitat 2009). With the 2008 global financial crisis, economic growth has slowed in many parts of the world, and it is likely that the capacity of governments to provide urban housing and services will similarly be reduced, as will the ability of people to access formal housing. Therefore, the future is very likely to be one of increasing urban informality.

It is important to consider not only the extent of informal settlement but also where it tends to be located within cities. The bulk of rapid urban growth in developing countries is now taking place in the peri-urban areas, as poor urban dwellers look for a foothold in the cities and towns where land is more easily available, where they can escape the costs and threats of urban land regulations, and where there is a possibility of combining urban and rural livelihoods. These kinds of areas are impossibly costly to plan and service in the conventional way, given the form of settlement. Even if that capacity did exist, few could afford to pay for such services. The attractiveness of these kinds of locations for poor households is that they can avoid the costs associated with formal and regulated systems of urban land and service delivery. However, because of this, environmental issues in these areas are particularly critical, in terms of both the natural hazards to which these settlements are exposed and the environmental damage that they cause.

# WHY INFORMAL SETTLEMENTS FORM AND PERSIST

There is a great deal of misunderstanding regarding how informal settlements form and emerge, and this, in turn, frequently leads to simplistic housing policies and strategies that may do no more than displace informal settlements from one location to another. Mitlin and Satterthwaite (2004, 15) argue that inadequate housing must be viewed as an aspect of urban poverty. They suggest that there are eight interlinked aspects of urban poverty: inadequate and unstable income; an inadequate and risky asset base (which is both material and nonmaterial, including education and housing); inadequate provision of public infrastructure and basic services; limited or no safety net for times when income fails; inadequate protection of poorer groups' rights through the law; and poorer groups' powerlessness within political systems. Occupants of informal settlements are caught in a vicious circle: they are unable to afford alternative living conditions, and the living conditions themselves trap them into ongoing poverty.

Households in informal settlements find themselves subject to a range of marginalizing forces, which propel them into these kinds of areas. The first set of forces is legal and regulatory, and often occurs through the urban planning system. Many cities in the Global South have inherited colonial planning legislation, originally designed for European or American contexts. Zoning ordinances stipulate building standards and materials for housing as well as tenure requirements. For example, in Cameroon, without an official building permit, an approved building plan, and land title, a house is regarded as informal (Njoh 2003, 142). Yet securing these involves five different government agencies and is a long and expensive process that most poor people cannot understand or afford. Inevitably, the bulk of housing in many African and Asian cities is classed as "informal."

The second set of forces is related to the urban land and property market. Many cities and towns in the Global South have experienced growing rates of property and land development in recent decades, often with the aim of constructing new shopping malls, sports stadiums, conference centers, golf estates, and so on. These projects usually seek out well-located land and frequently displace older and poorer residential areas, whose residents are unable to find alternative accommodation in the formal property market. Such households end up in informal settlements. This can also occur through developments initiated by the public sector. For example, the implementation of the 1979 master plan for Abuja, the capital of Nigeria, gave rise to extensive informal settlements that house a growing indigenous population as well as people employed in Abuja but unable to find housing. By 2006, 800,000 people had been evicted from this land that was "zoned for other purposes under the Master Plan" and, in some cases, has been allocated to private developers. Evicted nonindigenes were offered access to 500-square-meter plots at some distance from the city, but this required a payment of $2,612 and building a house based on certain planning standards within two years, or rights to the plot are lost (COHRE 2006).

The third set of forces is political. Households may find themselves in informal settlements as a result of political action or because they belong to a different ethnic or cultural group from those with political power. Yiftachel and Yacobi (2003), writing in the context of Israel/Palestine, describe how whole communities are overlooked by the planning process, as it is considered that they belong elsewhere. Defining these (Palestinian) settlements as informal allows the authorities to ignore them when it comes to providing urban services and urban rights, and as a result they are condemned to unserviced, deprived, and stigmatized urban fringes. In Zimbabwe in 2005, President Robert Mugabe ordered an eviction of 700,000 people from their homes in the capital of Harare, as part of what was called Operation Murambatsvina (also termed "Restore Order, Cleanup, and Drive out the Rubbish"). This eviction was carried out under British colonial planning legislation (still in force), but it was widely interpreted as a move against political opposition.

A fourth set of forces that can lead to informal settlements lie (ironically) in state strategies to implement low-income housing policies. Neoliberal housing policies followed by many countries in the Global South have promoted a belief in freehold tenure and have often taken the form of providing small, formal, and serviced units under private ownership. Certain influential housing "experts" (for example, Hernando de Soto) have argued that the urban poor who occupy land are sitting on "dead capital," and all that is needed to eradicate poverty is for them to raise bank finance against their property as security and use it to start small businesses. Unfortunately, it is not that simple to overcome poverty (Gilbert 2002), and experience has shown that poor households are rarely willing to risk their land and house by mortgaging it to formal financial institutions (Benda-Beckman 2003; Mitchell 2004). Nonetheless, governments persist with this approach, which means that accessing formal land is cumbersome, slow, and very expensive for poor households. Therefore, the demand for urban land by lower-income groups regularly outstrips supply, and such households have no option but to move to informal settlements.

These factors discussed above (and indicated in Table 20.1) show that the reasons households find themselves in informal settlements are complex and often the result of forces beyond their control. There are many myths which suggest that people who live in informal settlements do so in order to escape "law and order," are too lazy to secure "proper" jobs and homes, or only see themselves as temporarily in the urban area and thus have no interest in upgrading and improving their living conditions. There is little possibility of addressing the issue of informal settlements unless the full complexity of these areas is understood.

## LIVING IN AN INFORMAL SETTLEMENT

Occupants of informal settlements often find there are both advantages and disadvantages. As far as advantages are concerned, such places may be cheaper to live in than new housing estates or inner city locations, as long as "shacklords" or protection racketeers do not extort an extra income from households. Families may also find that land and housing is cheaper, but there are other costs, such as high transport costs if their settlement is on the urban periphery, and possibly high water and energy costs if these have to be obtained through small vendors. One advantage of self-built shelters is that they are often bigger than private rental units or government provided units, and spaces can be planned to suit family needs. Allowing space for a full extended family is often very important for sharing child-rearing, cooking, and care of the aged and sick. Space can be left outside of the shelter for growing food, storage, or rituals, and the house can be designed to accommodate income-generating activities, such as informal businesses or subletting. Table 20.1 shows the large proportion of people who had moved to an informal settlement for privacy, which reflects a need for more space. Informal settlements often create their own public spaces (a factor usually left out of formal residential areas) where community activities, selling, and interaction happens.

TABLE 20.1   Reasons for Moving to the Kayamandi Zone F Informal Settlement (Cape Town)

| Reasons for Moving | Number of Households in Sample | Percentage |
| --- | --- | --- |
| Overcrowding, lack of space, privacy | 87 | 59 |
| Evicted | 31 | 20 |
| High rent | 14 | 9 |
| Nowhere else to go/needed shelter | 8 | 5 |
| Conflict/violence | 4 | 3 |
| Death of partner/divorce | 2 | 1 |
| Don't know | 2 | 1 |
| Total | 148 | 100% |

Source: W. Smit, 2006, Planning in contemporary Africa, Informal settlements: A perpetual challenge, ed. M. Huchzermeyer and A. Karam, Cape Town: UCT Press, 109.

The problems of informal settlements are often related to the larger-scale services and infrastructure that cannot be provided to these households on their own. So access to drinking water and electricity is difficult, as is the disposal of solid waste and sewerage. These factors have obvious public health implications. Households also lack the capacity to respond to disasters, such as floods, fire, and strong winds. Often, informal settlements occur on land that has been avoided by formal developers because it is in some way undesirable: the land may be very steep, inaccessible, or liable to flood. For these reasons, informal settlements are often under greater threat from the effects of climate change than are other urban areas. Finally, these households may be under greater threat from criminals and gangs, given the usual lack of police services and criminals' ability to hide more easily in informal settlements. Informal settlements in Latin American cities have become notorious havens for organized crime, to the extent that gangs sometimes take control of areas and keep out all government functionaries.

Most households do not live in informal settlements by choice—they live there because there is no affordable or accessible alternative. Efforts by governments to remove these settlements simply displace them to other areas. For this reason, it is crucial to understand the wider socioeconomic and political factors that need to be addressed in housing policy, as well as the technical and physical ones.

# STRATEGIES

Government policies aimed at addressing the issue of informal settlements vary from country to country and have shifted over time. Huchzermeyer and Karam (2006, 22) have developed a typology of responses to informal settlements. They suggest six possible strategies, noting that numbers 4–6 result from a growing influence of civil society organizations in policy making:

1. Repressive—removal of informal settlements.
2. Deterministic—rigid prescription of a "good" solution, often with little understanding of people's livelihoods and socioeconomic reality. Such approaches can lead to displacement or the imposition of expensive alternatives on households.
3. Tolerant/ambivalent—often based on a cost-benefit analysis regarding votes before an election.
4. Transitional—temporary occupational rights in the informal settlement, with a view to future relocation, often with little consideration of the impact of uncertainty on people's fragile livelihoods.

5. Giving amnesty—immunity to eviction, possibly involving temporary or permanent occupation rights.
6. Transforming—upgrading infrastructure and facilities, formalizing land tenure and integrating the informal settlement into the surrounding urban fabric, while also seeking to address the larger socio-economic and legal framework. This approach would also include formally recognizing residents as having a right to the city (see the box "What Is Adequate Shelter?"), and allowing their organizations to have a role in planning and policymaking.

Strategies that seek to transform informal settlements need to consider such specific approaches to this process (see UN-Habitat 2009, Chapter 7).

Tenure arrangements based on freehold title may be problematic, as this is the most costly and complex form of tenure and can often conflict with traditional

## What Is Adequate Shelter?

In the UN-Habitat Agenda, all member states affirmed their commitment "to the full and progressive realization of the right to adequate housing, as provided for in international instruments" and recognized in this context "an obligation by Governments to enable people to obtain shelter and to protect and improve dwellings and neighborhoods."

The Agenda defines "adequate shelter" as

> More than a roof over one's head. It also means adequate privacy; adequate space; physical accessibility; adequate security; security of tenure; structural stability and durability; adequate lighting, heating, and ventilation; adequate basic infrastructure, such as water supply, sanitation and waste management facilities; suitable environmental quality and health-related factors; and adequate and accessible location with regard to work and basic facilities, all of which should be available at an affordable cost. Adequacy should be determined together with the people concerned, bearing in mind the prospect for gradual development. Adequacy often varies from country to country, since it depends on specific cultural, social, environmental, and economic factors. Gender-specific and age-specific factors, such as the exposure of children and women to toxic substances, should be considered in this context.

*Source:* UN Millennium Project, 2005, *Task force on improving the lives of slum dwellers: A home in the city*, London: Earthscan, 41.

tenure arrangements that are still in place and supported. Group titling may be one alternative, although this has not always been successful. An alternative may be to recognize and document previous and existing land transactions and agreements, drawing perhaps on written or verbal evidence. In some parts of Africa, this is being done using videotapes and GPS systems.

One of the more innovative approaches to informal transformation is in Brazil. Informal areas have been demarcated as ZEIs (zones of "special interest") where the free market in land is suspended. These programs concentrate on the right to adequate and affordable housing rather than on absolute property rights. A form of leasehold, the Concession of the Real Right to Use (CRRU), was adopted (typically thirty years, inheritable, and registered in the names of both partners where appropriate), and specific planning regulations (plot size, construction standards, and so on) appropriate for the existing low-income population were used.

A further vital component of upgrade is community involvement. This is important in part to gain an understanding of the particular dynamics of an informal settlement, in part to build confidence and organizing capacity, and in part to draw on community resources for upgrade, especially in situations where municipalities lack the funding and manpower to undertake these tasks. Where the public finance is lacking to install sewage treatment works or fresh-water pipes, it may be necessary to rely on small and localized infrastructure and service provision, for example, to undertake the digging of latrine pits and the sale of water by community-based vendors. There is a growing recognition among policy makers concerned with informal settlement that community involvement is crucial for success. The recent UN Millennium Project report on improving the lives of slum dwellers (2005, 3) placed as its top requirement "the recognition that the urban poor are active agents and not passive beneficiaries of development." In effect, this requires working with local communities to upgrade settlements and negotiating all planning decisions and infrastructure developments with them.

It is important to note a growing realization that upgrading existing settlements is only part of the answer. There also needs to be a program to open up new and well-located areas of land for settlement at a sufficient rate which preempts the formation of new informal settlements. Various strategies have been suggested to achieve this goal. The provision of new trunk infrastructure, together with the release of related land, can serve as an attraction to newly settling households. In a Land Banking approach, a municipality would buy up and hold land for future settlement, timing the release of this land to guide new settlement. This land can also be held by communities in a Community Land Trust arrangement. However, all of these strategies require well-functioning local governments and well-organized local communities who can work together, and often these requirements are lacking.

## SUMMARY

This chapter has argued that informal settlements are increasingly a phenomenon in cities (primarily, but not only) in the Global South, and as urbanization and poverty are set to increase in this part of the world, it can be expected that the extent of these kinds of settlements will continue to grow. In many cities, the dominant form of accommodation is now informal. However, the factors that give rise to these settlements are complex, and many causes are within the scope of government action if the political will exists. Particularly important are the planning and regulatory aspects of urban development, which compel the poor to break the law if they are to survive in the urban areas. Given the extensive literature and research on informal settlements where these aspects are identified, it is therefore of concern that housing policies in so many parts of the world still fail to reflect the dynamics of informality in the actions undertaken to address the issue.

This chapter has introduced readers to the complexities and dilemmas of informal settlements, and to some of the ideas that have been promoted to improve living conditions for their inhabitants. Many policy approaches have focused on a narrow understanding of why informal settlements emerge and persist: they have failed to appreciate the wide range of factors (regulatory, economic, and political) that underlie this urban form, and they have often relied on narrow solutions that attempt to address only the physical and infrastructure aspects of informal settlements. The chapter has argued that if the aim of policy is to promote "adequate" shelter (see the box "What Is Adequate Shelter?"), then a far more comprehensive and intersectoral approach is required.

The chapter suggests that a better understanding is needed of the demographic complexity of inhabitants of these areas as well as the various reasons that propel people into them and induce them to remain there. There are numerous disadvantages of living in informal settlements, but there are also advantages for people who are poor and unemployed. These understandings should inform the nature of interventions to upgrade and improve informal settlements.

## REFERENCES

Benda-Beckman, F. 2003. Mysteries of capital or the mystification of legal property? *Focaal: European Journal of Anthropology* 41:187–191.

Center on Housing Rights and Evictions (COHRE). 2006. Forced evictions: Violations of human rights. *Global Survey* 10. Geneva: COHRE.

Gilbert, A. 2002. On the mystery of capital and the myths of Hernando de Soto. *International Development Planning Review* 24(1):1–19.

Gilbert, A. 2007. The return of the slum. Does language matter? *International Journal of Urban and Regional Research*, 31(4):697–713.

Huchzermeyer, M., and A. Karam, eds. 2006. *Informal settlements: A perpetual challenge?* Cape Town: UCT Press.

Mitchell, T. 2004. The properties of markets: Informal housing and capitalism's mystery. Working paper no. 2, Cultural Political Economy Working Paper Series, Institute for Advanced Studies in Social and Management Sciences, University of Lancaster.

Mitlin, D., and D. Satterthwaite, eds. 2004. *Empowering squatter citizens: Local government, civil society and urban poverty reduction.* London: Earthscan.

Njoh, A. 2003. Planning in contemporary Africa: The state, town planning and society in Cameroon. Aldershot, UK: Ashgate.

Smit, W. 2006. Understanding the complexities of informal settlements: Insights from Cape Town. In *Informal settlements: A perpetual challenge?* ed. M. Huchzermeyer and A. Karam. Cape Town: UCT Press.

UN-Habitat. 2003. *The challenge of slums: Global report on human settlements.* Nairobi: UN Habitat. Also available online at http://www.unhabitat.org/pmss/listItemDetails.aspx?publicationID=1156.

UN-Habitat. 2008. *The state of the world's cities 2008/2009.* Nairobi: UN-Habitat.

UN-Habitat. 2009. *Planning sustainable cities: Global report on human settlements 2009.* London: Earthscan. Also available online at http://www.unhabitat.org/content.asp?typeid=19&catid=555&cid=5607.

UN Millennium Project. 2005. *Task force on improving the lives of slum dwellers: A home in the city.* London: Earthscan.

Yiftachel, O., and H. Yacobi. 2003. Control, resistance and informality: Urban ethnocracy in Beer-Sheva, Israel. In *Urban informality: Transnational perspectives from the Middle East, Latin America and South Asia*, eds. N. Al-Sayyad and A. Roy. Boulder, CO: Lexington.

# CHAPTER TWENTY-ONE

# URBAN AIR QUALITY

## JONATHAN M. SAMET

### LEARNING OBJECTIVES

- Identify the complex mixture and multiple sources of urban pollution—local, regional, and even transnational

- Discuss urban "hot spots" for a complex mixture of pollutants that convey high exposures

- Review air quality management strategies, which include controlling emissions at the source, reducing the volume of emissions, and decreasing population exposure

- Describe innovative solutions that are needed which involve urban planning and transportation management

# URBAN HEALTH

AIR pollution in cities has long been known to harm the health of urban dwellers. The density of combustion sources in urban environments produces pollution that is typically visible and readily evident, and levels were high enough in many places in the past to have posed a clear public health threat. The air pollution experience in London, long one of the world's largest cities, has been well documented (Brimblecombe 1987). As early as the reign of Edward I (1272–1307), the pollution of London by coal smoke prompted a royal proclamation banning burning of "sea-coal" in craftsmen's open furnaces (Brimblecombe 1987). In 1661, John Evelyn published *Fumifugium or the Aer and Smoake of London Dissipated*, documenting a worsening air pollution problem in London and describing approaches to improve air quality. However, air pollution was not effectively regulated in England until approximately two centuries later with the passage of the Smoke Nuisance Abatement Act and the Alkali Act, directed at industrial pollution.

During the twentieth century, excess mortality was documented in London at times when "fogs," episodes of atmospheric stagnation, occurred and air pollution levels were high. The most dramatic episode, the London Fog of 1952, caused thousands of excess deaths (Figure 21.1; Bell and Davis 2001). The high levels of smoke (an index of airborne particles) and sulfur dioxide during the fog—approximately two orders of magnitude higher than values

FIGURE 21.1  Weekly Mortality and Sulfur Dioxide Levels Before, During, and After the London Fog of December 1952

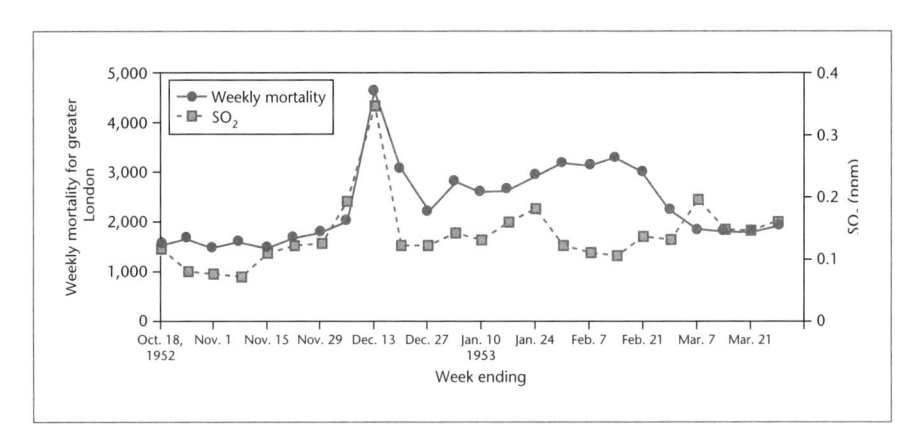

*Source:* M. L. Bell and D. L. Davis, 2001, Reassessment of the lethal London fog of 1952, *Environmental Health Perspectives* 109(Suppl 3).

permitted under the most recent World Health Organization (WHO) guidelines (WHO 2006)—reflected coal combustion for space heating, industrial emissions, and vehicles. This and other disasters during the twentieth century motivated research, including epidemiological studies, on the health effects of air pollution and the development of evidence-based approaches to air quality management.

Now, air quality has improved in most of the large cities in more developed countries, consequent to regulation, reduced emissions from vehicles, and a sharp decline in smokestack industries within urban areas. However, air pollution remains a threat to public health in many large cities in less developed countries, reflecting industry and power generation, high-emitting vehicles, burning of biomass fuels for space heating and cooking, and dust suspended by wind and traffic. The problems are particularly severe in the ever-increasing mega-cities, such as Bangkok, Beijing, Jakarta, and Mexico City. Mega-cities—urban agglomerations with populations of at least 10 million—now number nineteen, posing major challenges for assuring environmental quality (Table 21.1). Additionally, air pollution is no longer a localized problem, and air pollution within an urban area may be adversely affected by short- and long-range transport of pollutants, particularly particles. Crutzen and Ramanathan (2003) proposed the term "atmospheric brown 'clouds'" to refer to wide-reaching pollution by particles which may extend transnationally and across continents.

One problem particular to cities is exposure to emissions from traffic, as many homes are immediately adjacent to roadways or in proximity to major thoroughfares. Recent studies raise concern that proximity to traffic with associated exposure to fresh emissions may by itself threaten public health, adding risk beyond that coming from the general mixture of air pollution in cities (White and others 2005; Health Effects Institute 2009). Slow-moving traffic now chokes many mega-cities, leading to emissions from idling vehicles and high levels of exposure to those living and working along thoroughfares and to the people in vehicles.

This chapter provides a perspective on air quality and health in urban areas. There is already voluminous evidence on the health effects of air pollution, which has been the basis for air quality regulation. This evidence is periodically summarized by the U.S. Environmental Protection Agency (EPA) in its Integrated Science Assessment documents (National Center for Environmental Assessment 2009) and the World Health Organization's Air Quality Guidelines. Global Update 2005 provides a succinct review for major pollutants (WHO 2006). The chapter provides an introduction to the problem of air pollution in urban areas, covering sources and concentrations of pollutants and associated health risks.

TABLE 21.1  Annual Ambient Air Quality in Global Mega-cities

| Mega-City | Population (millions) | Total Suspended Particles | SO$_2$ | NO$_2$ |
|---|---|---|---|---|
| Tokyo, Japan | 35.7 | 40 | 19 | 55 |
| New York-Newark, USA | 19.0 | 27 | 22 | 63 |
| Mexico City, Mexico | 19.0 | 201 | 47 | 56 |
| Mumbai, India | 19.0 | 243 | 19 | 43 |
| São Paolo, Brazil | 18.8 | 53 | 18 | 47 |
| Delhi, India | 15.9 | 405 | 18 | 36 |
| Shanghai, China | 15.0 | 246 | 53 | 73 |
| Kolkata, India | 14.8 | 312 | 19 | 37 |
| Dhaka, Bangladesh | 13.5 | 516 | 120 | 83 |
| Buenos Aires, Argentina | 12.8 | 185 | 20 | 20 |
| Los Angeles-Long Beach-Santa Ana, USA | 12.5 | 39 | 9 | 66 |
| Karachi, Pakistan | 12.1 | 668 | 13 | 30 |
| Cairo, Egypt | 11.9 | 593 | 37 | 59 |
| Rio de Janeiro, Brazil | 11.7 | 139 | 15 | 60 |
| Osaka-Kobe, Japan | 11.3 | 34 | 19 | 45 |
| Beijing, China | 11.1 | 377 | 90 | 122 |
| Manila, Philippines | 11.1 | — | — | — |
| Moscow, Russia | 10.5 | 150 | 15 | 170 |
| Istanbul, Turkey | 10.1 | — | — | — |

Pollution Measurements (µg/m$^3$)

*Sources:* Population of mega-cities obtained from United Nations Department of Economic and Social Affairs, 2008, *World Urbanization Prospects: The 2007 Revision.* Air quality measurement data obtained from B. R. Gurjar and others, 2008, Evaluation of emissions and air quality in megacities, *Atmospheric Environment* 42(7), 1593–1606. Data not available for Manila and Istanbul.

# EXPOSURE TO AIR POLLUTION IN URBAN ENVIRONMENTS

The concept of personal exposure is central to characterizing the risks of urban air pollution. Exposure, defined as the contact of a person with the pollutant of concern, is calculated for air pollutants as the product of the concentration of the pollutant in the place(s) where time is spent with the time spent in that place,. Total personal exposure to a pollutant reflects the concentrations in the various places where time is spent, weighted by the time spent in each.

The microenvironmental model is useful for estimating personal exposure and for assessing the contributions of different environments to exposure; this concept defines total personal exposure as the sum of exposures received in the various microenvironments where time is spent. A microenvironment is defined as a place where time is spent that has a particular pollutant concentration profile during the time spent there; for example, a motor vehicle might represent a microenvironment during time spent commuting, and a restaurant where a meal is eaten would be another.

This model is useful for considering the numerous microenvironments relevant to considering exposures to urban air pollution and associated risks to health. Table 21.2 lists some of these microenvironments along with pollution sources. Within framework of the microenvironmental model, there are a number of specific microenvironments of particular relevance to the health of urban dwellers. The residence is particularly important because most people spend the majority of their time at home. In urban areas, the air contaminants in the home include those generated by indoor sources, such as cooking and smoking of tobacco, and the penetration of outdoor air pollutants indoors, including those pollutants generated by traffic and by nearby and more distant sources. The streets, which may have "hot spots" of air pollution generated by traffic or industrial sources, are another key and distinct microenvironment.

TABLE 21.2 Sources of Pollution in Urban Microenvironments

| Microenvironment | Sources | Pollutants |
|---|---|---|
| Home | Cooking, space heating, parked vehicles, hobbies, smoking, household products, pets, rodents, insects | PM, CO, $NO_x$, VOCs, allergens |
| Transportation environments | Vehicle and industrial emissions, road dust, background pollution, smoking | PM, including ultrafine PM, CO, $NO_x$, $O_3$, VOCs, aeroallergens, carcinogens |
| Streets | Vehicle emissions, road dust, background pollution | PM, including ultrafine PM, CO, $NO_x$, $O_3$, VOCs, carcinogens, lead |
| Work environments | Industrial processes, smoking, background pollution | PM, CO, VOCs, $NO_x$, carcinogens |
| Entertainment environments | Cooking and space heating, background pollution, smoking | PM, VOCs, carcinogens |

Note: PM = particulate matter; CO = carbon monoxide; $NO_x$ = nitrogen oxides; $O_3$ = ozone; VOCs = volatile organic compounds.

# MAJOR URBAN AIR POLLUTANTS AND HEALTH RISKS

This section provides a brief introduction to the principal air pollutants of concern in urban areas. Table 21.3 provides an overview of the major air pollutants in urban areas, their sources, principal adverse health effects, and U.S. standards and WHO guideline concentrations. While the pollutants are covered individually, following current regulatory approaches, they are present in a complex pollution mixture that varies spatially and temporally. The toxicity of the mixture may be determined by its overall composition and the interactions among its components and not fully captured by the risks of its components.

TABLE 21.3  Major Urban Air Pollutants: Sources, Health Effects, and Regulations[a]

| | Source Types and Major Sources | Health Effects | Regulations and Guidelines |
|---|---|---|---|
| Lead | Primary<br>Anthropogenic: Leaded fuel (phased out in some locations such as the U.S.), lead batteries, metal processing | Accumulates in organs and tissues. Learning disabilities, cancer, damage to the nervous system. | U.S. NAAQS:<br>Rolling 3-month average: 0.15 µg/m$^3$<br>Quarterly average: 1.5 µg/m$^3$<br>WHO Guidelines:<br>Annual: 0.50 µg/m$^3$ |
| Sulfur dioxide | Primary<br>Anthropogenic: Combustion of fossil fuel (power plants), industrial boilers, household coal use, oil refineries<br>Biogenic: Decomposition of organic matter, sea spray, volcanic eruptions | Lung impairment, respiratory symptoms. Precursor to PM. Contributes to acid precipitation. | U.S. NAAQS:<br>Annual arithmetic mean: 0.03 ppm (80 µg/m$^3$)<br>24-hour average: 0.14 ppm (365 µg/m$^3$)<br>WHO Guidelines:<br>10-minute average: 500 µg/m$^3$<br>24-hour average: 20 µg/m$^3$ |
| Carbon monoxide | Primary<br>Anthropogenic: Combustion of fossil fuels (motor vehicles, boilers, furnaces)<br>Biogenic: Forest fires | Interferes with delivery of oxygen. Fatigue, headache, neurological damage, dizziness. | U.S. NAAQS:<br>1-hour average: 35 ppm (40 mg/m$^3$)<br>8-hour average: 9 ppm (10 mg/m$^3$)<br>WHO Guidelines:<br>15-minute average: 100 mg/m$^3$<br>30-minute average: 60 mg/m$^3$<br>1-hour average: 30 mg/m$^3$ |

TABLE 21.3 (Continued)

| | Source Types and Major Sources | Health Effects | Regulations and Guidelines |
|---|---|---|---|
| Particulate matter[b] | Primary and secondary Anthropogenic: Burning of fossil fuel, wood burning, natural sources (e.g., pollen), conversion of precursors ($NO_x$, $SO_x$, VOCs) Biogenic: Dust storms, forest fires, dirt roads | Respiratory symptoms, decline in lung function, exacerbation of respiratory and cardiovascular disease (e.g., asthma), mortality. | U.S. NAAQS: PM10 24-hour average 150 µg/m³ PM 2.5 Annual arithmetic mean: 15 µg/m³ 24-hour average: 35 µg/m³ WHO Guidelines: PM10 Annual: 20 µg/m³ 24-hour average: 50 µg/m³ PM2.5 Annual: 10 µg/m³ 24-hour average: 25 µg/m³ |
| Nitrogen oxides | Primary and secondary Anthropogenic: Fossil fuel combustion (vehicles, electric utilities, industry), kerosene heaters Biogenic: Biological processes in soil, lightning | Decreased lung function, increased respiratory infection. Precursor to ozone; Contributes to PM and acid precipitation. | U.S. NAAQS for $NO_2$: Annual arithmetic mean: 0.053 ppm (100 µg/m³) Related to compliance with NAAQS for ozone. WHO Guidelines for $NO_2$: 1-hour average: 200 µg/m³ Annual: 40 µg/m³ |
| Tropospheric ozone | Secondary Formed through chemical reactions of anthropogenic and biogenic precursors (VOCs and $NO_x$) in the presence of sunlight | Decreased lung function, increased respiratory symptoms, eye irritation, broncho-constriction. | U.S. NAAQS: 1-hour average: 0.12 ppm (235 µg/m³). Applies in limited areas. 8-hour average: 0.075 ppm (147 µg/m³) WHO Guidelines: 8-hour average: 100 µg/m³ |
| "Toxic" pollutants ("hazardous" pollutants) (e.g., asbestos, mercury, dioxin, some VOCs) | Primary and secondary Anthropogenic: Industrial processes, solvents, paint thinners, fuel | Cancer, reproductive effects, neurological damage, respiratory effects. | EPA rules on emissions for more than 80 industrial source categories (e.g., dry cleaners, oil refineries, chemical plants) EPA and state rules on vehicle emissions |

(Continued)

TABLE 21.3 (Continued)

| | Source Types and Major Sources | Health Effects | Regulations and Guidelines |
|---|---|---|---|
| Volatile organic compounds (e.g., benzene, terpenes, toluene) | Primary and secondary<br>Anthropogenic: Solvents, glues, smoking, fuel combustion<br>Biogenic: Vegetation, forest fires | Range of effects, depending on the compound.<br>Irritation of respiratory tract, nausea, cancer.<br>Precursor to ozone.<br>Contributes to PM. | EPA limits on emissions<br>EPA toxic air pollutant rules<br>Related to compliance with NAAQS for ozone |
| Biological pollutants (e.g., pollen, mold, mildew) | Primary<br>Biogenic: Trees, grasses, ragweed, animals, debris<br>Anthropogenic systems, such as central air conditioning, can create conditions that encourage production of biological pollutants. | Allergic reactions, respiratory symptoms, fatigue, asthma. | |

*Source:* Modified from M. L. Bell and J. M. Samet, 2009, Air pollution, *Environmental health: From global to local*, Ch. 12, ed. H. Frumkin, San Francisco: Jossey-Bass.

NAAQS = National Ambient Air Quality Standards; WHO = World Health Organization; EPA = Environmental Protection Agency;
PM = particulate matter; $NO_x$ = nitrogen oxides; $SO_x$ = sulfur oxides; $NO_2$ = nitrogen dioxide; VOCs = volatile organic compounds.

[a] This table lists only a sample of the sources and health effects associated with each pollutant. Additionally, health effects may be the result of characteristics of the pollutant mixture rather than the independent effects of a pollutant. Additional legal requirements often apply, such as state regulations.
[b] Sources and effects of PM can differ by size.

### Particulate Matter

"Particulate matter" (PM) refers to a general type of pollution comprising solid or liquid particles suspended in air. While treated as a specific type of pollution, PM is itself a mixture, reflecting its many sources and chemical and physical processes that lead to particle formation from various gaseous pollutants. Particulate matter can be primary (directly emitted from the source) or secondary (formed in the atmosphere through physical and chemical conversion of gaseous precursors, such as nitrogen oxides [$NO_x$], sulfur oxides [$SO_x$], and volatile organic compounds [VOCs]). The sources of primary PM include the burning of fuel in stationary and mobile sources; unpaved roads and road dust; industry; wood burning stoves; and from natural sources such as pollen, dust, salt spray, and erosion. The composition of PM differs by geographic area, reflecting the source mix and other local characteristics, and it can vary with season, source, and meteorology. This variation may be a source of variability in risk to health.

Particles are generally categorized by size, using a measure called aerodynamic diameter. PM10 refers to particles with an aerodynamic diameter of 10 microns or less, but PM2.5, or "fine PM", has an aerodynamic diameter up to 2.5 microns, and "ultrafine" particles have an aerodynamic diameter up to 0.1 microns. "Coarse PM" (PM10–2.5) refers to particles with an aerodynamic diameter

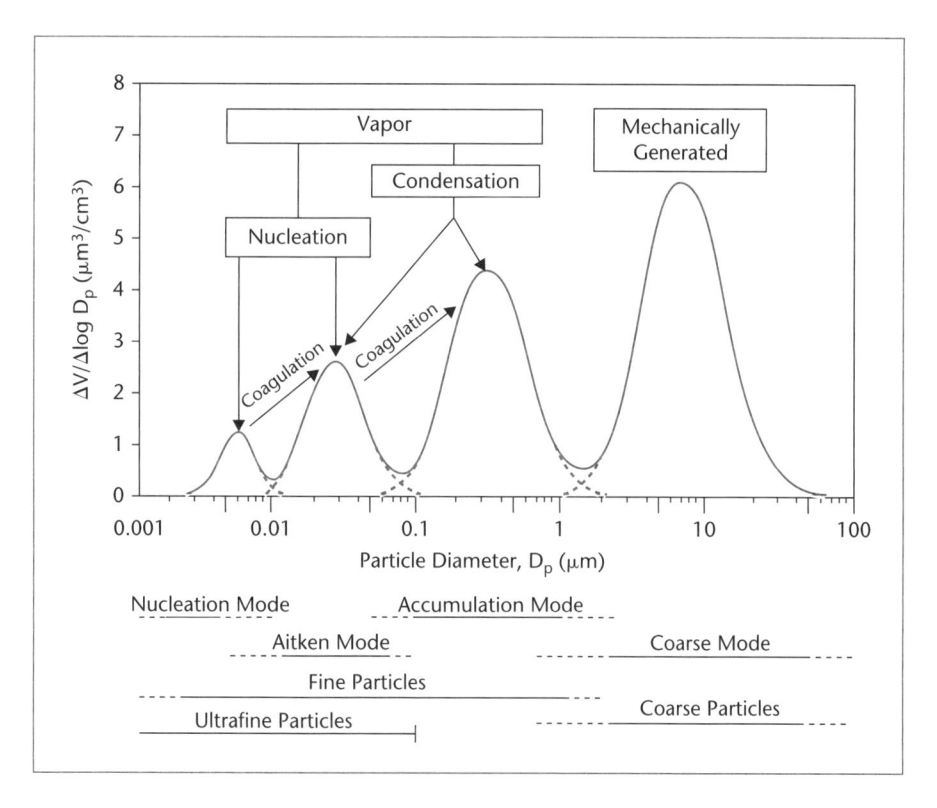

FIGURE 21.2 Modes of Particulate Matter

*Source:* U.S. Environmental Protection Agency, 2004, Air quality criteria for particulate matter, Vol I. Research Triangle Park, NC: USEPA, National Center for Environmental Assessment.

between 2.5 and 10 microns. In urban air, there are typically particles in three size modes: coarse (reflecting dust and bioaerosols), fine (reflecting secondary particles from combustion emissions), and ultrafine (reflecting fresh combustion emissions; Figure 21.2). Very small particles are present in fresh combustion emissions, but they quickly agglomerate and become larger through coagulation. A second size mode extends from about 0.1 to 1.0 microns, the size range that penetrates into the deep lung. The third mode comprises the larger or coarse particles.

Smaller particles are of special health concern because they penetrate more deeply into the lung. Such particles are typically generated through combustion processes and often reach high concentrations in urban environments. Levels of ultrafine particles tend to be quite high adjacent to heavily trafficked roads. Diesel exhaust, a combination of gases and particles, is of particular concern because of widespread diesel vehicle use in urban areas and because the diesel particles are in a size range that penetrates into the deep lung.

PM in outdoor air has been associated with a wide range of health effects, including increased hospital and emergency room admissions, respiratory symptoms, excess rate of decline in pulmonary function, exacerbation of chronic respiratory and cardiovascular diseases, and premature mortality (Pope and Dockery 2006; U.S. EPA 2008). Laboratory animals exposed to PM experienced a range of responses including inflammation and pulmonary injury as well as indication of cardiac dysfunction (Brook and others 2004; U.S. EPA 2008). Time-series studies—tracking day-to-day variation in health outcomes in relation to variation in PM levels—have shown that acute PM exposure is associated with higher risk for hospitalization and mortality, reminiscent of the London episodes, but occurring even at modern levels of PM exposure (Samet and others 2000). Cohort studies that involve long-term observation of people in cities having a range of pollution levels show that those people residing in cities with higher PM levels have greater mortality (Pope and Dockery 2006).

## Sulfur Dioxide

$SO_2$ is a water-soluble gas that was a primary component of the 1952 London Fog. Sulfur oxides are produced from the combustion of sulfur-containing fuels and materials, such as coal and metal ores and diesel. Some coal, such as that from the Eastern United States and parts of China, has particularly high sulfur content. Power plants are a main source of $SO_2$ emissions in many places, and industrial sources may be important in cities. In port cities, ships may be an important source since the sulfur content of marine fuels has been unregulated. Household use of coal can also contribute significant amounts of $SO_2$. In some areas, such as parts of China, coal is the primary fuel source for cooking and heating and causes high levels of $SO_2$ indoors and contributes to ambient air pollution. Sulfur dioxide levels have dropped in most cities in the more developed countries, as a result of declining smokestack industry, less coal burning locally, and changes in diesel fuel. In fact, Hedley and colleagues (2002) were able to show a benefit to mortality after reduction of the sulfur content of fuels in Hong Kong.

Sulfur dioxide threatens public health, both through its direct effect and its contribution to PM, particularly the sulfate component of PM. Because $SO_2$ is highly soluble in water, most inhaled $SO_2$ is absorbed by the mucous membranes of the upper airways with little reaching the lung; however, increased ventilation and oral breathing, such as from exercise or working outdoors, can raise the dose delivered to the lung (Schlesinger 1999). $SO_2$ exposure has been associated with reduced lung function, bronchoconstriction (increased airway resistance), respiratory symptoms, risk for hospitalizations from cardiovascular and respiratory causes, eye irritation, adverse pregnancy outcomes, and mortality. However, it is difficult to attribute these reported associations to $SO_2$ itself, because it is a precursor to PM and generally exists as a component of a complex, combustion-related pollutant mixture. Experimental studies, involving brief exposures of people with asthma to $SO_2$, suggest that some people with asthma may be highly sensitive to $SO_2$ itself and be at risk for initiation of an asthma attack on exposure. These results imply that urban dwellers with asthma may be at particular risk if they live or work adjacent to sources of $SO_2$.

## Nitrogen Oxides

Nitrogen oxides ($NO_x$) are highly reactive gases containing nitrogen and oxygen, such as nitrogen dioxide ($NO_2$) and nitrogen oxide (NO). $NO_x$ is produced through combustion sources which oxidize nitrogen in air. Sources of $NO_x$ in urban areas include motor vehicle engines, electric utilities, and industries. Indoor sources, many found in urban areas, can also contribute to exposure, including kerosene heaters, gas stoves and heaters, and tobacco smoke. Because $NO_2$ is strongly linked to mobile sources, it is often used as an indicator of traffic-related pollution.

Like ozone, $NO_2$ is nearly insoluble in water and can reach the lower respiratory tract. Health effects of $NO_2$ include irritation of the eyes, nose, and throat at higher concentrations; short-term decreases in lung function; and possibly increased respiratory infections and symptoms for children. Both NO and $NO_2$ are toxic gases, and $NO_2$ is regulated in the United States as a criteria pollutant under the Clean Air Act. Nitrogen oxides also have indirect but important roles as precursors. $NO_x$ is a precursor of tropospheric ozone and secondary particulate matter and plays a crucial role in the formation of acid precipitation. NO is also a greenhouse gas.

### Tropospheric Ozone

Ozone, a gas, is present in the troposphere, the lowest atmospheric layer up to approximately 10 to 15 kilometers above the earth's surface; it is also in the stratosphere, which extends from the troposphere to about 45 to 55 kilometers above the earth's surface. Stratospheric ozone forms the naturally occurring "ozone layer" that protects from ultraviolet radiation, while tropospheric ozone, sometimes called "ground level ozone," is a harmful pollutant. Tropospheric ozone is a colorless gas and a photochemical oxidant formed through complex chemical reactions, involving precursor volatile organic compounds (VOCs) and $NO_x$ in the presence of sunlight. As a result, pollution involving ozone is sometimes referred to as "photochemical smog" or "smog."

Ozone pollution, first identified in Los Angeles, is now a problem in many urban areas because motor vehicles are a major source of its precursors. After ozone precursors are emitted, they can travel downwind in an expanding plume and contribute to the formation of ozone, which itself travels with wind patterns. Therefore, elevated concentrations can result from the transport of ozone and its precursors up to hundreds of miles away; ozone is typically a regional problem, extending across large urbanized regions. Ozone levels are much lower indoors than outdoors, since ozone adsorbs to indoor surfaces and rapidly breaks down. Hence, personal exposure to ozone is dominated by ambient exposure.

Because ozone is not highly soluble in water, it reaches the lower respiratory tract, where it causes damage through oxidant injury. Short-term exposure to ozone for healthy adults has been associated with temporarily decreased lung function, increased resistance to airflow in the lung, and increased respiratory symptoms, such as coughing and wheezing. These changes are reflected by increases in clinic visits, emergency room visits, school absenteeism, and hospitalizations, following high-ozone days. Short-term variation in ozone concentrations has also been associated with daily mortality (Bell and others 2004). Long-term ozone exposure may contribute to the development of chronic lung diseases, such as asthma and bronchitis, and accelerate aging of the lungs. Ozone concentrations have also been linked to impaired lung development in children (Gauderman and others 2002) and with onset of childhood asthma (McConnell and others 2002).

### Carbon Monoxide

Carbon monoxide (CO) is a colorless, odorless gas formed by incomplete combustion of carbon-containing material, such as gasoline, natural gas, oil, coal, tobacco, and other organic materials. Motor vehicles contribute the majority of CO emissions to outdoor air, and consequently, CO concentrations tend to be higher in urban areas with high traffic density and during times of high traffic volume. Carbon monoxide levels may also be high in congested urban areas with stalled and slow-moving traffic. Biomass fuel burning also provides significant CO emissions in some areas, particularly where such fuels are commonly used for heating and cooking. Carbon monoxide has long been a problem in urban areas because of traffic; concentrations have dropped in many urban areas because of vehicle emissions controls, but standards are variable around the world, and undoubtedly CO exposures remain high in many urban areas. There are indoor sources as well, including heating and cooking devices and biomass fuel burning. These indoor exposures add to those outdoors.

When CO is inhaled, it binds to hemoglobin with high affinity to form carboxyhemoglobin (COHb). An increased level of COHb reduces the transport of oxygen to tissues and inhibits the release of oxygen (U.S. EPA 2009). The brain and heart are sensitive to low oxygen conditions and therefore to the effects of COHb on oxygen transport and delivery to tissues. Consequently, people with cardiovascular and respiratory disease are particularly susceptible to CO. Health responses to CO include visual impairment, fatigue, decreased dexterity, dizziness, and nausea. Mortality and severe neurological damage can result from extremely high CO levels, which can occur from CO poisoning from exposures indoors.

## Volatile Organic Compounds

Volatile organic compounds (VOCs) comprise a broad category of organic chemicals with a high vapor pressure: they readily evaporate at normal temperature and pressure. They include benzene, chloroform, formaldehyde, isoprene, methanol, monoterpenes, and hundreds of additional compounds that are of concern in urban environments as both irritants and carcinogens themselves and as precursors to PM and ozone. VOCs originate from natural sources (primarily vegetation, such as oak and maple trees); industrial processes such as chemical processing, solvents, and power plants; and transportation, including motor vehicles and off-road transportation sources, such as aircraft, construction equipment, and lawn mowers. In urban areas, there is a potential for "hot spots" around sources and traffic.

## Lead

Lead has long been a cause of adverse health effects in workers and in the general population. Exposure comes through both ingestion and inhalation; historically, lead in urban air largely came from leaded gasoline, containing lead as an anti-knocking agent. Fortunately, lead has now been removed from gasoline in most countries, and levels of airborne lead have dropped in urban areas in the

United States and elsewhere. However, lead remains in gasoline in some places such as Egypt, Algeria, and Serbia, although the United Nations Commission on Sustainable Development called for its elimination in 1994, and people living near industrial facilities that have lead in their emissions, for example, smelters and battery reprocessing plants, may still have unacceptable exposures.

Lead can be harmful even at low doses because it accumulates in the body, mostly in the bones, which continue to function as an internal source of exposure. The health effects of lead have been studied extensively. Exposure to lead can cause damage to the nervous system and kidneys and can interfere with red blood cell formation, reproductive function, and gastrointestinal function. Children and pregnant women are particularly vulnerable, because the developing nervous system is a target of lead toxicity. To date, a safe level of lead exposure has not been found, and adverse effects on neurocognitive development have been found in association with exposures in contemporary settings (Grant 2009).

### Air Toxics

Hundreds of other ambient air pollutants exist, which are often referred to as "air toxics." These include hydrochloric acid, mercaptans, parathion, naphthalene, biphenyl, vinyl bromide, methyl bromide, dioxin, and cadmium. Exposure to these pollutants can occur through inhalation, but they also enter other environmental media, such as water and food. Health effects of these air toxics include damage to the neurological, immune, respiratory, and reproductive (for example, reduced fertility) systems, as well as developmental problems and some cancers.

## PUBLIC HEALTH IMPLICATIONS OF URBAN AIR POLLUTION

Air pollution continues to contribute to morbidity and premature mortality in urban areas. Fortunately, dramatic episodes, like the London Fog of 1952, appear to have ended. However, there is still a potential for such episodes, particularly as mega-cities become larger and more common and traffic continues to grow. Even without such episodes, urban air pollution is estimated to make a substantial contribution to disease burden. In the most recent estimates of global disease burden (Cohen and others 2005), ambient PM2.5 air pollution was estimated to cause about 3 percent of mortality from cardiopulmonary disease in adults; 5 percent of mortality from trachea, bronchus, and lung cancer; and 1 percent of mortality from acute respiratory infection in children under age 5. In total, air pollution is estimated to cause 0.8 million (1.2 percent) premature deaths and 6.4 million

(0.5 percent) years of life lost (YLL). In spite of these substantial estimates, the contribution of urban air pollution to disease burden may be overlooked because air pollution has nonspecific consequences and increases risk and severity of diseases that have multiple other determinants. Consequently, risk assessment is generally used, as in the Global Burden of Disease project, to estimate the damage to public health and the costs of this damage. Policy makers may set aside such estimates as too uncertain to be used as the basis for decision making.

Traffic is a particular concern in urban areas. There is a rapidly enlarging body of evidence indicating that exposure to traffic emissions is associated with adverse health effects, beyond those conveyed by individual pollutants (Health Effects Institute 2009). This evidence has potentially profound implications, not only for public health but as a consideration in urban planning and transportation management (White and others 2005). Much of the evidence comes from epidemiological studies that have used a variety of indicators of exposure to traffic emissions, such as proximity of the residence to major roadways, air pollution models, and surrogate indicators, for example, $NO_2$. These measures are surrogates for exposure to combustion emissions from motor vehicles, a mixture that includes ultrafine PM along with nitrogen oxides and VOCs. A variety of health effects have been investigated: all-cause and cardiorespiratory mortality, asthma and respiratory symptoms in children and adults, lung function level, allergy, birth outcomes, and cancer.

Findings of a systematic review of this evidence, carried out by the Health Effects Institute (a nonprofit research organization in the United States), were reported in 2009. Overall, while calling for more research, the review did support a conclusion that "the evidence was 'sufficient' to infer a causal relationship between exposure to traffic-related air pollution and exacerbation of asthma and 'suggestive but not sufficient' to infer a causal relationship with onset of childhood asthma, non-asthma respiratory symptoms, impaired lung function, and total and cardiovascular mortality."

## AIR QUALITY MANAGEMENT IN URBAN ENVIRONMENTS

There are many approaches to improving urban air quality; air quality management is a topic that is too diverse for full treatment here. Air quality management strategies are based on a foundation of evidence that builds from sources of air pollution to patterns of population exposure, and then to associated health risks. Approaches include controlling emissions at the source, such as scrubbers at coal-fired power plants; reducing the volume of emissions, such as with increased use of public transportation to lower air pollutants from motor vehicles or emissions controls for automobiles; and decreasing population exposure, such as with the U.S. Environmental Protection Agency's (EPA) Air Quality Index, which provides a health warning on high air pollution days to encourage susceptible individuals to avoid outdoor exposure.

Reduction of the health effects of air pollution comes from actions at multiple spatial and institutional levels, ranging from personal decisions by individuals, to community and state plans, and to multigovernment agreements. Due to the transport of pollution across jurisdictional boundaries, many pollutants, such as ozone, need to be addressed through collaborative mechanisms. Since air pollution crosses national boundaries, agreements between governments may be needed. Actions by individuals may also contribute to improved air quality; use of mass transit instead of private automobiles and lessened use of wood-burning fireplaces may enhance air quality locally.

Management of urban air quality also needs to involve collaboration and planning by multiple public and private stakeholders. Within government, there needs to be overall leadership and support for maintaining and improving air quality and engagement of those involved in environmental management, planning and design, and transportation. Key stakeholders include the public, nongovernmental organizations concerned with the environment and health, transportation companies, and industry. The potential for conflicting interests and insufficient emphasis on public health is evident. Nonetheless, there are examples (see case studies) of successes in reducing urban air pollution. These case studies illustrate how changes in fuels and innovative transportation management can reduce pollution emissions. They also highlight the roles of advocacy and litigation, and the need for leadership.

## Case Studies

### London Traffic Congestion Charging Scheme

One approach to limiting urban air pollution is to restrict sources. In London, the mayor introduced the Congestion Charging Scheme in 2003, with the goal of reducing traffic in Central London. The zone was extended in 2007. With six years of experience, robust data are now available on the impact of the Congestion Charging Scheme on traffic and air pollution emissions, and estimates have been made of health benefits (http://www.tfl.gov.uk/assets/downloads/sixth-annual-impacts-monitoring-report-2008–07.pdf). Traffic has dropped in comparison to the baseline data by approximately 10–15 percent, though the decline is variable from year to year. Pollution emissions have also declined, although modestly (Tonne and others 2008). The estimated benefit to mortality attributable to reduced emissions in the original zone was also modest: 183 years of life per 100,000 in the charging zone and 18 years per 100,000 outside of the zone (Tonne and others 2008). Research is in progress with pollution and health data to further quantify the health benefits.

The London Congestion Charging Scheme represents an important model that may prove useful in other urban areas. While implemented primarily to deal with the clogging of Central London by traffic, it led to reduced emissions and pollution levels and potentially to health benefits. The ongoing assessment of its consequences for air pollution and health will offer guidance for other urban areas where such schemes may be considered.

• • •

## Public Health Litigation in Delhi

Delhi has long been among the world's most polluted cities. The sources of pollution are myriad and include mobile sources, industry, and power generation, along with biomass fuel-burning and suspension of dust. Public health litigation, which can be effective in India, led to improved air quality. A series of actions by the Indian Supreme Court prompted major changes in industry with the closure of major polluting industries and a shift in motor vehicles from diesel and gasoline to clean fuel technology, primarily compressed natural gas (CNG; Goyal and Sidhartha 2003). These directives addressed certain industries and fuels used for commercial vehicles, mandating a switch to concentrated natural gas (CNG). Several researchers have addressed the pollution and health consequences of these legal mandates. Levels of $SO_2$ declined substantially and those of PM to a lesser extent. There is also a co-benefit for greenhouse gas emissions (Reynolds and Kandlikar 2008).

• • •

## Public Transportation in Bogotá

Bogotá, Colombia, has been widely lauded for its urban planning and mass transportation. Among the innovations are a bicycle path system (Ciclorutas) and the Transmilenio system, a bus rapid transit system (Parra and others 2007). The bus system was an attempt to replace the less efficient private system that choked the city streets with many polluting vehicles. The public bus system operates in a separate lane. The buses are fueled by diesel, rather than natural gas, based on a stakeholder process and consideration of costs and risks to health (Valderrama and Beltran 2007). Nonetheless, the reduction of congestion should have air quality benefits.

Regarding target levels for pollutants in urban areas, the World Health Organization provides guidelines, most recently updated in 2005 (WHO 2006). In proposing its guidelines, the WHO acknowledged the wide range of pollution levels in cities around the world and the impossibility in some countries and cities of attaining standards as stringent as those in the United States and Europe. Consequently, it proposes targets that are above the guideline value and have acknowledged risks but are at progressively lower levels. The intent is to provide guidance for moving towards the WHO guidelines; attaining them may not be feasible in many urban areas in lower- and middle-income countries.

Having local evidence on public health consequences of air pollution may be critical for motivating action and for tracking the consequences for health of air quality management. Time-series studies, using routinely collected public health and air quality monitoring data, have been carried out for many cities around the world. They provide an indication of local risk, though the results may be imprecise and the findings need cautious interpretation in the context of broader evidence. The Health Effects Institute, through its Public Health and Air Pollution in Asia (PAPA) program, has enhanced capacity in a number of Asian countries to carry out such studies and periodically summarized the literature on the health effects of air pollution in Asia (Health Effects Institute 2004). Continued tracking of the benefits of air pollution management is needed to sustain impetus for improved air quality.

There are both direct and indirect benefits of urban air quality management. Many atmospheric pollutants affect air quality and human health through multiple pathways. For example, $NO_2$ affects health directly and also contributes to the formation of ozone; $SO_2$ contributes to the formation of particulate matter. Ambient air pollutants also figure into many other environmental problems. $NO_x$ and $SO_x$ are the primary causes of acid precipitation. Indoor air pollution levels are driven by both indoor sources and outdoor pollution through the penetration of outdoor air into homes. PM and ozone both reduce visibility. The same fossil fuel-burning processes that generate the ambient air pollutants also produce greenhouse gases, such as $CO_2$ and methane ($CH_4$), which contribute to global warming. So a potential co-benefit of urban air quality management is reduced greenhouse gas emissions.

Trends of air quality in the world's mega-cities cannot be readily predicted at present. Continued population growth and rising numbers of motor vehicles are of concern; fortunately, gains may be made as older, highly polluting vehicles are replaced and reduction of fuel combustion to limit greenhouse gas emissions should be beneficial in the longer term. Some cities already have levels well above accepted guidelines (Table 21.1), and careful tracking and proactive management are needed to avoid future air pollution disasters.

## SUMMARY

In the twentieth century, evidence-based research confirmed the health effects of air pollution. Regulation has improved air quality in most large cities in the more developed countries, but air pollution is still a threat in less developed countries, especially in their mega-cities. Major urban air polluters include lead, sulfur dioxide, carbon monoxide, particulate matter, nitrogen oxides, tropospheric ozone, "toxic" pollutants, volatile organic compounds, and biological pollutants.

In urban areas, traffic is a major cause of poor air quality. Because air pollution crosses jurisdictional boundaries, improvements in air quality require changes at every level—in individuals' behavior, community and state plans, and multigovernment agreements. The experiences of London, Delhi, and Bogotá show that changes in fuels and innovative transportation management can reduce pollution emissions. The World Health Organization is providing guidance for cities in less developed nations to lower their air pollution levels, and the Health Effects Institute is helping Asian nations study the effects of air pollution. Urban air quality management can benefit not only public health but also the environment.

## REFERENCES

Bell, M. L., and D. L. Davis. 2001. Reassessment of the lethal London fog of 1952: Novel indicators of acute and chronic consequences of acute exposure to air pollution. *Environmental Health Perspectives* 109(Suppl 3):389–394.

Bell, M. L., A. McDermott, Z. L., Zeger, J. M. Samet, and F. Dominici. 2004. Ozone and short-term mortality in 95 US urban communities, 1987–2000. *Journal of the American Medical Association* 292:2372–2378.

Bell, M. L., and J. M. Samet. 2009. Air pollution. In *Environmental health: From global to local*, 2nd ed., ed. H. Frumkin. San Francisco: Jossey-Bass.

Brimblecombe, P. 1987. *The big smoke: A history of air pollution in London since medieval times*. New York: Methuen.

Brook, R. D., B. Franklin, W. Cascio, Y. Hong, G. Howard, M. Lipsett, R. Luepker, M. Mittleman, J. Samet, S. C. Smith, Jr., and I. Tager. 2004. Air pollution and cardiovascular disease: A statement for healthcare professionals from the Expert Panel on Population and Prevention Science of the American Heart Association. *Circulation* 109(21):2655–2671.

Cohen, A. J., H. Ross Anderson, B. Ostro, K. D. Pandey, M. Krzyzanowski, N. Kunzli, K. Gutschmidt, A. Pope, I. Romieu, J. M. Samet, and K. Smith. 2005. The global burden of disease due to outdoor air pollution. *Journal of Toxicology and Environmental Health*, Part A 68(13–14):1301–1307.

Crutzen, P. J., and V. Ramanathan. 2003. Atmospheric chemistry and climate in the anthropocene: where are we heading? In Earth system analysis for sustainability, ed. H.-J. Schellnhuber, P. J. Crutzen, W. C. Clark, M. Claussen, and H. Held, 265–292. Cambridge, MA: MIT Press.

Gauderman, W. J., G. F. Gilliland, H. Vora, E. Avol, D. Stram, R. McConnell, D. Thomas, F. Lurmann, H. G. Margolis, E. B. Rappaport, K. Berhane, and J. M. Peters. 2002. Association between air pollution and lung function growth in southern California children: Results from a second cohort. *American Journal of Respiratory and Critical Care Medicine* 166(1):76–84.

Goyal, P., and Sidhartha. 2003. Present scenario of air quality in Delhi: A case study of CNG implementation. *Atmospheric Environment* 37(38):5423–5431.

Grant, L. D. 2009. Lead and compounds. In *Environmental toxicants: Human exposures and their health effects*, 3rd ed., ed. M. Lippmann, 757–809. Hoboken, NJ: Wiley.

Gurjar, B. R., T. M. Butler, M. G. Lawrence, and J. Lelieveld. 2008. Evaluation of emissions and air quality in megacities. *Atmospheric Environment* 42(7):1593–1606.

Health Effects Institute. 2004. Health effects of outdoor air pollution in developing countries of Asia. Special report 15. Boston: Health Effects Institute.

Health Effects Institute. 2009. Traffic-related air pollution: A critical review of the literature on emissions, exposure, and health effects. Special report 17. Boston: Health Effects Institute.

Hedley, A. J., C. M. Wong, T. Q. Thach, S. Ma, T. H. Lam, and H. R. Anderson. 2002. Cardiorespiratory and all-cause mortality after restrictions on sulphur content of fuel in Hong Kong: An intervention study. *Lancet* 360(9346):1646–1652.

McConnell, R., K. Berhane, F. Gilliland, S. J. London, T. Islam, W. J. Gauderman, E. Avol, H. G. Margolis, and J. M. Peters. 2002. Asthma in exercising children exposed to ozone: A cohort study. *Lancet* 359(9304):386–391.

National Center for Environmental Assessment. 2009. Air quality: EPA's Integrated Science Assessments (ISA). http://cfpub.epa.gov/ncea/cfm/recordisplay.cfm?deid=149164.

Parra, D., L. Gomez, M. Pratt, O. L. Sarmiento, J. Mosquera, and E. Triche. 2007. Policy and built environment changes in Bogotá and their importance in health promotion. *Indoor and Built Environment* 16(4):344–348.

Pope, C. A., III, and D. W. Dockery. 2006. Health effects of fine particulate air pollution: Lines that connect. *Journal of Air and Waste Management Association* 56(6):709–742.

Reynolds, C.C.O., and M. Kandlikar. 2008. Climate impacts of air quality policy: Switching to a natural gas-fueled public transportation system in New Delhi. *Environmental Science & Technology* 42(16):5860–5865.

Samet, J. M., F. Dominici, F. C. Curriero, I. Coursac, and S. L. Zeger. 2000. Fine particulate air pollution and mortality in 20 U.S. cities, 1987–1994. *New England Journal of Medicine* 343(24):1742–1749.

Schlesinger, R. B. 1999. Toxicology of sulfur oxides. In *Air pollution and health*, ed. S. T. Holgate, H. S. Koren, J. M. Samet, and R. L. Maynard, 585–602. New York: Academic Press.

Tonne, C., S. Beevers, B. Armstrong, F. Kelly, and P. Wilkinson. 2008. Air pollution and mortality benefits of the London Congestion Charge: Spatial and socioeconomic inequalities. *Occupational and Environmental Medicine* 65(9):620–627.

United Nations Department of Economic and Social Affairs. 2008. *World urbanization prospects: The 2007 revision*. New York: United Nations.

U. S. Environmental Protection Agency (EPA). 2004. *Air quality criteria for particulate matter*. Research Triangle Park, NC: U.S. EPA, National Center for Environmental Assessment.

U.S. Environmental Protection Agency (EPA). 2008. Integrated science assessment for particulate matter (first external review draft). Research Triangle Park, NC: U.S. EPA.

U.S. Environmental Protection Agency (EPA). 2009. Integrated science assessment for carbon monoxide (first external review draft). Washington, DC: U.S. EPA.

Valderrama, A., and I. Beltran. 2007. Diesel versus compressed natural gas in Transmilenio-Bogotá: Innovation, precaution, and distribution of risk. *Sustainability: Science, Practice, & Policy* 3(1):59–67

White, R. H., J. D. Spengler, K. M. Dilwali, B. E. Barry, and J. M. Samet. 2005. Report of workshop on traffic, health, and infrastructure planning. *Archives of Environmental and Occupational Health* 60(2):70–6.

World Health Organization (WHO). 2006. *Air quality guidelines: Global update 2005—Particulate matter, ozone, nitrogen dioxide and sulfur dioxide*. Copenhagen: World Health Organization.

# CHAPTER TWENTY-TWO

# URBAN PLANNING AND AESTHETICS

CAROLA HEIN

KALALA NGALAMULUME

KEVIN J. ROBINSON

## LEARNING OBJECTIVES

- Describe the role played by the aesthetics of the urban environment and urban planning in promoting or impeding public health

- Identify the multiple factors and agents that affect urban aesthetics

- Discuss how changes in aesthetic factors contribute to public health

- Summarize current discussions on aesthetics and public health in developed countries that center on "walkability" (that is, improved neighborhood design to increase physical activity)

- Discuss the growing global need for innovative aesthetic interventions for disadvantaged neighborhoods

- Summarize recent efforts to improve urban design policy and its impact on urban neighborhoods, communities, health, and well-being

THIS chapter focuses on the importance of aesthetics in the urban environment for public health from a historical and contemporary perspective and in a global context. In particular, it looks at the ways in which aesthetics are supportive of or detrimental to public health, with *health* defined as a "state of complete physical, mental, and social well-being and not merely the absence of disease or infirmity," in accordance with the World Health Organization (1946).

*Aesthetics*, a word with Greek origins meaning "perceptible to the senses," refers to the larger human experience of the environment through sound, smell, touch, movement, and vision. There is no absolute definition of appealing aesthetics. Rather, the specific appreciation of a space will vary according to personal taste, cultural preferences, socioeconomic background, academic training, or time period. The sensory perception of space can refer to abstract aesthetic principles as well as cleanliness and the absence of broken doors, windows, or litter; it can refer to open green spaces, old buildings, detailed design, or winding streets that integrate nature. It matters not whether these features belong to the natural environment, are the outcome of everyday life practices, or have been professionally planned. The experience of a space will also change in response to one's personal awareness in a given situation: vacationers may be more aware of urban aesthetics than people who cross the same spaces daily.

Numerous actors, public and private forces, planners and architects, as well as citizens shape the form and function of the city, since they exploit environmental features; develop infrastructure for transportation and the distribution of utilities; construct public spaces, buildings, and monuments; and establish particular systems of economic and social organization, making aesthetic decisions throughout. Urban planning, which allows us to intervene consciously in urban spaces, can be a tool to increase well-being and public health through multiple means, including sensory design.

This chapter examines the interrelation of urban form, aesthetics, and health. It highlights the role that environmental and technological factors, governance structures and policies, economic and social structures, and everyday use play in the creation of urban aesthetics. It provides examples from different periods and places around the world to illustrate the historic interaction among planning, aesthetics, and health. It then concludes by examining the role of urban aesthetics today, focusing on the issue of health improvement through aesthetics in different urban areas and socioeconomic contexts around the world.

# INTERRELATION OF URBAN FORM, AESTHETICS, AND HEALTH

Urban design can promote physical health and aesthetics in multiple ways, with specific approaches toward the improvement of the function or the form of the city being more prominent at particular times. For example, in the nineteenth century, planners and public health practitioners concentrated on urban interventions directly linked to hygiene, such as the construction of water and sewage infrastructure, waste disposal, and zoning according to income, which are discussed in other chapters of this book. Aesthetics had only an indirect role in these projects, whereas some planning doctrines, such as the American City Beautiful movement, came into existence around the same time with the specific goal of beautifying the city, but only for select, elite populations and without a direct focus on urban health improvement. At other times, public health and aesthetic concerns were part of the same planning concepts. Thus, in the early nineteenth century, functional and rational city planning ideas emerged, making public health a key theme of architectural design and aesthetics while placing a priority on improving living conditions through adequate provision of sunshine and fresh air, elements especially lacking in impoverished quarters of the city prior to this time. Recently, the discussion on aesthetics, urban planning, and community building in developed countries has again brought public health concerns to the fore of planning discussions as it focuses on the theme of physical movement in an everyday setting, often referred to as "walkability," which can improve physical health, community cohesion, safety, and the environment by encouraging everyday physical activity, such as walking or bicycling.

The aesthetics of the built environment can also affect mental health, since architecture and urban form facilitate orientation and confer a sense of safety and identity to the people who use the space. For example, as described by the American urban planner Kevin Lynch (1960), the design quality of buildings, public spaces, and infrastructure—from materials to the overall urban form—can provide "legibility" to the city, that is, facilitating identification as well as wayfinding and cognitive mapping. Psychological well-being, offered by neighborhood coherence, familiarity with local history, and small-scale development were aspects of urban design introduced in the late 1960s, especially under the impetus of Jane Jacobs's book *The Death and Life of Great American Cities* (1961). Furthermore, lighting, sound, temperature, air pollution, sensory boundaries, ergonomic fit, and crowding are all potential environmental stress factors that can positively or negatively impact mental health, as professors of human ecology, architecture, and psychology Gary Evans (1982), Craig Zimring (1982), and Ralph B. Taylor (1982) have argued.

A built environment that enlivens the senses and promotes well-being and safety may enhance social relationships and community structures and therefore public health. The British environmental psychologist David Canter (1997) has recognized place identity as key to describing the interaction among people's actions, conceptions, and the physical environment, and the work of Australian professor of architecture Kim Dovey (2008) has revealed that places as stabilized contexts of everyday life can serve as important tools to stabilize identity. Personal involvement in a place entails an emotional relationship and can contribute to the maintenance of public space and promote social interaction and improved health. The appearance and physical design of public spaces can contribute to social health by increasing community interaction. Community health—cohesion and a sense of well-being—can be positively influenced by aesthetically enriched places and objects. This is particularly the case when such places and objects are directed at the pedestrian, according to authors in the Norwegian architect Birgit Cold's (2002) edited volume *Aesthetics, Well-Being and Health: Essays within Architecture and Environmental Aesthetics.*

The assessment of aesthetics by design practitioners, however, is not always agreed upon by the general public or by specialists from other disciplines. For example, buildings considered aesthetically pleasing by specialists that are imposed on their occupants may adversely affect the mental health of those occupants, who may find living in these structures stressful. The absence of sensory stimulation in some districts—or aesthetic interventions that are reserved for specific population groups or areas—can be detrimental to the emotional health of excluded parts of the population; conversely, surroundings that give people high self-esteem help to make them healthy.

In spite of general agreement that aesthetics can impact health, the concrete relationship among urban aesthetics, planning, and public health remains difficult to ascertain. For example, although British policy scholar David Halpern (1995) agrees that built environments influence mental health, he nonetheless cautions that people with poorer mental health are generally economically less successful and tend to live in less pleasant areas, thus raising questions about which is the origin and which is the result. Urban design that encourages physical activity is also of less concern in developing parts of the world, where cities still struggle with the basic provision, maintenance, and distribution of public health services.

# FACTORS SHAPING URBAN AESTHETICS AND PUBLIC HEALTH

The sensory appearance of the built environment is the result of numerous natural and man-made features, political, economic and social organizational structures, and their particular interaction with each other, as the following sections highlight.

## Environmental Factors

A host of environmental factors—such as geography, geology, and climate—influence a city's overall aesthetics affecting the city's location, internal structure, social organization, and built form. Availability of fresh water and food sources, the accessibility of land, and the availability of natural connections to other cities also influence the sensory appearance of a city and the health of citizens, favoring some and disfavoring others. For example, the urban elite in many cities, including Edo (today's Tokyo) and Brussels, settled on the highlands, leaving the easily flooded lowlands to poorer classes, who were therefore forced to create high-density, multifunctional districts with little open space. Similarly, predominant wind patterns in European cities have led to the emergence of affluent areas in the western parts, where fresh air from western winds reaches the city, leaving the more polluted eastern parts to industry and working-class housing. Such examples exist around the world and raise questions of environmental and aesthetic justice as affluent groups live in environmentally privileged areas in safe and aesthetically pleasing settings with well-designed houses and extensive public spaces, which are recognized as having a positive impact on mental and physical health. Conversely, environmentally challenged areas—mountain slopes prone to landslides, for example—may be home to squatter settlements (as in Caracas, Venezuela) that are aesthetically displeasing and unclean.

## Technological Factors

Technological factors also play a role in urban aesthetics and public health as urban actors use them to overcome environmental challenges and human choices. For example, the development of technology for use in infrastructure, such as roads or railway lines, and also public utilities, such as water, gas, electricity, or communication lines, in construction technology or in building materials can affect the quality of living as well as shape settlements. New technology can lead to very different urban form and aesthetics and can provoke the complete overhaul of existing cities.

The insertion of underground fresh water and sewage lines in many nineteenth-century European cities was a big factor in eradicating diseases, such as cholera, that killed large parts of the population, while at the same time allowing for the construction of an aesthetically pleasing streetscape. The transformation of Paris under Napoleon III and Baron George Eugène Haussmann is a good example of such an intervention, since it included the insertion of underground infrastructure and the construction of large avenues bordered by carefully conceived facades of new apartment buildings—designed to bring more light and air into the crowded city and to house the bourgeoisie. Meanwhile, the later construction of subways contributed to the segregation of the urban population according to income (pushing the low-income population of Paris into the periphery, for example), improving public health for some parts of the population and worsening it for others.

In the last decades, new technology for heating, cooling, or irrigation may make formerly inaccessible areas available for healthy and appealing human living. For example, construction of the lush green public parks that promote outdoor living and leisure activity on the newly reclaimed waterfront of Abu Dhabi (a desert climate) would not have been possible without irrigation technology (as well as strong political leadership, extensive public funding, and private investment).

## Governance

Governance structures and the policies that specific governments adopt can determine the interrelated concerns of urban form, the distribution of various population groups, and the overall appearance of a city as well as public health. Furthermore, traditional methods of designing buildings and locating cities in harmony with nature have created particular design forms while responding to issues of public health. For example, in ancient China, the state carefully laid out capital cities, respecting the feng shui practice that includes prescriptions aimed at protecting the health of people in a house and a city, while creating the easily recognizable forms of the traditional Chinese capital city (such as a four-sided enclosure punctuated by gates, a hierarchical and clearly oriented space, a street grid, and a ward system), which take into account health issues, such as availability of water and cardinal directions. In some instances, a strong political focus on the display of aesthetics and symbolism at the expense of environmental features can lead to cities with limited livability and public health. Madrid became the capital of Spain simply because it was closer to the geographic center of the country, despite its location on a plateau that features cold winters, sharp winds, and consistently hot and dry summers. Local policy makers will further establish criteria for the urban design and aesthetics of the city, the size of streets and other public spaces, its zoning and building legislation, and the existence of health-care institutions, education, and public housing, all essential for public health.

Socioeconomic—and spatial but also urban design—segregation continues to be visible in cities around the world, where parts of the population are isolated socially and fiscally in business centers or where gated communities often lay in plain sight of (or are surrounded by) slums. Affluent areas produce taxes that allow for the creation of well-designed amenities, playgrounds, parks, and other structures. Private investment and design decisions can complement and partly steer political choices on how and where to invest public funding into open spaces, infrastructure, housing, or historic preservation. Compounded individual decisions can help revitalize decayed areas and develop new economic bases. For example, due to a combination of public policies, development strategies, and private investment, medieval European cities once characterized by diseases, hygiene problems, and warfare have become today's tourist attractions for their elaborately detailed architecture, small block structures, and walkability, where well-maintained public spaces are bordered by busy restaurants and boutiques. The Cittaslow Movement that appeared in Europe in the wake of the Slow Food movement of the 1990s is a good example of how public and private initiative can help to redefine the economic base of a city.

## Economic and Social Factors

The politics of economic inequalities typically determine the distribution of aesthetic assets that influence public health. Selected social groups may impose their will on the form and function of specific areas. For example, colonial powers, traders, and other elite populations that came to "new" lands brought foreign aesthetics and public health improvements to new settlements near existing cities that were often limited to foreign and elite populations. In Africa and India, for example, disease epidemics and the development of tropical medicine provided a justification to colonial state officials, physicians, and planners for initiating changes in residential patterns, from cohabitation with the indigenous populations to residential segregation along racial and class lines. While the "European towns" developed on the plateaus with wide streets, attractive business districts, better housing, leisure opportunities, and other amenities promoting public health, the slums were characterized by overcrowding, few job opportunities, crime, and inadequate or inaccessible community services and recreational facilities. Moreover, the slums served as labor reserves, where illegal activity inevitably occurred, some of it constituting the main sources of pollution and noise, further increasing the challenges to public health posed by these districts.

Aesthetic and functional improvement of living conditions for the affluent has occurred in cities around the globe since their inception. Decisions taken by private companies and individual actors led to the creation of new, appealing healthy townships and neighborhoods. For example, in order to escape the mosquitoes and dense living conditions that helped bring yellow fever to central Philadelphia, affluent individuals departed to the western periphery, the Main Line, laying the basis for today's wealthy suburbs with their handsome houses set in lush greenery.

Even the issue of walkability needs to be seen in a different light in the disadvantaged urban neighborhoods. Disparities in function and design aesthetics can actually make disadvantaged urban neighborhoods less conducive to walking, offsetting the advantages of high population density and land use mix. For example, in lower income neighborhoods, decaying building structures, intrusive land-uses, noise, air pollution, traffic hazards, and the absence of greenery and public spaces, as well as crime and violence, often make these areas less walkable and more conducive to the emergence of chronic diseases related to physical inactivity. Improved aesthetics may incite citizens to walk and engage more with the community, thus reducing real and perceived crime in a neighborhood.

## BRIEF HISTORY OF PLANNING, AESTHETICS, AND HEALTH

Although some of the urban health improvement mentioned above included socioeconomic segregation, the urban elite eventually came to understand that diseases needed to be eradicated among all classes of the urban population. As a result, a dozen International Sanitary Conferences were organized across Europe between 1851 and 1903 that addressed the threat of cholera; the construction of hospitals and better housing also became more important. With the realization that creating disease-free and aesthetically pleasing areas for the rich alone was not politically, morally, or even physically possible, planners and public health authorities introduced housing reforms to improve the provision of clean drinking water and living conditions, reduce population density, and allow sufficient air and light into buildings by controlling building height, lot depths, block sizes, access to ventilation, and street layout, simultaneously improving the overall sensory quality of the environment. Public health and urban design thus became intertwined. Simultaneously, urban reformers took up as their cause the challenges of mega-cities, slums, and public health: Ebenezer Howard proposed the garden city concept at the end of the nineteenth century, suggesting that carefully designed small towns of 30,000 residents be created in the countryside, where housing and working would come together, surrounded by wholesome nature, so as to combine the social and health advantages of city living and country living (Howard and Osborn 1902/1965).

From the 1920s to the 1950s, the desire to improve the living conditions of the working class by providing fresh air and sunshine, and to improve housing conditions, drove modernist aesthetics with its focus on public health. Architects and planners designed high-rise blocks in greenery, orienting their houses for maximum exposure to the sun and ventilating breezes. Tiny but separate kitchens for the lower-income group as well as tiny bathrooms were seen as great improvements by those who had earlier used outhouses, hall toilets, metal tubs in the kitchen, and public baths. European modernists led the movement toward industrialization of simple, well-designed products, including houses and city buildings. The Hufeisensiedlung (horseshoe-shaped settlement) in Berlin by Bruno Taut or the settlements by Ernst May in Frankfurt are examples of early attempts at promoting a functionalist aesthetic of public health and functional housing for the working classes. The CIAM movement (Congrès Internationaux d'Architecture Moderne) in the 1920s and 1930s further promoted themes of minimally decent, rationally planned housing units, combining public health improvement with the attempt to create an aesthetic for the modern industrialized world and for lower-income tenants. Jose Luis Sert's book *Can Our Cities Survive?* (1942) illustrates the perceived squalor of the city and the modernist proposals for improvement of public health.

After the Second World War, planners around the world used the opportunity provided by wartime destruction to implement the modernist proposals of the 1920s that had been guided by aesthetic principles, as well as the social engagement and health concerns that originated in the nineteenth century. By the 1950s, planners in the United States and around the world promoted urban transformation, based on modernist ideas, including high dependency on motor vehicles, segregated land uses (designed initially to separate workers' housing from polluting factories), disconnected streets so as to promote purely residential enclaves, low residential density (and thus limited public transport), and local employment. In the United States, this led to movements based around "slum clearance" (as in the projects promoted by Robert Moses in New York City), high-rise buildings, and extended open spaces in discrete zones.

Many of the districts characterized as slums showed aesthetic neglect, defined as the absence of upkeep. The visuals of decay of various low-income urban areas—often crowded, shadowed, damp, and polluted—displayed a depressive visual environment and posed challenges to public health, including the emergence and spread of new diseases or the reemergence of old diseases. Aesthetic neglect and poor health conditions were often due to public disinvestment. For example, the closure of firehouses in poor Black and Hispanic neighborhoods, such as the South Bronx in New York City, which had the most poorly maintained housing stock, the highest density, the highest unemployment, the greatest proliferation of illicit drugs, and the fewest per capita medical personnel and facilities, led to longer and more extensive fires in these areas. The cutbacks spread to other municipal services as well, such as policing, sanitation, public health, and welfare services, as well as housing inspections to enforce housing codes. According to U.S. Census data, between 1970 and 1980, 62 contiguous "health areas" in the South Bronx lost between 55 and 81 percent of occupied units largely due to the abandonment of housing following catastrophic fires (Wallace and Wallace 2001). As a result, given their meager resources, and the shortage of low-income housing, many of these families moved in with relatives, exacerbating the already overcrowded living situations commonly experienced by this population. Others were forced into the city's shelter system. Inadequate public health support, domestic overcrowding, and the illegal immigration of unhealthy individuals also led in part to the rise of tuberculosis in the 1970s and 1980s. Moreover, large-scale public planning projects, such as new urban highways (designed to promote suburbanization, a healthy choice for one part of the population) often exacerbated aesthetic neglect and public health problems, notably of decaying Black and Hispanic neighborhoods.

The modernist movement's focus on specific aspects of public health—air, sunshine, and greenery—and the resulting aesthetics of high rises in greenery, led to counter-movements both in regard to a less invasive restructuring of inner cities and the reimagining of the suburbs. Starting in the 1980s, attempts at reversing aesthetic neglect and transforming inner cities put greater emphasis on inner-city living and housing, multifunctional and walkable neighborhoods, and community participation aimed at functional and aesthetic improvement of the neighborhood, addressing several factors identified with improved public health. Examples include the 1987 Berlin International Building Exhibition (IBA), which promoted innovative architectural and urban design, and the renewal and beautification of the Barcelona waterfront in conjunction with the 1992 Olympics and other international events, where improved urban form, the reconnection of the city with its waterfront by channeling the coastal highway through a tunnel, and the fashioning of new beaches, parks, and neighborhoods have added to individual and collective well-being and have attracted numerous tourists who appreciate the newly created, architecturally innovative, and socially diverse spaces.

Suburbanization, despite its original focus on improving public health and its promotion of a captivating imagery of wide streets, large green yards, and freestanding homes, contributed to the development of the sedentary lifestyle. As planners abandoned the nineteenth-century model of dense, walkable, and multifunctional neighborhoods, they introduced a new health challenge into the built environment. Although suburbs featured lush greenery, low density, and pleasing design, their sprawling and mono-functional nature promoted car usage and created major health challenges (such as obesity, resulting from a more sedentary lifestyle), increased social isolation and reduced community interaction, therewith negatively impacting physical, mental, and social health.

Criticism of suburban sprawl provoked the rise of New Urbanism, an aesthetics-based planning movement, starting in the 1980s. It proposes higher-density communities with mixed-use zoning combining commercial and residential development, interconnected streets, bicycling paths, and access to public transport, as well as appropriate residential and employment densities, all of which could improve public health. Transit-oriented developments (TOD) emphasize walkable design with the pedestrian as a priority. TODs feature train stations as prominent features of town centers, and as regional nodes that would include offices, residential areas, stores, and civic uses. New Urbanists want these areas to be accessible by public transportation—trolleys, trains, and buses—and to accommodate users of bicycles, scooters, and rollerblades. These changes could reduce traffic congestion, car accidents, and pollution.

New Urbanism has already found numerous followers, as the Center for New Urbanism's website documents, but the use of these principles in gated communities at the edge of cities or in suburbs contributes to the sprawl in American cities and caters to affluent groups, contradicting the principles around which these areas were designed. New Urbanism promoters are therefore trying to apply their principles to inner-city developments, emphasizing neighborhood revitalization, balanced economic development, and social equity goals. In order to improve public health throughout the city, urban design policy has to take into account all population groups.

# URBAN AESTHETICS TODAY

Changes in the built environment can promote health in multiple ways. Politicians, planners, and health scholars have recently begun to focus on the redesign of neighborhoods to improve the sensory appeal and the legibility of the built environment and enhance identification with the local community, therewith encouraging increased physical activity during leisure time and commutes. For example, land use patterns, transportation structures, and urban design characteristics can promote walking, cycling, and sports activity. Vegetation and public parks, pleasant design of streets, bicycle lanes and walkways, small blocks, and proximity to multiple amenities, recreational facilities, and public transportation can also incite people of all ages to walk. Attractive architecture, appropriate maintenance of built structures, and urban design, with carefully placed urban furniture (such as outdoor seating), ornamental fencing, pedestrian lighting, public art, sidewalk commercial activity, and sports facilities may motivate neighbors to engage in more physical activity. Together with environmental interventions aimed at increasing residential density, reducing physical barriers to walking, developing social-support networks, and creating greener and more aesthetically pleasing environments, these design factors may help increase physical activity and walking for transport.

## Walkability and Community Enhancement

The design of streets and urban sites is a key element in urban transformation for increased walkability and physical exercise. In the United States, Portland,

Oregon, and Multnomah County, Oregon (where Portland is situated), recently joined forces to advocate for "safe, sound & green" streets under the auspices of Portland Oregon Street Repair, a plan that seeks to correct Portland's worst transportation problems through highway road improvements, street safety additions, and increased bicycle paths. Many measurement tools exist for promoting walkability, and several studies have found significant relationships between environmental characteristics (for example, number of destinations, aesthetics) and physical activity. Aesthetics alone, however, cannot be the solution. It needs to occur in the context of a new policy focus that restructures our cities, focuses on healthy transportation, high connectivity, high density, land use mix, and active communities (Frumkin, Lawrence, and Jackson 2004). While walkability may have a positive health impact on the individual, it also benefits the health of the community, as it reduces car usage and thus energy consumption and $CO_2$ emissions, therewith increasing sustainability. In general, the lower the density of a city, the higher are its emissions from the transport sector.

An example of community-building and public health improvement that does not conform to academic notions of urban beauty comes from Japan. Locals and foreigners with changing aesthetic principles have come to appreciate the chaotic design and traditional patchwork character of traditional high-density, small-scale neighborhoods with narrow roads that promote close-knit social ties in multifunctional and highly walkable neighborhoods, organized around local shopping streets and connected by an extensive network of public transportation. There has been a recent reevaluation of these districts, which some scholars today consider as exemplary for urban living. However, given their location in the cities' lowlands, their density and mostly wooden construction, these areas are admittedly challenged by fire, flooding, and/or wind damage and are thus public health hazards. Aesthetic improvements in such traditional areas that have recently been reappreciated can also lead to gentrification, again providing the affluent groups with the most recent aesthetic models and putting mental and physical health pressure on less dominant population groups who are displaced.

## Urban Retrofitting

Interestingly, rapid urban growth around the world presents opportunities for architectural and urban design for new neighborhoods as well as for the retrofitting of existing ones, thus potentially improving public health. Retrofitting of traffic systems—through the reduction of car lanes and the increase of cycling paths and walkways, the creation of walkable green neighborhoods in the middle of existing cities, and the widespread availability of rental bikes in cities such as Amsterdam and Paris—can encourage physical activity for everyday transportation. Several other recent initiatives in Europe aim at improving urban health while considering aesthetics. The Belfast Healthy Cities initiative, for example, considers urban design, and the Slow Cities movement refers to local aesthetic traditions (http://www.belfasthealthycities.com; Knox 2005).

Yet the discussion of the aesthetics of the built environment must include the socioeconomic issues of rich versus poor. Recent scholarship, in fact, considers aesthetic justice and aesthetic welfare. While current discussions address aesthetics, only parts of the population are affected by this discussion. For example, the historic, small red-brick Beard Elementary school in Detroit, built in 1886, looked picturesque to modern eyes. Nevertheless, it sat close to the Chrysler Freeway and industrial plants, was grievously overcrowded, had subpar recreational facilities, and lacked a cafeteria. Despite its aesthetic value, it was deemed obsolete, and a new school was initiated in 2000. The new building, however, was situated above soil contaminated with lead, arsenic, polychlorinated biphenyls (PCBs), benzo(a)pyrene, and trichloroethylene. This example highlights the necessity of assessing the politics of the built environment. Who gets the new school? Who gets the contaminated locale? Who gets the blacktop playground? Who gets the aesthetically pleasing playground equipment? These matters of urban form, function, and amenity distribution transcend those of aesthetics.

Aesthetic improvements are attractive for policy makers as they can often be implemented more quickly and at more modest cost than more fundamental shifts in population density, land use patterns, or other indicators of urban form. In addition, community stakeholders often support neighborhood aesthetic enhancements in order to improve the quality of life and attract consumers to local businesses, especially if local residents are actively included in the decision making from the beginning. Measures that could reduce the poor–non-poor disparities include planting trees, increasing the frequency of trash pickup and other sanitation services, increasing sidewalk commercial activity, increasing pedestrian convenience, implementing traffic-calming measures, reducing area and noise pollution, and promoting economic development. Other easily implemented urban design features, such as public art, murals, and lighting, can enhance the neighborhood's appearance, as well as its walkability, safety, and sustainability. Green spaces, parks, and community gardens can improve the appearance of decaying neighborhoods, incite community activities, offer more diverse nutrition to inhabitants, and increase environmental knowledge. Green roofs or local water-cleaning facilities can also enhance urban aesthetics and sustainability. However, there is no absolute, single aesthetic that can be considered good for health. Instead, any intervention needs to emerge from local considerations and as part of larger policy choices.

## SUMMARY

As the above discussion suggests, aesthetics and its influence on public health are linked to environmental, political, socioeconomic, and technological factors. The evidence, however, is very difficult to quantify. Further research is necessary to document and analyze the evidence to better understand causation and association. It is important to remember that aesthetics are related to multiple aspects of public health and that the importance of each one changes over time. A design that promotes public health at one point may become unhealthy at another time, and one that favors one segment of the population may be negative for others. Urban governance that integrates a concern for health into its policy making can assure the maximum health impact for its urban planning and aesthetic choices

## REFERENCES

Canter, D. 1997. The facets of place. In *Advances in environment, behavior, and design*. Vol. 4: *Toward the integration of theory, methods, research and utilization*, ed. G. T. Moore and R. W. Marans, 109–148. New York: Plenum.

Cold, B. 2002. *Aesthetics, well-being and health: Essays within architecture and environmental aesthetics*. London: Ashgate.

Dovey, K. 2008. *Framing places: Mediating power in built form*, 2nd ed. London: Routledge.

Evans, G. W., ed. 1982. *Environmental stress*. New York: Cambridge University Press.

Frank L., P. Engelke, and T. Schmid, eds. 2003. *Health and community design: The impact of the built environment on physical activity*. Washington, DC: Island Press.

Frumkin, H., F. Lawrence, and R. Jackson, eds. 2004. *Urban sprawl and public health. designing, planning, and building for healthy communities*. Washington, DC: Island Press.

Halpern, D. 1995. *More than bricks and mortar? Mental health and the built environment*. Abingdon, UK: Taylor and Francis.

Howard, E., and F. J. Osborn. 1965. *Garden cities of tomorrow*. Cambridge, MA: MIT Press. Originally published 1902.

Jacobs, J. 1961. *The death and life of great American cities*. New York: Vintage Books.

Knox, P. L. 2005. Creating ordinary places: Slow cities in a fast world. *Journal of Urban Design* 10(1):1–11.

Lynch, K. 1960. *The image of the city*. Cambridge, MA: The Technology Press and Harvard University Press.

Sert, J. L. 1942. *Can our cities survive?* Boston: Harvard University Press.

Taylor, R. B. 1982. Neighborhood physical environment and stress. In *Environmental stress*, ed. G. W. Evans. New York: Cambridge University Press.

Venturi, R., D. S. Brown, and S. Izenour. 1977. *Learning from Las Vegas*. Cambridge, MA: MIT Press.

Wallace, D., and R. Wallace. 2001. *A plague on your houses: How New York was burned down and national public health crumbled*. Brooklyn, NY: Verso (Haymarket Series).

World Health Organization. 1946. Preamble to the Constitution of the World Health Organization (as adopted by the International Health Conference). New York: World Health Organization.

Zimring, C. 1982. The built environment as a source of psychological stress: Impacts of buildings and cities on satisfaction and behavior. In *Environmental stress*, ed. by G. W. Evans. New York: Cambridge University Press.

# CHAPTER TWENTY-THREE

# HEALTHY URBAN GOVERNANCE

## SCOTT BURRIS
## DANIELLE OMPAD

### LEARNING OBJECTIVES

- Define and distinguish governance and government
- List and describe the characteristics of good governance
- Discuss the challenges of polycentric good urban governance
- Review the limits of governance

URBAN health promotion is not simply a matter of the right interventions or the necessary resources. Urban (and indeed global) health depends to an important extent on governance, the institutions and processes through which societies manage interventions and allocate resources. People throughout the world are experimenting with governance strategies to improve urban well-being, and there is a growing literature on governance and its impact on health (Burris 2004; Dodgson, Lee, and Drager 2002; Hein 2003; Navarro and others 2006). This chapter describes the concept of governance, explains why governance has become an important topic in public affairs, and how it matters to students of urban health. After offering examples of governance innovation in urban health, the chapter concludes with some observations on the limitations of local governance strategies.

Governance may be defined as "the management of the course of events in a social system" (Burris, Drahos, and Shearing 2005). In the urban setting, it is "the sum of the many ways individuals and institutions, public and private, plan and manage the common affairs of the city" (UN-HABITAT 2002). Governance today is characterized by a plurality of institutions (states, corporations, the World Trade Organization, institutions of civil society, criminal and terrorist gangs) forming more or less interconnected governance networks, a plurality of methods of power (force, persuasion, economic pressure, norm creation and manipulation), and rapid adaptive change.

Health governance may be more specifically defined as

> the actions and means adopted by a society to organize itself in the promotion and protection of the health of its population. The rules defining such organization, and its functioning, can . . . be formal (for example, Public Health Act, International Health Regulations) or informal (for example, Hippocratic Oath) to prescribe and proscribe behaviour. The governance mechanism, in turn, can be situated at the local/subnational (for example, district health authority), national (for example, Ministry of Health), regional (for example, Pan American Health Organization), international (for example, World Health Organization) and . . . the global level. Furthermore, health governance can be public (for example, national health service), private (for example, International Federation of Pharmaceutical Manufacturers Association), or a combination of the two (for example, Medicines for Malaria Venture). (Dodgson, Lee, and Drager 2002)

Studies of governance emphasize three main elements, or levers, of governance:

- *Institutions:* organizational sites where governing resources are gathered and mobilized (government agencies, corporations, foundations, NGOs, street gangs; Spiro 2007; Teubner 2004);

- *Methods of power:* tools that governors use to project influence (deliberation, bribes, military force, claims of legitimate right to rule, forum-shifting; Braithwaite 2004; Rose and Miller 1992); and
- *Constraints on governors:* limitations on the freedom of action of governors that may arise from laws (like constitutions or treaties) or competition from other governors (as in a market) or from culture (social norms; Braithwaite 2005; McGrew 2000).

## GOVERNANCE IS NOT JUST THE JOB OF GOVERNMENT

Governance is not just what the government does to manage the society; it embraces the work of every actor and agency that seeks deliberately to shape events in the neighborhood, city, nation, or world (Commission on Global Governance 1995; Keohane 2002; UN-HABITAT 2002). The distinction between the public sphere, which was the realm of the governors, and the private sphere, the realm of the governed, has eroded. States do not enjoy a monopoly on governance and themselves are often governed by nonstate actors. It now makes more sense to describe governance as polycentric, with power distributed among multiple agencies and sites of governance that govern through a variety of forms of power and largely in their own interests (Kempa, Shearing, and Burris 2005; Rosenau 2007; Teubner 2004).

This is apparent at the international level (Fidler 2004). International nongovernmental organizations (NGOs), such as Greenpeace and Doctors without Borders, are able to mobilize popular opinion against particular states to constrain and shape their action by issuing reports and by having access to global information media (Spiro 2007). Transnational corporations use their domestic political power to influence everything from the interpretation of health and safety regulations to negotiation of international treaties (Braithwaite and Drahos 2000). The World Health Organization, one of the weakest international agencies, was able to govern states' response to SARS because it could enroll the power of the global media to spread its message and of global businesses to withhold investment in countries that did not comply with its directives (deLisle 2004).

Polycentric governance is also true within states, where governments, corporations, and NGOs are now widely understood to be linked in governance networks, interfacing at all levels of social organization and through a variety of means (Burris, Drahos, and Shearing 2005; Castells 2000; Drahos 2004; Hein 2003; Rhodes 1997; Shearing and Wood 2003). The phenomenon has many faces. It is seen clearly in the widespread privatization of services that were formerly thought to be the work of governments—water supply, sewers, disease prevention, even policing—that is characteristic of neoliberal policies. It is seen in the increasingly common presence of "mass private property": shopping malls, business improvement districts, and gated communities that use legal concepts of private property and contract to create new zones of private governance (Shearing 2005). It is seen in contemporary practices of regulation, which increasingly depend upon private or hybrid public-private bodies to set standards, oversee compliance, and punish noncompliance (Black 2003). Of course, it is also seen in the manipulation of public opinion and government processes by well-organized or wealthy organizations.

# GOVERNANCE VERSUS GOOD GOVERNANCE

"Governance" is not synonymous with "good governance." Polycentric governance is a description, no more. Any given contemporary governance system may be inefficient, corrupt, or unresponsive to the needs of the governed. Governance can be "good" in at least two senses: it can deliver good results—in this case, healthy public policies and good health—and it can work through processes and institutions that meet broadly accepted standards of justice and due process. Ideally, governance is good in both of these ways, and many people believe that governance that fails the second criterion will normally have difficulty delivering on the first. We consider healthy urban governance to be governance that has as its focus the improvement of the health and well-being of the urban population and the reduction in inequity in health and its determinants, therefore promoting a process of healthy urbanization that results in the creation of healthy urban settings.

Good governance has some generic elements. Aside from efficiency in delivering good results, these include

- *Participation*: the degree of ownership and involvement that stakeholders have in the political system;
- *Fairness*: the degree to which rules are applied equally to everyone;
- *Decency*: the degree to which rules are formed and implemented without humiliating or harming particular groups of people;
- *Accountability*: the extent to which those with governing power are responsible and responsive to those affected by their actions;
- *Sustainability*: the extent to which current needs are balanced with those of future generations; and
- *Transparency*: the extent to which decisions are made in a clear and open manner. (Hyden, Court, and Mease 2003; UN-HABITAT 2002)

Many commentators express a strong normative preference for democracy as the essence of good governance. This reflects in part the evident virtues of democracy as a mode of governance, but it is also an empirical claim: modes of decision making that enroll more diverse knowledge and are tested in a governance competition are more likely to produce correct answers more of the time (Burris, Drahos, and Shearing 2005; Cohen and Sabel 1997; Manor 1999). Good governance should not be assumed to depend at all time and in all places on the kinds of institutions and procedures that have worked in Western liberal democracies (Hyden, Court, and Mease 2003).

## WHY GOVERNANCE IS AN IMPORTANT CONCEPT IN PUBLIC AFFAIRS

Many factors combine to explain the increasing salience of governance in public policy analysis (Braithwaite, Coglianese, and Levi-Faur 2007). There is, first, the plain fact that policy always reflects the preferences of those making it and the processes through which policy is enacted. The move to governance also reflects the ever-increasing complexity of regulation in a global economy. Using a governance approach makes it possible for scholars and governors to think more creatively and effectively about how to manage social processes. Traditional regulatory functions—standard-setting, oversight, and enforcement—can be separated from each other and from the government agencies that traditionally carried them out (Scott 2001). A wide variety of institutional actors can then be "enrolled" to carry out, alone or in collaboration, one or more of these regulatory functions (Black 2003). Depending upon the context, industries may do a better job setting standards than government does; government may need the assistance of NGOs to monitor adherence to those standards; and market sanctions triggered by publicity may be more efficient in enforcing standards than traditional penalties imposed by governments.

## WHY GOVERNANCE MATTERS TO HEALTH

Governance is a necessary consideration in any program to understand and influence the social determinants of health (Dodgson, Lee, and Drager 2002; Hein 2003). Urban settings demonstrate clearly the inequalities that plague the poor, who almost invariably live—and have always lived—downwind; downstream; downhill (unless the hills are dangerous, and then they live uphill); on marginal lands; in unsafe, polluted, and unhealthy neighborhoods that lack basic services; and where they work is in the least healthy and most dangerous workplaces

(Commission on Social Determinants of Health 2008). Health outcomes are affected by the physical infrastructure in cities, differential access to urban services afforded by different neighborhoods, and the social and economic relationships embedded in the way people live, learn, work, and play. The articulation among these determinants of health is shaped by instruments of urban governance—such as land use planning, zoning, building and design codes, public participation—as well as specific investment decisions (such as in public housing, land acquisition, infrastructure development, transportation, and services; Freudenberg, Galea, and Vlahov 2006).

Governance as a social practice tends to reflect existing social structure and to act as one of the social mechanisms that sort people for unequal health outcomes. Governance systems influence health by upholding and facilitating existing distributions of resources like power, money, property, services, and knowledge. Those with the power to shape events in the community are able over time to organize matters in ways that benefit them and externalize undesirable effects on those less able to exert influence. The use of zoning to push insalubrious land uses away from "better" neighborhoods to lower socioeconomic status (SES) areas is a common urban example (Maantay 2001): those wielding legal power can use it to shift exposure to unhealthy conditions onto those with less power. There is also a theoretical basis and some evidence suggesting that participation in governance may be healthy for individuals and communities (Kawachi and Berkman 2000).

# ELEMENTS AND EXAMPLES OF HEALTHY URBAN GOVERNANCE

At the local level, the greatest challenges in a polycentric system of governance are (1) mobilizing dispersed knowledge, capacity, and resources through effective and efficient institutions that promote collective interests, and (2) leveraging local knowledge and capacity to influence regional, national, and global governance to promote the kind of economic and political conditions in which a city and its residents are most likely to be able to thrive. In this section, we review examples of governance reforms or innovations that have tried, and in some cases succeeded, in meeting these challenges.

## Housing

Over one billion urbanites live in substandard housing without basic sanitary services (Milbert 2006 300). Quality housing for the poor frequently turns on the rules and practices governing land tenure. In developed countries, ownership is governed by a system of land titling within the legal system governing property rights. Such systems also exist in most if not all developing countries, but may not be the chief source of "property rights," particularly in slum and squatter areas (de Soto 2000; Porio and Crisol 2003). Rather, "ownership" may arise from a combination of local norms, law enforcement controls limiting violent expropriation, and political or other legal factors limiting the ability of title "owners" to regain control of their land (Porio and Crisol 2003). Although both formal and informal systems can protect land tenure, as a general matter, informal governance of poor people's property has substantial disadvantages. Uncertainty about ownership and tenure is not only a potential source of individual and community stress (Macintyre and others 2001), but it also deprives poor people the opportunity to convert property into capital for investment or home improvement, and it undermines the incentive to improve housing stock and neighborhood amenities (de Soto 2000).

Reforms in property governance have most notably consisted of simplifying land title registration systems and developing finance mechanisms to mediate the movement of legal title between "squatters" and "owners." Zoning rules must also sometimes be addressed, where the land in question is substandard. The most widely known land titling program was initiated in Lima, Peru, by the Peruvian economist Hernando de Soto in an unusual process where the governance of extralegal land registration was essentially vested in an NGO, which designed and then implemented a new system that was eventually absorbed back into state law and administration (Kagawa and Turkstra 2002).

Financing has been used as a means of dealing with community conflict while also mobilizing community action. In Thailand, modest results from a government-led effort at top-down housing improvement in the 1990s led to a decentralized approach where community-based organizations were given responsibility and spending authority to plan and implement housing upgrades in their own neighborhoods under the auspices of a government-created and funded but independent public agency, the Community Organizations Development Institute (CODI). CODI has a partnership structure, with a board of government and civil society representatives, but works primarily through organizations and networks in the target communities. The theory is that "when low income households and their community organizations do the upgrading, and their work is accepted by other city actors, this enhances their status within the city as key partners in solving city-wide problems" (Boonyabancha 2005).

## Entrepreneurship and Business

Simplifying the governance of entrepreneurship—the administrative procedures required to legalize small businesses often operated informally by poor urban entrepreneurs (Bromley 1990; Jansson and Chalmers 2001; Johnson and Kaufmann 2001; Loayza 1996)—can allow poor people to more effectively use, and add to, their resources. In less-developed countries, bureaucratic procedures frequently are so complex and expensive that poor business owners choose to sacrifice the benefits and protections of operating within the formal business sector to avoid high costs (Johnson, Kaufmann, and Zoido-Lobaton 1998; Loayza 1996). In the informal sector, entrepreneurs are typically unable to readily expand their businesses, legally enforce contracts, access new or lower-interest financing, obtain insurance, or benefit from government programs (Jansson and Chalmers 2001; Loayza 1996). Their employees work without the protections of government safety and health standards. The economy stagnates because it lacks new investment. Society is foreclosed from enjoying the improved income distribution, social security coverage, and tax revenue-funded programs that would result from increased investment (Jansson and Chalmers 2001).

Addressing this problem has involved new legislation or decrees, public-private reform partnerships, and increased intragovernmental cooperation (Jansson and Chalmers 2001). One of the best-known examples of administrative simplification improving the lives of the urban poor again took place in Lima under the influence of de Soto, who measured and then undertook to systematically remove the barriers to operating businesses legally (Loayza 1996). Evidence suggests that debureaucratization—for example, eliminating or reducing license requirements, centralizing the regulatory process—results in greatly increased formalization of small- and medium-sized businesses.

## Policing and Security

Civil order, in particular freedom from violence, is an important element of health and a fundamental aim of good governance. Community policing, which usually involves the formation of boards, committees, or other forms of partnership to give communities more influence on security, has been a widely used tool for the better governance of security (Fung 2001; Groenewald and Peake 2004; Seagrave 1996). Because formal legal systems, whether criminal or civil, are cumbersome and expensive, innovators in poor countries have turned to models that take security and conflict resolution out of the hands of the government justice system and put them into the hands of the community. Particularly notable are nonstate systems of local dispute resolution, such as those reported in Bangladesh, Philippines, and South Africa (Braithwaite 2000; Dupont, Grabosky, and Shearing 2003; Golub 2003; Roche 2002), and special courts designed to empower women in cases of domestic abuse (Magar 2003). Alternative dispute resolution can strengthen communities while reducing recidivism rates in some areas, providing higher levels of security than traditional public institutions.

## The Participatory Approach to Public Expenditure Management

The local government budget is an excellent mirror of policies and priorities. Public spending is often characterized by lack of transparency, inefficiency, elite capture, and corruption. Direct engagement of citizens in government budget planning, overseeing public expenditures, and monitoring delivery of goods and services is emerging as a potent tool for better governance. Broadly known as Participatory Public Expenditure Management (PPEM), this approach helps to operationalize participation in local governance to improve transparency, accountability and effectiveness in public resource management (World Bank 2004).

The PPEM cycle offers different entry points for citizens to hold people in power accountable: (1) voicing their needs in decision making; (2) reviewing government decisions to assess whether public policies and budgets address social priorities; (3) engaging in administrative and procurement oversight to identify bottlenecks and leakages in resource flow, tendering, bidding, and contracting; and (4) monitoring and evaluating delivery of services, public goods, and local governance performance.

Participatory budgeting is probably the most internationally known form of PPEM. Over the last two decades, participatory budgeting has grown from a Brazilian experiment to an international model for participatory urban governance. More than two hundred cities in Brazil have adopted a form of participatory budgeting. Peru, the Philippines, and the state of Kerala in India have adopted legal provisions mandating that citizens directly voice their priorities in the local government annual budgeting process. The practice of participatory budgeting is expanding exponentially in more than twenty countries, with more advanced decentralization and democratization (Avritzer 2000; Baiocchi 2000; Cabannes 2004). While there is evidence that participatory budgeting affects governance and empowerment, the same cannot be said for well-being. A recent study of participatory budgeting in Brazilian municipalities found participatory budgeting was associated with a less than one percent decrease in the proportion of the population living in extreme poverty and was not associated with widespread improvements in well-being on a variety of indicators, including infant mortality, literacy, and life expectancy (Boulding and Wampler 2010).

## Microgovernance and Networks

Communities suffer relatively poor health (and other problems, like crime) when they cannot effectively manage the course of local events, making the creation of new local institutions of governance itself a health intervention. Communities' well-being can be strengthened by supporting—or creating—institutions that enable collective efficacy (Morenoff, Sampson, and Raudenbush 2001; Sampson

2002; Sampson and Raudenbush 1999). On this view, interventions that promote new forms of "microgovernance" are a potentially important tool for promoting health problems in poor communities.

The Sonagachi Project is a leading example of a project that combines explicit health goals with a deeper effort to mobilize local efficacy. Sonagachi was introduced as an HIV prevention intervention in Calcutta in the early 1990s. Organized as a worker's collective, it deployed a mentality of worker's rights and occupational safety among sex workers, using simple community organization techniques like peer education. It has grown to thousands of members, significantly improved sex workers' relations with madams, pimps, and the police (Biradavolu and others 2009), and has been given substantial credit for the unusually low rates of HIV among Calcutta sex workers compared to other major Indian cities (Basu and others 2004). An evaluation comparing Sonagachi's model to a standard STI prevention program illustrated how governance interventions go beyond narrow health outcomes: the Sonagachi model was no more effective in preventing STIs than the standard approach, but Sonagachi participants had a more optimistic outlook and a greater willingness to seek health care (Gangopadhyay and others 2005).

Microgovernance projects like sex worker collectives can be hypothesized to enable communities to manage the course of events in at least three ways. First, they create an institution where resources and situated knowledge can cohere and people can define their own needs and priorities for change. Second, they can reconfigure relations of governance within the community. A new institution can fill governance gaps or challenge the dominance of institutions that do not perform well enough. Sex work collectives have helped members challenge unhealthy policing practices and discrimination in social services. Third, microgovernance institutions can reconfigure relations between the community and the larger system it inhabits. The Sonagachi Project and other sex worker collectives in India have enabled sex workers to enter into the national debate about HIV/AIDS and sex work policy.

## LIMITS OF GOVERNANCE

Strong local governance has its pitfalls (Fung 2001; Johnson, Deshingkar, and Start 2005). Those with greater resources of experience, money, or skill can game the local system as they can a national government (Dahl 1961). The voices of the poorer, weaker, and more socially marginal can be ignored. Women may be denied the chance to speak at all. Urban settings often have large populations of "illegal" internal or international migrants whose right to participate is contested (Shearing and Wood 2003). Urbanites do not necessarily, or even most of the time, organize themselves and vote as urban dwellers, but rather act as members of ideological or ethnic blocks organized around national political issues that may reflect and worsen divisions at the local level (Devas 1999).

Urban governors are part of a system that works best as it approaches the ideal of a "virtuous circuit." At any level of social organization, governing institutions require the capacity to mobilize and coordinate local resources, but from a global governance perspective, vertical coordination and participation are essential. The best of interventions organized at the global level will suffer if the national, provincial, and especially the local institutions of governance are bypassed or lack the capacity for effective implementation. Even the imposition of "good" solutions in a top-down manner, without real decision-making participation by those most affected, is paternalistic and illegitimate from a democratic perspective.

Good governance requires the interplay of power and constraint to forestall dysfunctional phenomena such as capture. Good national and international governance can be a source of norms and a recourse for those excluded from local decision making (Johnson, Deshingkar, and Start 2005). National governments provide the "policy environment" in which local government and governance can innovate, or not (Barten and others 2002; de Vries and others 2001). It is not even clear that empowering urban areas leads to greater attention to urban inequities: "Although central governments are unlikely to be generally more 'pro-poor' than local governments, it may be easier for central governments to insist on pro-poor use of grant resources than for local governments to use their own resources in that way" (Devas 1999).

Local governments typically are short not just on cash but on properly trained bureaucrats with the skills and incentives to use their power productively. The strategies we have discussed here are hardly new to local health advocates; the problem is that lack of resources can limit efficacy at every step. Improving skills in governance, and widening the repertoire of strategies will make poor urbanites more effective, but local governors also need access to the resources controlled by higher levels of governance.

## SUMMARY

This chapter introduces the concept of "governance" as an important tool for urban health. Governance has become an important area of research and action in the enterprise of promoting human health, welfare, and development. Governance may be defined broadly as "the management of the course of events in a social system" (Burris, Drahos, and Shearing 2005). It consists of "the many ways individuals and institutions, public and private, plan and manage the common affairs" of a polity, large or small

(UN-HABITAT 2002). Therefore, the term embraces both the governing activities of governments and the many modes through which nongovernmental entities exercise more or less governing control in important social matters (Rosenau 2007).

The increasing use of governance as a framework for policy analysis reflects, in part, the obvious importance of good governance—that is, transparency, accountability, honesty, and capacity to recognize and adapt to change. Good policies rarely emerge from poorly managed systems of governance; even the best conceived and well-funded policy initiatives cannot meet their goals if their implementation is corrupt, grossly inefficient, or incompetent. But there are other relevant and important drivers of the focus on governance. Contemporary governance is characterized by the fragmentation of state sovereignty and the consequent multiplication in the number of agencies and forms of power that are active in the management of social systems. Today, private foundations may have as much or more control over global health policy than nation-states or the World Health Organization, and NGOs battle multinational corporations over the price nation-states will pay for pharmaceuticals. To describe governance as purely a function of governments is now, simply, inaccurate. Where top-down command fails, effective horizontal coordination becomes vital; where important decisions are made by private actors outside government, new ways must be found to ensure that governance respects social, civil, and political rights. Scholars, activists, and governors of all sorts are actively looking for new institutions and processes of governance that may help them achieve their goals more efficiently.

People can learn to improvise better, but no amount of research or technology transfer will turn governance from an art into a science. It will be difficult to prove that any particular form or process of governance causes urban health to improve, yet we have more than enough reasons to prefer good governance over the alternative. Good governance is valuable not just for the ends it promotes but for the process of collective cultural imagination it represents. Urban settings are places where the world can be reimagined, where efforts at reform create the context for new ideas and further action, and where new norms are formed (Castells 1983; Lake 2006). The world's urban settings present an enormous opportunity to define and implement healthy public policy through governance innovation.

# REFERENCES

Avritzer, L. 2000. Public deliberation at the local level: Participatory budgeting in Brazil. Paper presented at Experiments for Deliberative Democracy Conference, Wisconsin.

Baiocchi, G. 2000, January. Participation, activism, and politics: The Porto Alegre experiment and deliberative democratic theory. Paper presented at the Experiments for Deliberative Democracy Conference, Wisconsin.

Barten, F., R. P. Montiel, E. Espinoza, and C. Morales. 2002. Democratic governance—Fairytale or real perspective? Lessons from Central America. *Environment and Urbanization* 14(1):129–144.

Basu, I., S. Jana, M. J. Rotheram-Borus, D. Swendeman, S. J. Lee, P. Newman, et al. 2004. HIV prevention among sex workers in India. *Journal of Acquired Immune Deficiency Syndrome* 36(3):845–852.

Biradavolu, M. R., S. Burris, A. George, A. Jena, and K. M. Blankenship. 2009. Can sex workers regulate police? Learning from an HIV prevention project for sex workers in southern India. *Social Science and Medicine* 68(8):1541–1547.

Black, J. 2003. Enrolling actors in regulatory systems: Examples from UK financial services. *Public Law* (Spring):63–91.

Boonyabancha, S. 2005. Baan Mankong: Going to scale with "slum" and squatter upgrading in Thailand. *Environment and Urbanization* 17(1):21–46.

Boulding, C., and B. Wampler. 2010. Voice, votes, and resources: Evaluating the effect of participatory democracy on well-being. *World Development* 38:125–135.

Braithwaite, J. 2000. The new regulatory state and the transformation of criminology. *British Journal of Criminology* 40:222–238.

Braithwaite, J. 2004. Methods of power for development: Weapons of the weak, weapons of the strong. *Michigan Journal of International Law* 26(Fall):297–330.

Braithwaite, J. 2005. Responsive regulation and developing economies. *World Development* 34(5):868–932.

Braithwaite, J., C. Coglianese, and D. Levi-Faur. 2007. Can regulation and governance make a difference? *Regulation and Governance* 1(1):1–7.

Braithwaite, J., and P. Drahos. 2000. *Global business regulation*. Cambridge: Cambridge University Press.

Bromley, R. 1990. A new path to development? The significance and impact of Hernando de Soto's ideas on underdevelopment, production, and reproduction. *Economic Geography* 66(4):328–348.

Burris, S. 2004. Governance, microgovernance and health. *Temple Law Review* 77:334–362.

Burris, S., P. Drahos, and C. Shearing. 2005. Nodal governance. *Australian Journal of Legal Philosophy* 30:30–58.

Cabannes, Y. 2004. Participatory budgeting: A significant contribution to participatory democracy. *Environment and Urbanization* 16(1):27–46.

Castells, M. 1983. *The city and the grassroots: A cross-cultural theory of urban social movements*. Berkeley: University of California Press.

Castells, M. 2000. Materials for an exploratory theory of the network society. *British Journal of Sociology* 51(1):5–24.

Cohen, J., and C. Sabel. 1997. Directly deliberative polyarchy. *European Law Journal* 3(4):313–342.

Commission on Global Governance. 1995. *Our global neighbourhood: The report of the Commission on Global Governance and Democratic Accountability*. Oxford.: Oxford University Press.

Commission on Social Determinants of Health. 2008. *Closing the gap in a generation: Health equity through action on the social determinants of health*. Geneva: World Health Organization.

Dahl, R. 1961. *Who governs? Democracy and power in an American city*. New Haven: Yale University Press.

deLisle, J. 2004. Atypical pneumonia and ambivalent law and politics: SARS and the response to SARS in China. *Temple Law Review* 77:193.

de Soto, H. 2000. *The mystery of capital: Why capitalism triumphs in the West and fails everywhere else*. New York: Basic Books.
Devas, N. 1999. *Who runs cities? The relationship between urban governance, service delivery and poverty*. Birmingham: University of Birmingham School of Public Policy.
de Vries, J., M. Schuster, P. Procee, and H. Mengers. 2001. *Environmental management of small and medium sized cities in Latin America and the Caribbean*. Washington: Institute for Housing and Urban Development Studies.
Dodgson, R., K. Lee, and N. Drager. 2002. *Global health governance: A conceptual review*. London: London School of Hygiene and Tropical Medicine.
Drahos, P. 2004. Intellectual property and pharmaceutical markets: A nodal governance approach. *Temple Law Review* 77:401–424.
Dupont, B., P. Grabosky, and C. D. Shearing. 2003. The governance of security in weak and failing states. *Criminal Justice* 3(4):331–349.
Fidler, D. 2004. Constitutional outlines of public health's "new world order." *Temple Law Review* 77:247–289.
Freudenberg, N., S. Galea, and D. Vlahov, eds. 2006. *Cities and the health of the public*. Nashville: Vanderbilt University Press.
Fung, A. 2001. Accountable autonomy: Toward empowered deliberation in Chicago schools and policing. *Politics and Society* 29(1):73–103.
Gangopadhyay, D. N., M. Chanda, K. Sarkar, S. K. Niyogi, S. Chakraborty, M. K. Saha, and others. 2005. Evaluation of sexually transmitted diseases/Human Immunodeficiency Virus intervention programs for sex workers in Calcutta, India. *Sexually Transmitted Diseases* 32(11):680–684.
Golub, S. 2003. *Non-state justice systems in Bangladesh and the Philippines*. London: United Kingdom Department for International Development.
Groenewald, H., and G. Peake. 2004. *Police reform through community-based policing philosophy and guidelines for implementation*. New York: International Peace Academy.
Hein, W. 2003. Global health governance and national health policies in developing countries: Conflicts and cooperation at the interfaces. In *Globalization, global health governance and national health policies in developing countries: An exploration into the dynamics of interfaces*, ed. W. Hein and L. Kohlmorgan, 33–71. Hamburg: Deutschen Uebersee-Instituts.
Hyden, G., J. Court, and K. Mease. 2003. *Making sense of governance: The need for involving local stakeholders*. London: Overseas Development Institute.
Jansson, T., and G. Chalmers. 2001. *The case for business registration reform*. Washington, DC: Inter-American Development Bank.
Johnson, C., P. Deshingkar, and D. Start. 2005. Grounding the state: Devolution and development in India's panchayats. *Journal of Development Studies* 41(6):937–990.
Johnson, S., and D. Kaufmann. 2001. Institutions and the underground economy. In *A decade of transition: Achievements and challenges*, ed. O. Havrylyshyn and S. M. Nsouli. Washington, DC: International Monetary Fund.
Johnson, S., D. Kaufmann, and P. Zoido-Lobaton. 1998. Government in transition: Regulatory discretion and the unofficial economy. *American Economic Review* 88(2):387–392.
Kagawa, A., and A. Turkstra. 2002. The process of urban land tenure formalization in Peru. In *Land, rights and innovation*, ed. G. Payne, 57–75. London: ITDG Publishing.

Kawachi, I., and L. Berkman. 2000. Social cohesion, social capital and health. In *Social epidemiology*, ed. L. Berkman and I. Kawachi, 174–190. New York: Oxford University Press.
Kempa, M., C. Shearing, and S. Burris. 2005. Changes in governance: A background review. http://www.healthgov.net.
Keohane, R. 2002. Global governance and democratic accountability. In *Taming globalization: Frontiers of governance*, ed. D. Held and M. Koenig-Archibugi, 130–159. Oxford: Polity Press.
Kretzmann, J. P., and J. L. McKnight. 1993. *Building communities from the inside out: A path toward finding and mobilizing a community's assets*. Evanston, IL: Institute for Policy Research.
Lake, R. W. 2006. Recentering the city. *International Journal of Urban and Regional Research* 30(1):194–197.
Loayza, N. V. 1996. The economics of the informal sector: A simple model and some empirical evidence from Latin America. Washington, DC: World Bank.
Maantay, J. 2001. Zoning, equity, and public health. *American Journal of Public Health* 91(7):1033–1041.
Macintyre, S., R. Hiscock, A. Kearns, and A. Ellaway. 2001. Housing tenure and health inequalities: A three-dimensional perspective on people, homes and neighbourhoods. In *Understanding health inequalities*, ed. H. Graham. Buckingham: Open University Press.
Magar, V. 2003. Empowerment approaches to gender-based violence: Women's courts in Delhi slums. *Women's Studies International Forum* 26(6):509–523.
Manor, J. 1999. *The political economy of democratic decentralization*. Washington, DC: The World Bank.
McGrew, A. 2000. Power shift: From national government to global governance? *A globalising world? Culture, economics, politics*, ed. D. Held. London: Routledge.
Milbert, I. 2006. Slums, slum dwellers and multilevel governance. *European Journal of Development Research* 18(2):299–318.
Morenoff, J. D., R. J. Sampson, and S. W. Raudenbush. 2001. Neighborhood inequality, collective efficacy, and the spatial dynamics of urban violence. *Criminology* 39(3):517–559.
Navarro, V., C. Muntaner, C. Borrell, J. Benach, Á. Quiroga, M. Rodríguez-Sanz, and others. 2006. Politics and health outcomes. *Lancet*. 368(9540):1033–1037.
Porio, E., and C. Crisol. 2003. Property rights: Security of tenure and the urban poor in metro Manila. *Habitat International* 28:203–219.
Rhodes, R.A.W. 1997. Understanding governance: Policy networks, governance, reflexivity and accountability. Buckingham: Open University Press.
Roche, D. 2002. Restorative justice and the regulatory state in South African townships. *British Journal of Criminology* 42:514–533.
Rose, N., and P. Miller. 1992. Political power beyond the state: Problematics of government. *British Journal of Sociology* 43(2):173–205.
Rosenau, J. N. 2007. Governing the ungovernable: The challenge of a global disaggregation of authority. *Regulation and Governance* 1(1):88–97.
Sampson, R. J. 2002. Transcending tradition: New directions in community research, Chicago style. *Criminology* 40(2):213–231.
Sampson, R. J., and S. W. Raudenbush. 1999. Systematic social observation of public spaces: A new look at disorder in urban neighborhoods. *American Journal of Sociology* 105(3):603–651.
Scott, C. 2001. Analysing regulatory space: Fragmented resources and institutional design. *Public Law* 2001:329–353.

Seagrave, J. 1996. Defining community policing. *American Journal of Police* 15(2).
Shearing, C. 2005. Reflections on the refusal to acknowledge private governments. In *Democracy and the governance of security*, ed. J. Woods and B. Dupont, 11–32. Cambridge: Cambridge University Press.
Shearing, C., and J. Wood. 2003. Nodal governance, democracy, and the new "denizens." *Journal of Law and Society* 30(3):400–419.
Spiro, P. J. 2007. NGOs in international environmental lawmaking: Theoretical Models. In *Oxford handbook of international law*. Oxford: Oxford University Press.
Teubner, G. 2004. Societal constitutionalism: Alternatives to state-centered constitutional theory? In *Transnational governance and constitutionalism: International studies in the theory of private law*, ed. C. Joerges, I.-J. Sand, and G. Teubner, 3–28. Oxford and Portland, Oregon: Hart.
UN-HABITAT. 2002. *The global campaign on urban governance: Concept paper*, 2nd ed. Nairobi: UN-HABITAT.
World Bank. 2004. Social accountability: An introduction to the concept and emerging practice (Social Development Paper No. 76). Washington, DC: World Bank.

# CHAPTER TWENTY-FOUR

# GLOBAL BUSINESS AT THE LOCAL LEVEL

## NICHOLAS FREUDENBERG

### LEARNING OBJECTIVES

- Describe the impact of the business practices of multinational corporations on the health of cities

- Analyze the pathways by which business decisions on marketing, product design, retail distribution, and pricing can influence health

- Explain the unique characteristics of cities that make them attractive to multinational corporations

- Compare the strengths and limitations of market, government, and moral strategies to modify health-damaging business practices

- Discuss the role of researchers, policy makers, and public health professionals, and advocates in modifying business practices that harm health

THE social life of cities and the health of their populations depend on three foundational sectors: civil society, government, and business. In recent years, public health researchers have considered the impact of government and civil society on the health of urban populations (Commission on Social Determinants of Health 2007), analyzing their influences on living conditions, disparities in health, aging, and other health processes. Remarkably little attention, however, has been devoted to the influence of business on health, despite evidence that it is a large and growing social determinant of health (Freudenberg and Galea 2008).

This chapter considers the impact of business on the health of urban populations. It focuses on the intersection of three trends that have shaped cities in the last century: urbanization, globalization, and the growth of multinational corporations (MNCs). By 2030, two-thirds of the world's population will live in cities (United Nations 2006). Globalization describes the movement of capital, trade, and services across national borders. In the last sixty years, the value of world merchandise exports has increased more than one hundredfold (World Bank 2006). Multinational corporations (MNCs) transcend national boundaries, investing, buying, and selling around the world to maximize their return on investment. At the start of the twenty-first century, 51 of the 100 largest economies in the world were corporations, and the combined sales of the world's top 200 corporations were larger than the combined economies of all countries excluding the biggest ten (Anderson and Cavanagh 2000). To illustrate the size and impact of multinational companies, in 2008, the Coca Cola Company (2009) had revenues of almost $32 billion, employed 94,000 people (86 percent of whom lived outside the United States), sold 400 brands in 200 countries, and served 1.5 billion drinks a day.

This chapter describes the pathways by which business decisions affect the health of city dwellers in more- and less-developed countries (LDCs and MDCs), examines the strategies that have been used to strengthen the health-promoting capacities of business and reduce its health-damaging practices, and considers the roles public health professionals play in enhancing the positive and reducing the negative impact of business on health.

# HOW BUSINESS DECISIONS AFFECT THE HEALTH OF CITY DWELLERS

In a market economy, businesses play a key role in the distribution of needed goods and services. The decisions about which ones will be provided by government (such as clean air, sanitation, education, police), which by civil society (such as caring for the sick, child care, civic education), and which by businesses are political decisions that change with time and place. In the last few decades, in part as a result of what some have called the Washington Consensus or the neoliberal agenda (Szreter 2003), goods and services such as education, health care, and security that were previously considered a government responsibility have been increasingly privatized and transferred to the market sector.

In much of the world, businesses have the main responsibility for providing housing, employment, food, pharmaceuticals, transportation, and most other consumer goods. In the United States, markets also allocate most health care. Thus, businesses have a major influence on determining who gets the basic necessities of life even though these decisions are influenced by government and civil society.

Businesses influence health via a number of pathways, as illustrated in Table 24.1, which shows both salutogenic (healthy) and pathogenic (unhealthy) influences. Business practices such as marketing, product design, retail distribution, and pricing influence access and availability of healthy and unhealthy products and services. Corporate political practices such as campaign contributions, lobbying, and sponsored scientific research can either promote or undermine equitable and health-promoting policies. By their employment practices, benefits, and working conditions, businesses also influence health. Although MNCs employ only a fraction of the world's workforce, their practices often set the standards for other employers. In this century, business's consumer practices influence a far larger portion of the world's population than their employment practices do, suggesting that public health needs to focus on the health impact of consumption as well as production.

While business practices influence the health of all populations, their impact on urban populations may be greater. First, as people are concentrated in cities, urban density ensures that any global social determinant of health will have a disproportionate impact on cities. Second, cities are attractive for business because of their population density, availability of labor, established channels of communication, and marketing infrastructure. Thus, cities are now centers for both global production and consumption. For most businesses, making a profit in a densely populated urban area is easier than in less-dense rural areas. Not only do cities attract wealthier people, but even dense poverty offers more business opportunities than dispersed rural poverty. As poverty becomes increasingly concentrated in rural areas in the Global South, business opportunities may become even more concentrated in cities. Third, the diversity of urban populations allows businesses to segment markets, creating multiple profitable niches for entrepreneurs. Finally, cities are the control centers for multinational corporations. Increasingly, these companies play a central role in shaping urban culture and daily living, especially in the world's largest cities (Miles and Miles 2004).

TABLE 24.1    Salutogenic and Pathogenic Business Influences on Health

| Salutogenic Influences | Health Impact | Pathogenic Influences | Health Impact |
|---|---|---|---|
| Provide affordable and safe housing | Reduced injuries and accidents; improved mental health and child development; improved respiratory health | Provides unsafe or unhealthy housing or leaves sectors of the population homeless | Increased accidents and injuries; higher rates of mental health problems |
| Provide secure, safe and adequately compensated employment | Reduced occupational illness and injuries; income enables purchase of other necessities of life; benefits support meeting work and family responsibilities; improved social cohesion | Provides unsafe or insufficient employment; sectors of population under- or unemployed | Increased occupational illnesses and injuries; wages not sufficient to support well-being; increased mental health problems |
| Provide healthy, affordable food | Reduced hunger, obesity, and diet-related diseases; improved child health and development | Provides unhealthy, low-cost food | Increased obesity and diet-related diseases |
| Provide affordable, accessible, and effective health care | Preventable conditions avoided; improved management and reduced complications of chronic diseases; improved quality of life | Provides unaffordable or poor quality health care or no health care | Increased preventable conditions, premature mortality; higher rates of avoidable hospitalization |
| — | — | Provides easy access to affordable unhealthy products such as tobacco, alcohol, illicit drugs, or guns | Increased tobacco, alcohol and drug-related diseases; increased gun injuries and deaths |
| Promote democratic governance by following ethical business practices and transparent and ethical involvement in political processes | Increased social cohesion, governance makes population well-being a priority | Exerts disproportionate influence on political system to lower taxes or avoid regulation | Reduced public resources for health and human services; less effective health and environmental regulation |
| Support independent science and discloses knowledge on products | Government able to make informed decisions on health policy | Obfuscates and covers up scientific knowledge that threatens profit | Unsafe products and practices continue |

# THE IMPACT OF MULTINATIONAL CORPORATIONS ON URBAN HEALTH

Market economies are complex systems where individuals and organizations operate according to mostly unwritten rules within networks that are linked horizontally and vertically (Lindblom 2001). Most observers agree that multinational corporations (MNCs) now sit at the top of the business hierarchy (Chandler and Mazlich 2005); nevertheless, MNCs must negotiate relationships with governments, retailers, consumers, and workers, although often with more muscle than their partners.

To better understand the impact of MNCs and their local affiliates on urban health, a brief review follows on selected evidence regarding the health consequences of two business sectors—food and beverages, and firearms—on the health of urban populations. These sectors were selected because of their influence on health, their importance to the global economy, their distinct role in cities, and the availability of empirical studies on their health impact. Many other business sectors—such as alcohol, employment, energy, health care, housing, illicit drugs, pharmaceuticals, transportation, and tobacco—also influence health but will not be considered here.

## Food and Beverages

Over the past century, the food and beverage industry has made important contributions to improved health. Its success in bringing quantities of food to cities has all but eliminated malnutrition and nutritional deficiency diseases in many parts of the world; food safety standards have improved; and in the last century, the cost of food has declined (CDC 1999), making it more affordable to those in need. More recently, some food companies have tried to reformulate products to meet consumer demands for healthier diets (Yach 2009).

However, the practices of the food sector have also led to serious health threats facing the world today. Some observers estimate that if current trends in obesity and diabetes continue, future generations will have shorter life spans, reversing a century of public health progress (Olshansky and others 2005). The ubiquitous availability, low cost, and aggressive marketing of food high in fat, sugar, sodium, and calories have been linked with many chronic diseases (Lobstein 2002; Hawkes 2006, Nugent 2004), making the practices of the food industry a determinant of the world's most burdensome conditions. A growing body of literature links the practices of the food industry to diet-related health problems (Swineburn and others 2008; Story and others 2008; Ludwig and Nestle 2008). More recently, gyrating food prices and windfall profits for some global food companies have led to growing rates of hunger and food riots in cities around the world (Klapper 2008).

For example, like other countries, Mexico has seen a dramatic increase in obesity and diabetes in the last decade. While obesity has many causes that operate at multiple levels, the rapid rise in obesity and diabetes in urban Mexico shows how new trade agreements favored by business groups can lead to changes in the practices of MNCs that can then contribute to health problems. It also illustrates how these global changes interact with national and local trends to influence health.

In 1994 Mexico and the United States signed the North American Free Trade Agreement (NAFTA) (Hawkes 2006). The agreement removed trade barriers between the United States, Canada, and Mexico, making it easier for Mexico to export flowers and tropical fruits and for U.S. companies to sell Mexicans low-cost corn and processed food and to invest in the Mexican food industry. Between 1988 and 1997, U.S. businesses increased their investment in the Mexican food processing industry from $210 million to $5.3 billion, a twenty-five-fold increase (Hawkes 2006) that had a major impact on the types of food available in Mexico.

Most NAFTA-inspired, direct U.S. investment in the Mexican food industry supported production of processed food. Between 1995 and 2003, sales of processed food increased by 5 to 10 percent annually, contributing to troublesome changes in the Mexican diet. Between 1992 and 2000, calories from soft drinks increased by almost 40 percent. By 2002, the average Mexican was drinking 487 Coca Cola servings per year, more than the average U.S. consumption (Hawkes 2006). More than one-third of Mexican adolescents drank soda daily, and urban adolescents consumed significantly more than semiurban or rural teens (Ortiz-Hernández and Gómez-Tello 2008). In many countries, sweetened sodas have played a key role in the obesity epidemic.

Between 1988 and 1999, the total energy intake from fat in Mexico increased from 23.5 percent to 30.3 percent (Hawkes 2006; Rivera and others 2004). The increase in urban Mexico City was 32 percent, compared to only 22 percent in the poorer, more rural South. In this same period, the national prevalence of overweight/obesity increased by 78 percent (Rivera and others 2002). The overall prevalence of diabetes in Mexico increased by 30 percent between 1993 and 1999, imposing a substantial economic burden on the country.

Urbanization can contribute to a higher prevalence of obesity by increasing access to energy-dense fatty foods, especially for low-income groups moving from rural areas (Jimenez-Cruz, Bacardi Gascon, and Jones 2002). Between 1970 and 2000, the proportion of the Mexican population living in urban areas increased from 58 percent to 75 percent. And longitudinal studies suggest that the rapid transition from rural to urban and from high rates of early malnutrition to later childhood overnutrition serve as independent risk factors for obesity, diabetes, and adult cardiovascular disease (Jimenez-Cruz and Bacardi Gascon 2004). Therefore, the particular consequences of NAFTA facilitated gains in weight, especially in the growing urban low-income population. When food markets then made high-calorie, low-nutrient foods readily available to newly urbanized, mostly sedentary people, the stage was set for rapid weight gain.

At the municipal level, changes in the economy and food availability led to price increases. Between 1992 and 2000, the cost in pesos per megacalorie of food tripled in both urban and rural areas, but the cost remained twice as high in urban as in rural areas—making low-cost, low-nutrient foods more attractive, especially for the poor (Arroyo, Loria, and Mendez 2004). Aggressive marketing of high-calorie, low-nutrient snack foods and drinks, especially to urban children and young adults—industry's best hope for increased market share—further encouraged consumption (Hawkes 2006). With dense populations, established media markets, and numerous retail outlets, cities made particularly suitable venues for fast food and soda advertising. Often, ad campaigns were planned by increasingly globalized advertising companies. In Mexico City, the first McDonald's restaurant opened in the early 1980s; twenty years later, there were two hundred Golden Arches outlets in the city (Williams, Stern, and Gonzalez-Villalpando 2004).

In this case, changes in the practices of global food companies interacted with local factors to create an obesogenic environment that contributed to the explosive growth of obesity and diabetes in a genetically vulnerable population. As a result of dense urban markets that facilitated aggressive food advertising, a growing urban middle class that could afford more processed food, a working-class population whose food choices became more limited and less healthy, and declines in physical activity, the obesity and diabetes epidemics left a deep footprint in Mexico's cities. Others have described similar dynamics in Thailand, India, and Brazil (Hawkes 2006; Patel 2008)

## Firearms

For many cities, gun violence threatens public health and safety. Each year, guns kill about 200,000 people around the world, and another 100,000 die in conflict zones. For every individual killed by firearms, three are wounded, often with injuries that require lifetime care. What role do the practices of the gun industry play in this health burden, and what is their unique impact on urban health? Given the leading role that small arms play in cities, the focus here is on the practices of the MNCs making these weapons rather than the producers of the heavier weapons used in larger-scale international conflicts.

Small arms include pistols, revolvers, submachine guns, rifles, and assault rifles—all weapons that an individual can easily carry and use. Unlike major weapons, which are kept in government stockpiles, most small arms are in the hands of civilians, which makes them hard to regulate and trace. Unlike major weapons, few internationally recognized rules regulate small arms. In most countries, civilians can legally possess such weapons, making them widely available. How gun makers manufacture, advertise, and distribute small arms, both nationally and globally, influences their impact on health. How governments choose to regulate guns can mitigate or exacerbate adverse impacts.

There are 640 million small arms in the world, one for every ten people. Civilians own 59 percent of these firearms; government armed forces hold 38 percent, and the police and other armed groups hold the remainder. The Small Arms Survey (2007) estimates that U.S. civilians own one-third of all small arms in the world, making the United States the largest market for gun manufacturers.

More than 1,000 companies in at least 98 countries are currently involved in small-arms production. Between 1998 and 2003, the United States exported about 350,000 firearms per year, making it the world's largest exporter. Commercial interests drive the majority of gun exports. The total small arms production market is worth $7 billion per year; at least $1 billion of that may be generated from illegal transfers and sales (Gabelnic, Haug, and Lumpe 2006).

Death and injuries due to firearms disproportionately affect the Global South. During the 1990s, the poorest countries in the world were flooded with small affordable arms (Southall and O'Hare 2002). As the Cold War ended, small-arms makers and distributors found new markets for cheap weapons in Africa, the Middle East, and other regions. Increased competition in the small-arms industry brought prices down, making these weapons accessible to a larger market. In Kenya, AK47 rifles, a weapon easy to use and maintain, making it a favorite for gangs, paramilitary forces, and lone thugs, can now be obtained for as little as one chicken (Lumpe 2003).

Small-arms brokers often supply both sides of a conflict, selling in both legal and illegal markets. These brokers often evade the law by selling through intermediate countries, transferring production from one country to another or obtaining fraudulent export licenses (Southall and O'Hare 2002). In return for weapons, brokers receive narcotics, money, or precious minerals, expanding black markets and funding other criminal enterprises. Between 1986 and 1996, two million children were killed in armed conflict and six million were injured or permanently disabled (Stohl 2001). Women suffer disproportionately from the widespread availability of small arms; even though they are almost never the buyers, they are often the victims of gun violence (Southall and O'Hare 2002). Once a country is awash in weapons used in conflict, these weapons remain in the area, often aggravating a culture of violence that increases the need for protection, which further increases the number of weapons in civilian hands.

International arms trade both reflects and exacerbates global disparities in health. In 2000, the ten nations that were the largest consumers of guns in national conflicts had child mortality rates 10 to 100 times higher than the ten countries exporting the most arms in the prior decade. Guns did not cause most of these deaths, but they served as a powerful deterrent to addressing other health problems (Southhall and O'Hare 2002).

The gun trade has a greater impact on urban areas because fear of crime and armed criminal and political urban groups makes cities a reliable and profitable market (Small Arms Survey 2007). Some evidence suggests that rapid urbanization is especially conducive to higher levels of gun violence, perhaps because of the associated conflicts and inequities (Small Arms Survey 2007).

By its nature, controlling the small-arms trade requires a global solution. However MNCs in the gun trade lobby the governments of developed producer nations to oppose international regulation. Nevertheless, preventing gun violence has become an important international concern. In 2001, the United Nations held the first global conference on small arms that resulted in the adoption of a non-binding agreement encouraging governments to exercise tighter control over small and light weapons (United Nations 2001). Its passage began a process of negotiating a global standard for the import, export, and transfer of all conventional arms. Gun rights groups and gun lobbies (and the U.S. government) have strongly opposed this wider focus, preferring an exclusive emphasis on the illegal trade in small arms and no restrictions on their marketing or distribution practices.

While the gun industry prefers to transfer the health, human, and economic costs of these illegal guns to the public, gun-control advocates insist that gun makers have a cradle-to-grave responsibility for the costs of their products. Gun-control advocates are also increasingly reframing gun violence as a public health concern, rather than solely an issue of violence prevention. Until recently, local efforts to control gun violence have focused on changing the behaviors of gun users rather than manufacturers. Recently, however, the U.S.–based Mayors Against Illegal Guns (2008), a bipartisan coalition that now includes 225 members from more than forty states, has advocated for changes in national laws that would require gun manufacturers to provide greater oversight of the retail distribution of their products.

## STRATEGIES TO INFLUENCE HEALTH-RELATED PRACTICES OF BUSINESS

The preceding review and other sources (Simon 2006; Hawkes 2006; Siebel 2000) illustrate that the food and firearms industries employ common strategies to realize their business objectives of maximizing profit, increasing market share, and reducing financial risk. These include selecting countries with weaker regulations for investment; seeking to maximize consumption of their products by advertising and widespread retail distribution; creating multiple, similar products to market to distinct populations segments; using their political clout to lower their taxes, avoid regulation, and enable transfer of public health and environmental costs of their products to consumers and taxpayers; and making use of public relations experts, the media, scientists, and philanthropy to create a favorable economic, social, and political climate.

The review also shows that both urbanization and globalization magnify the impact of corporate practices on health. Urbanization concentrates populations and markets, making it easier for businesses to reach more consumers more efficiently, while globalization provides new markets for products, labor, and capital. In fact, a relatively few corporations now have the power to reach most of the world's population, ensuring that a significant portion will be exposed to their goods.

Clearly, the growth of corporations has unleashed an unprecedented flow of products, and for a growing portion of the world's population, these have improved the quality of life, raised living standards, and reduced suffering. However, these and other industries also play a central role in creating the health and environmental problems that most threaten population health in the twenty-first century: chronic diseases, injuries and accidents, global warming, and unsustainable development.

Whether public health professionals celebrate or decry the health impact of corporations, the pragmatic question remains: how can those dedicated to improving population health best contribute to enhancing the positive impact of MNCs and reducing the harmful ones? This section reviews and assesses three broad approaches to changing corporate practices.

## Market Responses

Some observers believe that, if corporations engage in harmful or inefficient practices, ultimately the "invisible hand" of the market will "punish" them, forcing them to change or go bankrupt. Milton Friedman (1970) claimed that "the social responsibility of business is to increase its profits" and those corporate managers who engage in unprofitable altruism are violating their obligations to shareholders. A more activist version asserts that government can play a limited role by making markets more efficient by providing information that helps consumers make informed choices, for example, posting calorie content on the menus of restaurant chains.

From a consumer perspective, boycotts also use market forces to change business practices by reducing demand for a product. For example, the international boycott of Nestlé's baby formula products led to marketing changes for a product associated with infant illnesses and deaths (Wise 1998). It also contributed to passage of a global code, setting standards for the promotion of human milk substitutes.

Some advantages of market solutions are that they may generate less opposition from businesses, making them more feasible, and that they may be less intrusive, making them more justifiable to some constituencies. But market solutions take time and therefore lives. The failure of markets to prevent the 10 million deaths from tobacco over the twentieth century shows that markets may not be able to account for the addictive properties of a substance such as nicotine.

Market theorists have identified certain conditions for markets to function effectively: access to information on products for all parties, competition rather than monopoly, and equal enforcement of existing market rules (Lindblom 2001). In practice, businesses often seek to modify these characteristics for their advantage, making market theory an uncertain guide for action.

## Government Responses

Another approach asserts that government has a responsibility to protect public health by setting ground rules—regulations—that require corporations to avoid activities that harm health. The advantages of public-sector action are that in many cases only government has the resources, expertise, and authority to compete with business interests and that governments are, in theory, accountable to the public. In practice, all levels of governments set standards for business behavior, and although stakeholders may disagree about the particulars, few contest that government has the right and responsibility to set some ground rules.

But the rise of MNCs has made it more difficult for government to control business behavior. The rise of global competition has precipitated what some have called a "race to the bottom," as governments compete to create more welcoming and less burdensome conditions for global capital (Reich 2007). Some governments also have become so business-friendly that they view their primary mandate as supporting economic growth, therefore diminishing their capacity to protect public health.

## Moral and Political Responses

A third approach favors moral and political appeals to corporations to develop practices that protect health and the environment and promote social justice. In the last few decades, corporate social responsibility (CSR) has emerged as a business ethic that has motivated some companies to change their environmental, employment, and other practices (Vogel 2005). For the most part, CSR has not emphasized public health goals (Ahn 2005), although recently, some food activists have called on MNCs to assume more responsibility for the health consequences of their practices (Ludwig and Nestle 2008), and many relevant companies are involved in regimes to minimize the negative impact of their activities on the environment.

Proponents of this approach argue that by appealing directly to businesses, it may be possible to circumvent the lengthy delays that government action often entails. Also by making moral arguments, advocates hope to mobilize broader constituencies for action, including shareholders, faith organizations, and the media.

Critics worry that the social responsibility approach predisposes to compromise, and businesses, because of their greater power, make symbolic rather than substantive concessions (Simon 2006). Since social responsibility campaigns also are often based in a single nation, health advocates fear they may simply push unhealthy practices into less powerful nations, magnifying harm and increasing global health disparities.

Although debates about the relative merits of these three approaches to making business practices more salutogenic occur in global, national, and local settings, cities are an important crucible for forging solutions. With their dense populations, concentrations of businesses, history of social movements (Pickvance 2003), and hands-on connections to the daily living conditions that shape health (Freudenberg, Galea, and Vlahov 2005), cities provide a laboratory for testing bottom-up and top-down; market, government, and moral; and cooperative and adversarial strategies for encouraging healthier business practices. However, since cities are embedded in national and global contexts, they have limited capacity to alter higher-level influences on their own and must link to efforts at higher levels.

## HOW PUBLIC HEALTH PROFESSIONALS CAN INFLUENCE THE HEALTH IMPACT OF BUSINESS

Public health professionals play a variety of roles, including researcher, public official, policy maker, and advocate. How have urban health professionals used these roles to encourage health-enhancing business practices?

### Researchers

By considering business practices as a modifiable determinant of health, researchers can seek answers to these types of questions:

- What changes in business practices offer promising opportunities for primary prevention of chronic conditions, homicide, and other urban conditions?
- To what extent do business practices (for example, retail distribution, pricing) contribute to inter- and intra-urban health disparities?
- What are promising strategies for modifying business practices to improve health, and how can we most efficiently identify, evaluate and disseminate effective strategies?

## Health Officials

Health officials are responsible for monitoring population health, enforcing standards, and acting to "assure the conditions of health." By including business practices in their scope of interest and by developing metrics to assess change, they can produce the evidence that policy makers need to respond appropriately. In recent years, health officials have challenged the tobacco and food industries to play a more constructive role (Chapman 2007; Brownell and Horgen 2004). Developing successful strategies will require careful scientific and political analyses. For example, the New York City Health Department was able to overcome opposition to its proposal to ban trans fat from restaurant food by beginning with a voluntary educational campaign, then mobilizing public support to pass a mandatory ban when restaurants failed to change (Okie 2007).

## Policy Makers

Increasingly, policy makers, including elected officials, create the environments that shape health. To act effectively to modify harmful business practices, decision makers need evidence, political support, and the backbone to stand up to special interests. To acquire evidence, they will need to commission researchers and public health officials to collect and analyze data. For example, after a U.S. senator requested the Institute of Medicine (IOM) to assess the impact of food marketing on children's obesity, several senators used the IOM's conclusion to build support for legislation to reduce industry practices that contribute to obesity (IOM 2005).

Policy makers also need to mobilize diverse constituencies to support efforts to change harmful business practices. These can include business groups (Simon and Fielding 2006), health providers, advocacy groups, social movements, and consumers (Freudenberg, Bradley, and Serrano 2009). By learning how to frame issues to appeal to diverse sectors, organize coalitions, and operate effectively across government levels, public officials can increase their ability to bring about policy change (Oliver 2006).

In some cases, cooperative strategies seem to work. For example, after a report summarized the evidence on the adverse cardiovascular consequences of high-salt diets, the government of the United Kingdom persuaded the British food industry to reduce salt in processed food (Scientific Advisory Committee on Nutrition 2003), reducing exposure to sodium. In other cases, public officials take a more adversarial stance, as illustrated by the agreement that U.S. state attorneys general negotiated with the tobacco industry (Schroeder 2004). In other cases, health professionals may choose to become business policy makers, offering opportunities to make key decisions but also confronting health professionals with significant ethical challenges (Yach 2009).

Finally, policy makers sometimes need help in withstanding the onslaught that business interests launch when they perceive a threat to their interests. Resources that can help supply the needed backbone are strong professional ethics standards, coalitions and social movements that are less constrained from acting in the political arena, public opinion that often supports officials who stand up to special interests, and advocacy groups that can make failure to act to control business as unpleasant as taking action. In South Africa, for example, the Treatment Action Campaign, an organization of people with HIV infection, anti-apartheid activists, and global health organizations convinced a sometimes reluctant South African government to support their efforts to force the drug company Glaxo to lower the price of antiretroviral medications so that more South Africans could afford this therapy (Friedman and Mottiar 2004).

## Advocates

Health professionals have a long tradition of acting as advocates for healthier policies, and they have played a variety of roles in campaigns and movements to change corporate practices (Wiist 2006). In a campaign to stop the release of a new brand of cigarettes designed to appeal to African Americans, Black physicians in Philadelphia helped to mobilize other citizens and to win the media attention that forced RJ Reynolds to withdraw Uptown cigarettes (Robinson and Sutton 1994). In this and other cases, health professionals provided information, educated policy makers, used the media and lobbied for legislation in order to support changes in harmful business practices.

## A New Kind of Public Health Campaign

In the past, public health officials and advocates have focused on increasing healthy choices for individuals. But in most cases, given the overwhelming disparity in resources available to businesses promoting unhealthy choices, these public health campaigns have had only modest effects. To have an impact on population health, health officials and advocates may need to tackle business practices more directly. This may include restricting marketing of unhealthy products, removing public subsidies or tax breaks for dangerous goods, and requiring companies to pay the full costs of harms associated with their practices. Only by asserting the right of government to protect public health can the public sector compete effectively against businesses that will always have more financial resources than any single health campaign. By conducting research on the most effective strategies for changing harmful business practices, by developing public health standards that include monitoring the health impact business practices, and by advocating for policies and programs that encourage businesses to promote health more and undermine it less, public health professionals can help to make the slogan "Healthy Cities for All" a reality.

## SUMMARY

This chapter describes the impact of the business practices of multinational corporations on the health of cities. It analyzes the pathways by which business decisions on marketing, product design, retail distribution, and pricing can influence health, using the food and beverage and the firearms industries as examples. The chapter explains the unique characteristics of cities that make them attractive to multinational corporations, including population density, concentrations of wealth, diverse marketing niches, and well-developed media and marketing infrastructures. The chapter goes on to compare the strengths and limitations of market, government, and moral strategies to modify health-damaging business practices. Finally, it discusses the role of researchers, policy makers, and public health professionals and advocates in modifying business practices that harm health.

## REFERENCES

Ahn, R. 2005. Corporate social performance in the context of global public health: Framework and analysis. PhD dissertation, Harvard School of Public Health.
Anderson, S., and J. Cavanagh. 2000. Top 200: The rise of corporate global power. Global Policy forum. http://www.globalpolicy.org/socecon/tncs/top200.htm.
Arroyo, P., A. Loria, and O. Mendez. 2004. Changes in the household calorie supply during the 1994 economic crisis in Mexico and its implications for the obesity epidemic. *Nutrition Reviews* 62:S163–S168.
Brownell, K. D., and K. B. Horgen. 2004. *Food fight: The inside story of the food industry, America's obesity crisis and what we can do about it.* New York: McGraw Hill.

Centers for Disease Control and Prevention (CDC). 1999. Safer and healthier foods. *MMWR* 48(40):905–913.

Chandler, A. D., and B. Mazlich, eds. 2005. *Leviathans: Multinational corporations and the new global history.* New York: Cambridge University Press.

Chapman, S. 2007. Public health advocacy and tobacco control: Making smoking history. London: Oxford.

Coca-Cola Company. 2009. Annual report 2008. http://www.thecoca-colacompany.com/ourcompany/index.html.

Commission on Social Determinants of Health. 2007. The civil society report. Geneva: World Health Organization. http://www.who.int/social_determinants/resources/cso_finalreport_2007.pdf.

Dauvergne, P. 2008. The shadows of consumption: Consequences for the global environment. Cambridge: MIT Press.

Ellison, K. 2002. Going for a Sunday drive: Evangelical campaign focuses on environmental awareness. *Washington Post*, November 8:A03.

Freudenberg, N., S. P. Bradley, and M. Serrano. 2009. Public health campaigns to change industry practices that damage health: An analysis of 12 case studies. *Health Education & Behavior*, December 12.

Freudenberg, N., and S. Galea. 2008. The impact of corporate practices on health: Implications for health policy. *Journal of Public Health Policy* 29(1):86–104.

Freudenberg, N., S. Galea, and D. Vlahov. 2005. Beyond urban penalty and urban sprawl: Back to living conditions as the focus of urban health. *Journal of Community Health* 30(1):1–11.

Friedman, M. 1970. The social responsibility of business is to increase its profits. *New York Times Magazine*, September 13. http://www.colorado.edu/studentgroups/libertarians/issues/friedman-soc-resp-business.html.

Friedman, S., and S. Mottiar. 2004. A moral to the tale: The treatment action campaign and the politics of HIV/AIDS. Centre for Civil Society, University of KwaZulu-Natal. http://www.ukzn.ac.za/ccs/files/Friedman%20Mottier%20TAC%20Research%20Report%20Short.pdf.

Gabelnic, T., M. Haug, and L. Lumpe. 2006. *A guide to the U.S. small arms market, industry and exports, 1998–2004.* Geneva: Smalls Arms Survey.

Gerth, J. 1998. Where business rules: Forging global regulations that put industry first. *New York Times*, January 9.

Gonzalez-Villalpando, C., M. P. Stern, M. E. Gonzalez, M. D. Rivera, J. Simon, I. S. Andrade, and S. M. Haffner. 1999. The Mexico City diabetes study: A population-based approach study of genetic and environmental interactions in the pathogenesis of obesity and diabetes. *Nutrition Reviews* 5:S72–S77.

Guay, T., J. P. Doh, and G. Sinclair. 2004. Nongovernmental organizations, shareholder activism, and socially responsible investments: Ethical, strategic, and governance implications. *Journal of Business Ethics* 52:125–139.

Hawkes, C. 2006. Uneven dietary development: Linking the policies and processes of globalization with the nutrition transition, obesity and diet-related chronic diseases. *Global Health* 2(4). http://www.globalizationandhealth.com/content/2/1/4.

Institute of Medicine (IOM). 2005. *Food marketing to children and youth: Threat or opportunity?* Washington, DC: National Academy Press.

Jimenez-Cruz, A., and M. Bacardi Gascon. 2004. The fattening burden of type 2 diabetes on Mexicans. *Diabetes Care* 27:1213–1215.

Jimenez-Cruz, A., M. Bacardi Gascon, and E. Jones. 2002. Fruit, vegetable, soft drink, and high-fat containing snack consumption among Mexican children. *Archives of Medical Research* 33:74–80.

Klapper, B. S. 2008. Red Cross warns of food riots over soaring prices. *Breitbart Newswires*, May 27. http://www.breitbart.com/article.php?id=D90U76PG0&show_article=1.

Lindblom, C. E. 2001. *The market system: What it is, how it works and what to make of it*. New Haven: Yale University Press.

Lobstein, T. 2002. Food policies: A threat to health? *Proceedings of the Nutrition Society* 61(4):579–585.

Ludwig, D. S., and M. Nestle. 2008. Can the food industry play a constructive role in the obesity epidemic? *JAMA* 300(15):1808–1811.

Lumpe, L. 2003. In arms way: Taking aim at the global gun trade. *Amnesty International Magazine*, Winter. http://www.amnestyUSa.org/amnesty-magazine/winter-2003/in-arms-way-taking-aim-at-the-global-gun-trade/page.do?id=1105529.

Mayors Against Illegal Guns. 2008. The movement of illegal guns in America: The link between gun laws and interstate gun trafficking. http://www.mayorsagainstillegalguns.org/downloads/pdf/trace_report_final.pdf.

Miles, M., and S. Miles. 2004. *Consuming cities*. Basingstoke, UK: Palgrave Macmillan.

Nugent, R. 2004. Food and agriculture policy: Issues related to prevention of noncommunicable diseases. *Food and Nutrition Bulletin* 25(2):200–207.

Okie, S. 2007. New York to trans fats: You're out! *New England Journal of Medicine* 356(20):2017–2021.

Oliver, T. R. 2006. The politics of public health policy. *Annual Review of Public Health*; 27:195–233.

Olshansky, S. J., D. J. Passaro, R. C. Hershow, and others. 2005. A potential decline in life expectancy in the United States in the 21st century. *New England Journal of Medicine* 352(11):1138–1145.

Ortiz-Hernández, L., and B. L. Gómez-Tello. 2008. Food consumption in Mexican adolescents. *Revista Panamericana de Salud Pública* 24(2):127–135.

Patel, R. 2008. *Stuffed and starved: The hidden battle for the world's food system*. New York: Melville.

Pickvance, C. 2003. From urban social movements to urban movements: A review and introduction to a symposium on urban movements. *International Journal of Urban and Regional Research* 27(1):102–109.

Reich, R. B. 2007. *Supercapitalism: The transformation of business, democracy and everyday life*. New York: Knopf.

Rivera, J. A., S. Barquera, F. Campirano, I. Campos, M. Safdie, and V. Tovar. 2002. Epidemiological and nutritional transition in Mexico: Rapid increase of non-communicable chronic diseases and obesity. *Public Health Nutrition* 5:113–122.

Rivera, J. A., S. Barquera, T. Gonzalez-Cossyo, G. Olaiz, and J. Sepulveda 2004. Nutrition transition in Mexico and in other Latin American countries. *Nutrition Reviews* 62:S149–S157.

Robinson, R. G., and C. D. Sutton. 1994. The coalition against Uptown cigarettes. In Making news, changing policy: Case studies of media advocacy on alcohol and tobacco issues ed. P. A. Wright and D. Jernigan, 89–108. Rockville, MD: Center for Substance Abuse Prevention.

Schroeder, S. A. 2004. Tobacco control in the wake of the 1998 master settlement agreement. *New England Journal of Medicine* 350:293–301.

Scientific Advisory Committee on Nutrition. 2003. *Salt and health*. London: The Stationery Office.

Siebel, B. J. 2000. The case against the gun industry. *Public Health Reports* 115(5):410–418.

Simon, M. 2006. *Appetite for profit: How the food industry undermines our health and how to fight back.* New York: Nation Books.
Simon, P. A., and J. E. Fielding. 2006. Public health and business: A partnership that makes cents. *Health Affairs* 25(4):1029–1039.
Small Arms Survey. 2007. *Small arms survey 2007: Guns and the city.* Geneva: Small Arms Survey.
Southall, D. P., and B. A. O'Hare. 2002. Empty arms: The effect of the arms trade on mothers and children. *BMJ* 325(7378):1457–1461.
Stohl, R. 2001. *Putting children first: Building a framework for international action to address the impact of small arms on children.* New York: United Nations.
Story, M., K. M. Kaphingst, R. Robinson-O'Brien, and K. Glanz. 2008. Creating healthy food and eating environments: Policy and environmental approaches. *Annual Review of Public Health* 29:253–272.
Swinburn, B., G. Sacks, T. Lobstein, and others. 2008. The "Sydney Principles" for reducing the commercial promotion of foods and beverages to children. *Public Health and Nutrition* 11(9):881–886.
Szreter, S. 2003. The population health approach in historical perspective. *American Journal of Public Health* 93(3):421–431.
United Nations. 2001. Programme of action to prevent, combat and eradicate the illicit trade in small arms and light weapons in all its aspects. New York: United Nations. http://disarmament.un.org/cab/poa.html.
United Nations. 2006. World urbanization prospects: The 2005 revision. New York: United Nations.
Vogel, D. 2005. *The market for virtue: The potential and limits of corporate social responsibility.* Washington, DC: Brookings Institution Press.
Wiist, W. H. 2006. Public health and the anticorporate movement: Rationale and recommendations. *American Journal of Public Health* 96:1370–1375.
Williams, K., M. P. Stern, and C. Gonzalez-Villalpando. 2004. Secular trends in obesity in Mexico City and in San Antonio. *Nutrition Review* 62(7 Pt 2):S158–162.
Wise, J. 1998. Companies still breaking milk marketing code. *BMJ* 316(7138):1115.
World Bank. 1986. *Urban transport.* Washington, DC: World Bank.
World Bank. 2006. *Global economic prospects 2007: Managing the next wave of globalization.* Washington, DC: World Bank.
Yach, D. 2009. PepsiCo marketing policy. *Public Health and Nutrition* 12(7):1024–1025.

# CHAPTER TWENTY-FIVE

# CITIZEN ACTION FOR URBAN POVERTY REDUCTION IN LOW- AND MIDDLE-INCOME NATIONS

### DAVID SATTERTHWAITE

## LEARNING OBJECTIVES

- Understand the current and potential role of grassroots organizations formed by the urban poor in reducing poverty in most low- and middle-income nations
- Discuss some of the most effective strategies and responses of these organizations in shifting their engagement with government for improving urban health
- Describe how national governments and international agencies have obstructed and supported the potential of these local-government urban-poor organization partnerships to reduce poverty

ALMOST all discussions of poverty reduction in urban areas in low- and middle-income nations share a concern for how best to address the needs of low-income dwellers—for instance, for housing, health care, and water, and sanitation. But for most such discussions, the focus is on the role of governments, aid agencies, or international NGOs. Little consideration is given to the role of the urban poor groups themselves—even in defining their needs. For the international agencies, there are the Millennium Development Goals (MDGs) that they have signed up for, which list the needs that have to be addressed. Although these help emphasize aspects of development that are important to low-income urban dwellers—such as health care, adequate livelihoods, and access to schools and to safe drinking water—again they were not involved in defining this list of needs and priorities. Urban-poor groups also get no say in whether or not they are defined as being "poor" (or in many nations even being classified by government as "extremely poor" or "destitute"). The definition of "poverty" (and from this, "urban poverty") and its measurement and monitoring is something entrusted to specialists.

The conventional approaches to poverty reduction—state-managed, professionally directed, and sometimes funded by international donors—have not met the needs of large sections of the urban population, despite six decades of "development." This can be seen in the very large numbers of urban dwellers who live in poverty. Most cities in low- and middle-income nations have large sections of their population living in poor quality housing in tenements and informal settlements, often three or more people to a room. Most of these people also have very inadequate provision for water. They do not have water piped to their home and at best they get it from public standpipes (which usually means a long walk and a queue) or water vendors that are expensive (Hardoy, Mitlin, and Satterthwaite 2001; UN-HABITAT 2003b). Most have no toilet in their home so they have to rely on public toilets that are usually poorly maintained, or they defecate in the open or into plastic bags or waste paper (often termed "wrap and throw"—or in some cities, "flying toilets").

In most informal settlements, there is no government health care and very inadequate provision for schools. There is also no rule of law—and many residents of informal settlements find it difficult to access government services or get onto the voters register because this requires an official address or identity card that they cannot get. Most of this housing is built by urban-poor households, outside formal rules and regulations, usually without legal tenure of the land they occupy

---

This chapter is based on the author's editorial "The social and political basis for action on urban poverty reduction" in *Environment and Urbanization*, 2008, 20(2), 307–318.

and without financial support from formal organizations. Around 800 million urban dwellers face these kinds of conditions. One of the most obvious consequences is very high levels of infant, child, and maternal mortality among urban populations in many nations (often ten or more times what they should be) with especially high levels among urban-poor groups (APHRC 2002; Satterthwaite 2007). The failure of development to reach urban poor groups can also be seen in the very high incidence of hunger and malnutrition among urban populations in many nations (Cohen and Garrett 2010). This failure is even evident in well-established democracies, where democratic pressures might have been expected to address these issues. It is also the case in cities and nations that have had rapidly growing economies (for instance, see Solinger 2006 for the growth in urban poverty in China, despite the nation's very rapid economic growth over more than two decades). While the proportion of the urban population living in poverty and lacking basic services varies considerably from nation to nation, even in successful middle-income nations, urban poverty is still a serious problem affecting large numbers of individuals and households (Satterthwaite 2004).

But in many nations, the urban poor are organizing themselves to address their needs through collective processes and activities. Sometimes, this is organizing and acting independent of the state. More often, it is organization to make demands on the state—for instance, to obtain something (support for upgrading existing housing with services, tenure of land they occupy or land sites on which they can build housing), or to prevent something (typically, eviction from their homes). But increasingly, there is a recognition of the value of combining these approaches—with urban-poor organizations taking autonomous action to demonstrate to governments and aid agencies what they are capable of. This article is interested in how low-income groups organize to take action and make demands, especially the means to allow them to have influence (which usually involves mass organization and collective political action). There is also an interest in how they mobilize, how they seek to represent and be accountable to their members—and how they plan and act, and build alliances.

## URBAN CONTEXTS

Urbanization can and should be beneficial to health. The unit costs of providing most of the infrastructure and services important for health (piped water, good sanitation, drainage, solid waste collection, health care, schools, emergency services) are cheaper in urban areas. Economies of scale or of proximity can be exploited, which is evident in the high life expectancies and low infant and child mortality rates achieved by many cities (Hardoy, Mitlin, and Satterthwaite

2001; UN-HABITAT 2008). Better housing and living conditions, access to safe water and good sanitation, efficient waste management systems, safer working environments and neighborhoods, food security, and access to services, such as education, health care, public transportation, and child care are examples of social determinants of health that can be addressed through good urban governance (Kjellstrom and Mercado 2008). But these are achieved only when there are city governments with the competence, capacity, and willingness to ensure that everyone in their jurisdiction has these. Where governments lack the capacity or the interest in serving low-income groups, the lack of infrastructure and services means the concentration of people, enterprises, and waste greatly exacerbates health problems.

Urban contexts influence not only what is needed but also what citizens can do and how state agencies respond. By concentrating people, urban areas provide the physical geography that helps urban-poor groups develop collective organizations. These collective organizations may focus on addressing particular local needs. Or they may come together to become movements. But the concentration of people and enterprises in urban areas also creates land markets that exclude low-income groups from all but the more dangerous and worst-located housing sites. So they have to rely on getting access to land outside the legal, formal market. Getting such access or getting tenure of land they already occupy usually requires collective organization and action.

Urban centers also mean close physical proximity between citizens and local governments, and this helps explain examples of more participatory and accountable urban governments in some nations (Campbell 2003; Cabannes 2006; Almansi 2009). But in most nations, city and municipal governments lack the fiscal and institutional base to meet citizens' needs. Physical proximity is also no advantage for urban-poor groups when city authorities view them or their settlements as "the problem" that constrains the city's development and capacity to attract new investment.

Urban concentration can also serve state bodies that repress organizations formed by the urban poor or manage them in ways that diffuse their influence and effectiveness. Urban areas also concentrate and make visible both absolute poverty and inequality. Inequality becomes particularly visible in cities with sustained economic success but where local governments have proved incapable or unwilling to address the housing and basic service needs of their growing populations. This is also a reminder of how much urban poverty reduction depends on changes in the relationships between the urban poor and city or municipal governments. Improved living conditions depend on state action and investment.

There is also the issue of how urban contexts have changed over the last few decades, especially dramatic reductions in the proportions of the urban labor force working in formal enterprises and being able to join trade unions. This means far less scope for trade unions to be the collective organizations through which the urban poor can organize and make demands. It also means no national collective body that represents workers and can negotiate on wage levels and working conditions. The casualization and informalization of the labor force may help to explain why most organizations of the urban poor are constructed around collective consumption needs rather than around workplace-based demands. Higher and more stable incomes are obviously a priority for all low-income groups, but what means collective organization can use to address this are not evident. The state cannot influence income levels in economies where almost all low-income groups work in the informal economy; they may also have little influence on this even when a significant proportion work in the formal sector. But the state can deliver on access to land for housing, land tenure, infrastructure, and services.

## HOW URBAN-POOR GROUPS GET THEIR NEEDS ADDRESSED

There is one key question for the urban poor: What action will be most effective in getting their needs addressed and avoiding repressive actions by the state? At least three different actions can be identified: autonomous action, claim making, and coproduction.

We probably greatly underestimate the scale and scope of community action autonomous of the state in informal settlements, as this takes place outside of any official program and usually without external funding. One example of this is the community-managed funding and construction of sewers in urban centers in Pakistan that was stimulated and supported by a local NGO (the Orangi Pilot Project Research and Training Institute). This has reached hundreds of thousands of low-income urban dwellers (Hasan 2006).

But there are limits in what community organization and action can do without government support. There is often no water source locally that can be tapped by community action (or else local groundwater is contaminated), and a neighborhood surrounded by other urban communities has nowhere to dispose of its solid and liquid wastes or channel storm and surface runoff. Cities need larger systems of trunk infrastructure for water, sanitation, drainage, and roads, which community organizations cannot construct. A case study on the different ways of providing waste-collection services in low-income communities in Siem Reap (Cambodia) that are not served by the official municipal waste-collecting services showed that organizing and funding the actual collection of waste is less problematic than organizing (and paying for) the secondary collection that takes the collected wastes to the dumpsite (Parizeau, Maclaren, and Chanthy 2008). A case study of fifteen disaster-prone informal settlements in El Salvador showed the difficulties of getting effective communitywide measures as households sought to strengthen their homes, but they could not agree on the communitywide measures that would have been more effective. In part, this was because of the lack of support from government agencies (Wamsler 2007).

Citizen groups often focus on making demands on the state. For instance, in Dhaka, the Bastee Basheer Odhikar Surakha Committee (BOSC) was founded in 2000 to provide the way that the urban poor could put pressure on city and ward governments—and go beyond the conventional confrontational protests that had previously been the way that the poor had sought to influence government (Banks 2008). This committee brought benefits to some informal settlements and has worked well with some local politicians; women have also commented on how they appreciated the committees that have allowed women to participate. But the impact is limited by the weakness of the ward and city government (Banks 2008). In addition, urban poor groups usually have to compete with citizen groups organized by middle- and upper-income groups to get government attention, and sometimes the demands of middle- and upper-income groups are to get urban poor groups evicted from their neighborhood (Baud and Nainan 2008; Bhan 2009).

Conventional democratic processes fail to deliver for the urban poor in most cities, although democracies generally allow more scope for urban-poor organizations to organize, to make claims, and to protest. In part, this is related to how little local politicians and civil servants within each district and city can deliver—because they lack the power, funding, and revenue-raising capacity. In part, it is related to the difficulty that urban-poor groups have to hold them to account, as discussions with women in one ward of Dhaka noted: "Without this vote we have no importance to them. Only during election times do they come and seek our votes" (Banks 2008, 371).

Since urban-poor groups have very little "market" power and often limited possibilities as individuals or households of getting state entitlements, this makes collective organization the only means of increasing their power. But in many locations and settlements, it is difficult to build collective organizations because of diversity among the urban poor in (among other things) political allegiances and ethnic ties. There are often language or religious barriers to collective organization. In India, there are also all the divisions created by caste, as well as religion and language.

Another key issue is how the state responds to urban-poor organizations and how this affects these organizations (Mitlin 2006). The state's response to citizen demands may be authoritarian, with strong repression of any protest or demonstration (especially where these are deemed to be illegal). At its most extreme, the state organizes or supports murder, unlawful arrest, and torture for individuals as a means of controlling such organizations (see Arputham 2008; Arévalo 1997). This can even extend to control of the Internet—as in Egypt, in response to the way that bloggers have created a new geography of protest on the Web and through the organization of meetings and street protests (Fahmi 2009).

There are often authoritarian responses within democratic states—for instance, in response to illegal land occupation or as large-scale evictions of urban-poor settlements clear space for infrastructure or commercial developments (see Bhan 2009; du Plessis 2005). Or the state's response may be bureaucratic, requiring urban poor organizations to go through conventional bureaucratic channels to make demands and access entitlements—or protest against unfair treatment. The informal nature of the homes, settlements, and livelihoods of many of the urban poor makes it difficult or impossible for them to use such measures—for instance, getting some entitlement may depend on living in a legal registered address or producing documents such as birth certificates, which they do not have. Such bureaucratic responses discriminate against those who do not fit within formal views of entitlements and proof of such entitlements, and they may also include civil servants' hostility to the poor (see, for instance, Sabry 2005). Even when the state recognizes the need to provide alternative accommodation for those its redevelopments are displacing, it almost always sets limits on who gets rehoused—typically providing only for those who have proof they have lived there for many years and excluding tenants. Or the promised access to housing within the redevelopment may be provided at prices that those displaced cannot afford.

Alternatively, the state may use clientelism to preempt the potential of community organizations or larger collective organizations or social movements, to negotiate changes in public policies. Here, politicians develop relations with leaders that allow these leaders to "deliver" something to their organization or movement (or they simply co-opt community leaders through, for instance, bringing them onto the government payroll). In Dhaka's low-income settlements, the *mastaans* have a role that is somewhere between that of a local strongman and a leader, an intermediary between local government and the population, and a vote mobilizer (Banks 2008). This co-option may be less explicit as the political party in power sets priorities for support only for those districts or community organizations that support them.

In most cities, the state's position is a complex (and often changing) mix of these responses. One aspect of pro-poor political change in urban areas is the space made by politicians (including mayors) or senior civil servants for urban-poor groups and/or the efforts to work directly with them. Certainly, decentralization and the return to democracy, or strengthening of local democracy over the last twenty years, have provided space for the election of many innovative mayors in South America, including those committed to working with urban-poor groups (see Almansi 2009; López Follegatti 1999; Roy, Arputham, and Javed 2004; Sisulu 2006). Local government reforms, such as those associated with participatory budgeting, have sought to make relations between the state and citizens (including the urban poor) more transparent and direct. If participatory budgeting allows each district within the city to influence public investments there, it also acts as an incentive for new neighborhood associations to emerge and for older ones to broaden their membership base (Abers 1998).

## FROM PROTEST TO COPRODUCTION

There are a growing number of examples of urban-poor citizen organizations that work with the state. Many are examples of what is termed "coproduction" of housing and services by organizations of the poor and the state (Mitlin 2008b). These can deliver immediate benefits and form the basis for better citizen–local government relationships. Here, relationships between low-income citizens and the state are influenced by the way low-income citizens organize. For instance, can citizen organizations retain independence and autonomy as they work in partnership with the state, or do they need to become clients for these partnerships to work? As they work with the state, does the state treat them as partners or as contractors? And to what extent is this relationship managed through intermediaries—for instance, NGOs who may have little accountability to low-income groups and who may allow these groups little role in determining what is done?

One of the most detailed accounts of how and why citizen groups shifted from protest to coproduction is provided by Jockin Arputham, the founder of the National Slum Dwellers Federation in India, as he describes the ways that citizen groups, formed by the urban poor, have sought to change government policies over the last forty years (Arputham 2008). It is based on his own work as a community organizer and one who has been jailed many times: he had to leave India during the Emergency (the period between 1975 and 1977 when the Indian government headed by Mrs. Gandhi suspended civil rights). His work included building a coalition of grassroots organizations within Janata colony in Mumbai (where he lived) to prevent its demolition; this managed to delay the demolition for many years but not prevent it. This large settlement, with some 70,000 inhabitants who had a legal right to be there, had the misfortune to come up against the power and political influence of India's nuclear research establishment, which wanted to expand on the land occupied by these 70,000 people.

Arputham also describes the building of federations of slum dwellers, first in Mumbai, then in many other cities, and finally the India-wide National Slum Dwellers Federation. At first, these federations focused on protest and on making demands on the state—especially to prevent evictions and to get services. Their strength came from their numbers, their capacity to mobilize mass protests and, in some instances, their capacity to get support from the courts. But the strategy of the Federation changed. It was recognized that demands on state organizations have limited value if these organizations are incapable of fulfilling such demands, and that even large coalitions or social movements of the urban poor have limited capacity to effect pro-poor change if both bureaucrats and politicians see them as the opposition—as the troublemakers. The National Slum Dwellers Federation and its partner federation Mahila Milan (a federation of savings groups formed by women pavement and slum dwellers) offered government agencies (especially local agencies) the knowledge, strengths, and capacities of their members. These are mass organizations, with hundreds of thousands of members.

This change in tactic by the federations has led to many government-supported programs being undertaken by these federations and by the Mumbai-based NGO SPARC (Appadurai 2001; Burra 2005; Patel, d'Cruz, and Burra 2002). The federations have organized and managed the design, construction, and management of hundreds of community toilets with washing facilities that serve hundreds of thousands of low-income households. The federations in Mumbai have worked with the police to set up and manage police stations in hundreds of "slums" that work with and are accountable to community organizations (Roy, Arputham, and Javed 2004). There is also an ambitious house-building program. These illustrate a scale of action that is far beyond what civil society organizations usually engage in and far beyond what government agencies would usually support.

This did not mean that the National Slum Dwellers Federation and Mahila Milan lost their capacity for independent action or that they were co-opted by the state—as can be seen in the current struggles over how the large informal township within Mumbai, Dharavi, will be developed (Patel and Arputham 2007, 2008). This struggle over Dharavi illustrates how the homes and livelihoods of the urban poor are threatened both by state power and market power. Dharavi contains the homes and livelihoods of hundreds of thousands of low-income groups, yet as Mumbai has expanded, what was once a peripheral location has become a desirable central location for new commercial and residential developments. The state is prevented from simply bulldozing Dharavi and transferring the land to developers by democratic pressures, even if this is the preferred solution for developers, advisors, and politicians. But what is at issue is the proportion of Dharavi's residents and enterprises that will be rehoused and their influence over the form and location of this rehousing. Without collective organization, the residents of Dharavi would have little possibility of influencing this.

Mitlin (2008b) examines how these partnerships between the state and urban-poor federations in housing and basic services (coproduction) serve as a route to political influence for grassroots organizations. Coproduction means the agreement by the state that local groups (in this case, urban-poor federations) can be directly involved in the implementation of state policies. Over the last fifteen years, national and citywide federations of slum or shack dwellers or homeless people have developed in many nations—in part drawing on the experiences and organizational models of the Indian federations, in part rooted in their own local traditions (especially savings groups). There are national federations of slum/shack dwellers in at least sixteen nations, and savings groups are developing federations in many more. These federations have also long supported each other and have set up an umbrella organization, SDI (Slum/Shack Dwellers International), that they manage with the support of local NGOs. This also means that federations that are members of SDI have a collective voice in their relations with international agencies. They have also received financial support from some external funding agencies, where the member federations themselves determine how this funding is used (Mitlin and Satterthwaite 2007).

The federations choose coproduction because this gives them an active role in designing, implementing. and managing responses to their needs. Their experience is that even when the state responds positively to their demands, these responses rarely serve their needs. Even in instances where the state has allocated considerable resources to urban poverty reduction—for instance, in housing subsidies or in public toilets and washing facilities—what is built by government bodies or the contractors they hire is often inappropriate or of poor quality, unless urban-poor organizations have the capacity to shape what is provided and how it is designed and managed. The government of South Africa has supported one of the world's largest and most generous subsidy programs to support low-income households to get their own housing, but much of what has been built has been of poor quality and often in inappropriate locations because low-income households had little influence on what is built and where it is located. The South African Federation of the Urban Poor was able to change the way a proportion of the subsidies were allocated, so federation members, not contractors, designed and built the homes. This meant larger and better quality homes. In India, the quality and management of public toilets in "slum" areas improved greatly when grassroots organizations were able to influence their location and took over their design, construction, and management (Burra, Patel, and Kerr 2003).

Therefore, coproduction is the way that the federations show politicians and civil servants their capacity as partners. It extends participatory democracy by extending to urban-poor groups not only the right to influence decisions about priorities and the allocation of resources but also the right to design, implement, and manage responses (Mitlin 2008b). Coproduction also allows the development of solutions (house designs, building materials, plot layouts, infrastructure standards) that bridge the gap between what works for the poor and the formal rules and regulations governing land use and building and infrastructure (see Mitlin and Muller 2004; Manda 2007).

Many national or city federations of slum or shack dwellers are now working with government organizations on coproduction—as a means both to address immediate needs and to secure effective relations with state institutions. In many instances, this allows the homes and neighborhoods that federation members build to shift from being illegal and outside state provision to becoming formal, legal parts of the city. In some nations, it has also encouraged and supported a shift in state policy to "slum" upgrading, especially in Thailand, where a national government agency (the Community Organizations Development Institute) has supported hundreds of community-designed and managed solutions (Boonyabancha 2005, 2009).

Each of the national or city urban-poor federations could be considered as an urban social movement organization. But the way that the federations interact with the state, including their combination of autonomous organization (to give them strength and demonstrate what can be done), pressure on the state (including protests but seeking constructive partnership), avoidance of alignment with political parties, and engagement with the state on issues of collective consumption *and* citizen rights falls outside conventional categories used in discussing urban social movements. So too does their use of tangible projects as entry points for mobilization, learning, and engaging with the state. The transnational network that they learn from, that provides mutual support, that lobbies, and that negotiates collectively with international agencies could be considered a new social movement. But new social movements are more oriented toward issue and identity politics rather than toward international lobbying for collective consumption. To date, the discussions on urban social movements have concentrated on more explicitly political strategies to contest power and influence—the very strategies that the organizations and federations of slum dwellers in India used throughout the 1970s. In addition, the urban poor federations are also different from urban social movements that developed with key roles within them for trade unions and particular political parties. They are also unusual because of the central role in their organization played by savings groups, mostly composed of and managed by women.

## WHAT IS THE ROLE OF INTERNATIONAL AGENCIES?

Urban poverty reduction has received a very low level of support from aid agencies and development banks (Satterthwaite 2001; Stren 2008). Proponents of urban poverty reduction have found it difficult to make a convincing case when competing for funding with issues that are more popular with voters in high-income nations—alleviating climate change, tackling HIV/AIDs, preventing famines, and stopping child labor and violence against women (Stren 2008).

That urban development is important in addressing all these concerns should be obvious, but apparently it is not. The kinds of pragmatic local responses that can bring significant benefits to low-income groups, such as upgrading, have difficulty competing for the high moral ground with issues such as rights, personal liberties, and environmental crises (Stren 2008). Development assistance agencies have also moved away from supporting local initiatives to channeling funding to national governments in large part because this reduces (or is meant to reduce) their staff costs. The failure of development assistance to learn how to support and engage with urban-poor groups and local governments helps explain why the scale and depth of urban poverty has grown so rapidly.

Official development assistance agencies were not set up to support citizen groups. They were set up in an era when it was assumed that development assistance should be channeled through "recipient" governments. If it is now accepted that representative organizations of the urban poor are important in addressing urban poverty, the official development assistance agencies have structures that make it difficult to respond to this. And "recipient governments" do not want funding to go directly to urban-poor organizations.

Aid agencies and development banks have little accountability to the poor; most have no relations at all with the poor's own organizations. Where they have programs funding "urban poverty reduction," there is rarely any role for urban-poor organizations in their design and implementation. The urban poor face bureaucratic and often clientelist barriers in accessing resources from these agencies that are often similar to those they face when accessing government resources. Access to funding is also often mediated by professionals who inhibit rather than support urban-poor groups' decisions.

There are some precedents showing how international funding can support organizations and federations of the urban poor directly. Many of these examples are from international NGOs, but there are also examples from international foundations and some official bilateral agencies. Most international funding agencies that seek to support urban-poor groups have struggled to reconcile the kinds of funding that best match the needs and priorities of the federations with conventional funding conditions and requirements. However, there is considerable progress in developing how international funding can strengthen and support federations of the urban poor while also being accountable to the funders—especially through funding channeled to urban-poor funds that national federations set up and manage (Mitlin 2008a).

## SUMMARY

Poverty reduction is generally seen as something designed and implemented by governments and professional organizations and supported by international agencies. Little attention has been given to actions taken by "the poor," whether this is working autonomously (outside of government), organizing to make demands on government (claim making) or coproduction, where they work with government. Yet there are a growing number of initiatives undertaken by urban-poor organizations themselves—many now work at city level and some at national level. In sixteen nations, these are undertaken by national federations of savings groups formed by slum or shack dwellers. Many urban-poor organizations have also shifted their engagement with government from making demands to offering partnerships in designing and implementing initiatives, because there is not much point in making demands on government agencies incapable of fulfilling these and because these urban-poor organizations and federations have demonstrated that they can design and implement cheaper and more effective responses. Many national governments and international agencies have not recognized the potential of these local government–urban-poor organization partnerships to reduce poverty. And even where they do, many are inhibited by bureaucratic constraints or clientelist political structures.

## REFERENCES

Abers, R. 1998. Learning democratic practice: distributing government resources through popular participation in Porto Alegre, Brazil. In *Cities for citizens*, ed. M. Douglass and J. Friedmann, 39–65. Chichester, UK: Wiley.

Almansi, F. 2009. Rosario's development; Interview with Miguel Lifschitz, mayor of Rosario, Argentina. *Environment and Urbanization* 21(1):19–35.

APHRC. 2002. *Population and health dynamics in Nairobi's informal settlements*. Nairobi: African Population and Health Research Center (APHRC).

Appadurai, A. 2001. Deep democracy: Urban governmentality and the horizon of politics. *Environment and Urbanization* 13(2):23–43.

Arévalo T. P. 1997. May hope be realized: Huaycan self-managing urban community in Lima. *Environment and Urbanization* 9(1):59–79.

Arputham, J. 2008. Developing new approaches for people-centred development. *Environment and Urbanization* 20(2):319–337.

Banks, N. 2008. A tale of two wards: Political participation and the urban poor in Dhaka city. *Environment and Urbanization* 20(2):361–376.

Baud, I., and N. Nainan. 2008. "Negotiated spaces" for representation in Mumbai: Ward committees, advanced locality management and the politics of middle-class activism. *Environment and Urbanization* 20(2):483–500.

Bhan, G. 2009. This is no longer the city I once knew: Evictions, the urban poor and the right to the city in Millennial Delhi. *Environment and Urbanization* 21(1):127–142.

Boonyabancha, S. 2005. Baan Mankong: Going to scale with "slum" and squatter upgrading in Thailand. *Environment and Urbanization* 17(1):21–46.

Boonyabancha, S. 2009. Land for housing the poor by the poor: experiences from the Baan Mankong nationwide slum upgrading programme in Thailand. *Environment and Urbanization* 21(2):309–330.

Burra, S. 2005. Towards a pro-poor slum upgrading framework in Mumbai, India. *Environment and Urbanization* 17(1):67–88.

Burra, S., S. Patel, and T. Kerr. 2003. Community-designed, built and managed toilet blocks in Indian cities. *Environment and Urbanization* 15(2):11–32.

Cabannes, Y. 2006. Children and young people build participatory budgeting in Latin American cities. *Environment and Urbanization* 18:195–218.

Campbell, T. 2003. *The quiet revolution: Decentralization and the rise of political participation in Latin American cities*. Pittsburgh: University of Pittsburgh Press.

Cohen, M., and J. Garrett. 2010. The food price crisis and urban food (in)security. *Environment and Urbanization* 22(2).

du Plessis, J. 2005. The growing problem of forced evictions and the crucial importance of community-based, locally appropriate alternatives. *Environment and Urbanization* 17(1):123–134.

Fahmi, W. S. 2009. Bloggers' street movement and the right to the city: (Re)claiming Cairo's real and virtual spaces of freedom. *Environment and Urbanization* 21(1):89–107.

Hardoy, J. E., D. Mitlin, and D. Satterthwaite. 2001. *Environmental problems in an urbanizing world: Finding solutions for cities in Africa, Asia and Latin America*. London: Earthscan.

Hasan, A. 2006. Orangi Pilot Project: The expansion of work beyond Orangi and the mapping of informal settlements and infrastructure. *Environment and Urbanization* 18(2):451–480.

Kjellstrom, T., and S. Mercado. 2008. Towards action on social determinants for health equity in urban settings. *Environment and Urbanization* 20(2):551–574.

López Follegatti, L. 1999. Ilo: A city in transformation. *Environment and Urbanization* 11(2):181–202.

Manda, M.A.Z. 2007. Mchenga—Urban poor housing fund in Malawi. *Environment and Urbanization* 19(2):337–359.

Mitlin, D. 2006. The role of collective action and urban social movements in reducing chronic urban poverty. Working paper 64. Manchester: Chronic Poverty Research Centre, Manchester University.

Mitlin, D. 2008a. Urban poor funds: Development by the people for the people. Poverty Reduction in Urban Areas Series, Working Paper 18. London: IIED.

Mitlin, D. 2008b. With and beyond the state: Co-production as a route to political influence, power and transformation for grassroots organizations. *Environment and Urbanization* 20(2):339–360.

Mitlin, D., and A. Muller. 2004. Windhoek, Namibia: Towards progressive urban land policies in Southern Africa. *International Development Planning Review* 26(2):167–186.

Mitlin, D., and D. Satterthwaite. 2007. Strategies for grassroots control of international aid. *Environment and Urbanization* 19(2):483–500.

Parizeau, K., V. Maclaren, and L. Chanthy. 2008. Budget-sheets and Buy-in: The need for political and community support in the financing of a community-based waste management project. *Environment and Urbanization* 20(2):445–464.

Patel, S., and J. Arputham. 2007. An offer of partnership or a promise of conflict in Dharavi, Mumbai? *Environment and Urbanization* 19(2):501–508.

Patel, S., and J. Arputham. 2008. Plans for Dharavi: Negotiating a reconciliation between a state-driven market redevelopment and residents' aspirations. *Environment and Urbanization* 20(1):243–254.

Patel, S., C. d'Cruz, and S. Burra. 2002. Beyond evictions in a global city: People-managed resettlement in Mumbai. *Environment and Urbanization* 14(1):159–172.

Roy, A., J. Arputham, and A. Javed. 2004. Community police stations in Mumbai's slums. *Environment and Urbanization* 16(2):135–138.

Sabry, 2005. The social aid and assistance programme of the government of Egypt: A critical review. *Environment and Urbanization* 17(2):27–42.

Satterthwaite, D. 2001. Reducing urban poverty: Constraints on the effectiveness of aid agencies and development banks and some suggestions for change. *Environment and Urbanization* 13(1):137–157.

Satterthwaite, D. 2004. The underestimation of urban poverty in low- and middle-income nations. Poverty Reduction in Urban Areas Series, Working Paper 14. London: IIED.

Satterthwaite, D. 2007. In pursuit of a healthy urban environment in low- and middle-income nations. In *Scaling urban environmental challenges: From local to global and back*, ed. P. J. Marcotullio and G. McGranahan. London: Earthscan.

Sisulu, L. 2006. Partnerships between government and slum/shack dwellers' federations. *Environment and Urbanization* 18(2):401–406.

Solinger, D. J. 2006. The creation of a new underclass in China and its implications. *Environment and Urbanization* 18(1):177–194.

Stren, R. 2008. International assistance for cities in developing countries: Do we still need it? *Environment and Urbanization* 20(2):377–392.

UN-HABITAT. 2003a. *The challenge of slums: Global report on human settlements 2003*. London: Earthscan.

UN-HABITAT. 2003b. *Water and sanitation in the world's cities: Local action for global goals*. London: Earthscan.

UN-HABITAT. 2008. *State of the world's cities 2008/9*. Nairobi: UN–HABITAT.

Wamsler, C. 2007. Bridging the gaps: Stakeholder-based strategies for risk reduction and financing for the urban poor. *Environment and Urbanization* 19(1):115–142.

# CHAPTER TWENTY-SIX

# HEALTHY CITIES: LESSONS LEARNED

## AGIS TSOUROS
## GEOFF GREEN

### LEARNING OBJECTIVES

- Identify six qualities, four elements, and six strategic goals for Healthy Cities
- Describe how these qualities, elements, and strategic goals were applied in the WHO European Region
- Describe the five phases of Healthy Cities
- Identify five critical success factors for Healthy Cities in Europe

THE World Health Organization (WHO) Healthy Cities project was established as a long-term international development project that aimed to place health high on the agenda of local decision makers in Europe. Recognizing the importance of local action and the specificity of urban settings in health, it emphasizes the convening power and the public health leadership role of municipal governments. This chapter provides an overview of the WHO European Healthy Cities Network (WHO-EHCN), tracing its origins in a paradigm global shift in the concept of health development; summarizing its essential features as applied over five phases; identifying critical success factors for maintaining the vitality of the network; and concluding with the innovation and coherence that have sustained the network for over twenty years.

## CREATION OF THE HEALTHY CITIES PROJECT

Healthy Cities was officially launched in 1987–1988 by the European Region of WHO as a vehicle to bring a strategy of "Health for All" to the local level of governance in member states. In the previous decade, a series of global and European policy and strategy documents—including the Alma-Ata Declaration of primary health care (WHO 1978), the Global Strategy for Health for All (WHO 1981), and the Ottawa Charter for Health Promotion (WHO 1986)—had laid the foundations of a new approach to public health. Supported by evidence on the wider social, economic, and environmental root causes of ill health, as well as evidence on inequities in health between and within countries, these documents provided legitimacy for action for health across many sectors. Health is "everybody's business" emerged as the new public health slogan in the late 1980s, signaling a redoubled effort to move away from the narrow perception of health as merely the absence of disease, a definition already rejected by the founding charter of WHO (1946), but sustained by many in the medical profession. Local action was recognized as an important dimension of national health policies, while local governments were identified as key stakeholders in implementing both Health for All and the Agenda-21 strategy originating in the Rio Declaration on sustainable development (United Nations 1992).

From its beginning, the Healthy Cities program recognized that health is determined by a range of personal, social, economic, and environmental factors: health behavior and lifestyle, income and social status, education, employment and working conditions, access to health services, and culture and the condition of the physical environment (Tsouros 1990). Though these factors influence health in all contexts, summarized generically as a social model of health (Dahlgren and Whitehead 1992), some specific threats to health are concentrated in cities and towns, including poverty, violence, social exclusion, unemployment, pollution, substandard housing, unmet needs of vulnerable groups, inequalities, and lack of public participation. Municipal governments and their local partners have significant responsibilities and powers to address these wider determinants of health (Green 1998).

Cities participating in the WHO European Healthy Cities Network continuously and actively explore ways of implementing WHO strategies at the urban and local levels. They have potential to provide essential public health leadership, to create the preconditions for healthier living and participatory governance, and to facilitate intersectoral action. Further, in times of economic downturns, city governments have a key role to play as advocates and guardians of the health needs of the people who are most vulnerable and socially disadvantaged.

Though the Healthy City program has evolved over twenty years in response to new urban health challenges and to WHO's recent European and global strategies, at its core is a coherent set of enduring qualities, elements, and goals. A Healthy City seeks to enhance the physical, mental, social, and environmental well-being of the people who live and work there. A Healthy City has not necessarily achieved a particular health status. Rather, its leaders are conscious of health as a core urban quality and are striving to improve it. They have given an explicit political commitment to improving their citizens' health. They acknowledge major health challenges and the economic, physical, and social factors which influence them. They are prepared for institutional reforms and innovative action for health and sustainable development. Any city can be a Healthy City if it is committed to health and has a structure and process to work for its improvement. The box shows the qualities of a Healthy City.

## The Qualities of a Healthy City

1. A clean, safe physical environment of high quality (including housing quality)
2. An ecosystem that is stable now and sustainable in the long term
3. A strong, mutually supportive and nonexploitive community
4. A high degree of participation and control by the public over the decisions affecting their lives, health, and well-being
5. The meeting of basic needs (for food, water, shelter, income, safety at work) for all the city's people
6. Access to a wide range of experiences and resources, with the chance for a wide variety of contact, interactions, and communication

*(Continued)*

> 7. A diverse, vital, and innovative economy
> 8. The encouragement of connectedness with the past, with the culture and biological heritage of city dwellers, and with other groups and individuals
> 9. A form that is compatible with and enhances the preceding characteristics
> 10. An optimum level of appropriate public health and sick care services accessible to all
> 11. High health status (high levels of positive health and low levels of disease)
>
> *Source:* World Health Organization, "Introducing Healthy Cities," 2005. http://www.euro.who.int/healthy-cities/introducing/20050202_4.

Special attention has been given to identifying and investing in preconditions for change through a carefully thought-out start-up process. Having a good understanding of city power and decision-making structures, identifying and convincing the key stakeholders, negotiating resources for the project, and producing briefings and supporting evidence for different groups are some of the important actions in exploring and preparing the ground for the launch and the sustainable future of the project. The WHO publication *Twenty Steps for Developing a Healthy Cities Project* has provided strategic guidance (WHO Regional Office for Europe 1997).

In brief, the Healthy Cities approach consists of six strategic goals and four elements for action. The six strategic goals are these (Tsouros 1990):

- To promote policies and action for health and sustainable development at the local level and across the WHO European Region, with an emphasis on the determinants of health, people living in poverty, and the needs of vulnerable groups
- To strengthen the national standing of Healthy Cities in the context of policies for health development, public health, and urban regeneration with emphasis on national-local cooperation
- To generate policy and practice expertise, good evidence, knowledge, and methods that can be used to promote health in all cities in the region
- To promote solidarity, cooperation, and working links between European cities and networks and with cities and networks participating in the Healthy Cities movement
- To play an active role in advocating for health at the European and global levels through partnerships with other agencies concerned with urban

issues and networks of local authorities, and to increase the accessibility of the WHO European Network to all Member States in the European Region.
- The summary in the box "Healthy Cities: The Four Elements for Action" includes political commitment to basic Healthy Cities principles and strategies; establishment of Healthy City project infrastructure; commitment to specific goals, products, changes and outcomes; and investment in formal and informal networking and cooperation.

## Healthy Cities: The Four Elements for Action

1. Explicit political commitment at the highest level to the Healthy Cities principles and strategies, for example:
   - Endorsement of WHO Health for All, Agenda 21, and Healthy Cities political declarations (for Phase V the Zagreb Declaration)
   - Achieving strong and sustainable political support from local stakeholders
   - Mayor's letter
   - Council Resolution
   - Partnership with relevant statutory and nonstatutory agencies and departments
2. Commitment to developing a shared vision for the city, with a health development plan and work on specific goals, themes, and products, for example:
   - City Health Development Plan
   - City Health Profile
   - Local targets and policies
   - Reduction of health inequalities
   - Healthy urban planning initiatives
   - Local strategy for healthy and active living
   - Access to care and support for vulnerable groups
   - Systematic monitoring and evaluation
3. Establishment of new organizational structures and processes to manage change, for example:
   - Intersectoral Steering Group
   - Coordinator and administrative support
   - Resources
   - Project management processes and infrastructure
   - Increase public participation
   - Health Governance

*(Continued)*

> 4. Investment in formal and informal networking and cooperation, for example:
>    - Attendance of Coordinator and politician at Business Meetings and Technical Conferences
>    - Attendance of Mayor at Mayors' Meetings
>    - Electronic communication
>    - Participation in networking activities
>
> Source: A. Tsouros, 1995, "WHO Healthy City projects: State of the art and future plans," Health Promotion International 24(S1).

# ORGANIZATIONAL STRUCTURE OF THE WHO EUROPEAN HEALTHY CITIES NETWORKS

The European network of cities supported by WHO consists of three main components. First is a network of cities whose mayors have signed a formal commitment to the WHO requirements for any current five-year phase (WHO Regional Office for Europe 2009). WHO leads and coordinates this WHO European Healthy Cities Network (WHO-EHCN), supported by a Network Advisory Committee. Designed as a laboratory for cutting-edge public health, WHO-EHCN is characterized both by continuity and expansion. Membership increased from 34 cities in Phase I (1987–1992) to 37 in Phase II, then to 56 in Phase III and 79 in Phase IV(2003–2008). Eighteen of the "pioneer" cities of Phase I retained membership into Phase IV, a span of twenty years, and the majority of "new-blood" cities in Phases II and III sustained their membership into Phase IV. About 100 cities are expected to sign up for Phase V (2009–2013).

The second component is subnetworks, task forces, or city action groups. A group of cities in the WHO-EHCN work together on selected themes or topics. The concept of subnetworks was introduced in Phase IV to allow cities that are advanced or strongly committed in certain core theme areas to work more intensely for the benefit of WHO-EHCN as a whole. Subnetworks are also responsible for developing and testing guidance materials and organizing training in their respective areas of expertise.

The third component, beyond the WHO-EHCN at the heart of the European movement, is more than 1,400 European cities in 29 countries under the umbrella of the Network of European National Healthy Cities Networks (the NETWORK; Lafond and others 2003; Lafond and Heritage 2009). National networks are established and run independently in member states. The NETWORK provides a forum for cooperation between and within these networks. National networks represent an integral part of the Healthy Cities movement in Europe, and they follow the principles and goals of the WHO Healthy Cities program, adjusting their priorities and work according to national and local public health policies and priorities. National networks are accredited by WHO, applying criteria renewed in every phase. WHO leads and coordinates the NETWORK, supported by an advisory committee whose members are elected from among the national coordinators and lead national networks politicians.

## CONTENT AND THEMES OF THE PHASES OF THE EUROPEAN HEALTHY CITIES PROGRAM

Though retaining constant goals and a core infrastructure over all five phases, the European Healthy Cities movement has evolved by responding to the changing sociopolitical, demographic, and organizational contexts of Europe. The WHO-EHCN developed and expanded over two decades against a background of major changes in the region, including enlargement of the European Union, the dissolution of the USSR and Yugoslavia, significant migration, and of course, globalization. In the decade following the fall of the Berlin Wall, over twenty European states changed their constitutions and enhanced the powers and competences of local government (Green 1998).

The shape and content of WHO-EHCN has also been influenced by lessons learned from previous phases and, most importantly, by advances in scientific evidence relevant to health and sustainable development. Particularly noteworthy is a better understanding of the determinants of health, summarized in the popular WHO-EHCN publication *Social Determinants of Health* (Wilkinson and Marmot 1998, 2003). Scientific knowledge on the extent to which socioeconomic factors influence health outcomes led the WHO global Commission on Social Determinants of Health to claim that health inequalities could be closed in a generation (WHO 2008).

In the first phase (1988–1992) of the WHO European Network, 35 cities focused mainly on creating new structures and mechanisms to manage change, building foundations for health promotion work, based on the contribution of different sectors (Draper and others 1993). In the second phase (1993–1997), 39 cities strongly emphasized developing healthy public policies and drawing up comprehensive city health plans targeting equity (Ritsatakis 2009), accountability, lifestyles, and sustainable development. In the third phase (1998–2003), 55 cities strived to make a transition from health promotion to integrated city health development plans—creating partnership-based policies stressing equity, the social determinants of health, Local Agenda 21, community development (Heritage and Dooris 2009), and regeneration initiatives. City health development planning provided cities with a means to build strategic partnerships for health (Green, Acres, and others 2009) and to develop a platform to encourage all sectors to focus their work on health and the quality of life.

In Phase IV (2003–2008), 79 cities focused on investing in health, further consolidated their work on city health-development planning, and worked intensively on four core developmental themes (Green and Tsouros 2008):

1. *Healthy urban planning:* integrating health considerations into spatial planning strategies and initiatives (Barton and others 2009)
2. *Health impact assessment:* providing a structured framework for mapping how a nonhealth policy, program, or project affects health (Ison 2009)
3. *Healthy aging:* addressing the needs of older people related to health, care, and the quality of life, with special emphasis on active and independent living, creating supportive environments and ensuring access to sensitive and appropriate services (WHO 2003)
4. *Active living and physical activity:* this theme was added during Phase IV to support the WHO European Office address the obesity epidemic, recognizing that cities have a key role in this domain (Edwards and Tsouros 2006)

This period of innovation is symbolized by development of an anthropocentric model that puts citizens at the heart of sustainable development. By the end of Phase IV, many cities had integrated environment and health in sophisticated plans and programmes for sustainable development, best exemplified by Helsingborg in Sweden (Figure 26.1; Helsingborg Department for Sustainable Development 2009).

The overarching theme for Phase V (2009–2013) is health and health equity in all local policies. Health in All Policies (HiAP) recognizes that population health is not merely a product of health sector programs but largely determined by policies and actions beyond the health sector. (Ståhl and others 2006). Developed by the European Union in Association with WHO, HiAP addresses policies such as those influencing transport, housing, and urban development, the environment, education, agriculture, finance, and tax and economic development. In implementing health and health equity in all local policies, Phase V will build on previous city-health development planning and draw on the conclusions and recommendations of the global Commission on Social Determinants of Health.

Within the overarching theme of health and health equity in all policies, Phase V focuses on three core themes:

## FIGURE 26.1  Helsingborg Plan for Sustainable Development

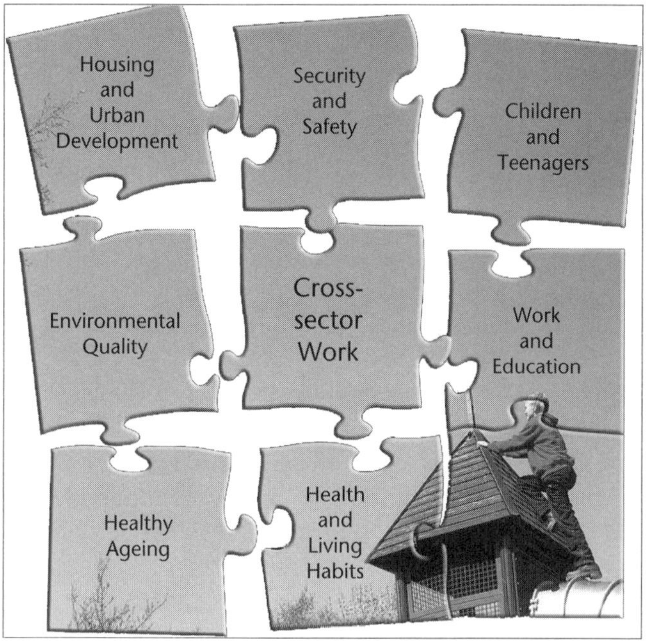

*Source:* Helsingborg Department for Sustainable Development, *Plan for Sustainable Development in Helsingborg 2009*, Helsingborg Municipal Executive Committee's Delegation for Sustainable Development, Helsingborg, Sweden, 2009.

1. *Caring and supportive environments*: a healthy city should be above all a city for all its citizens, inclusive, supportive, sensitive, and responsive to their diverse needs and expectations
2. *Healthy living*: a healthy city provides conditions and opportunities that support healthy lifestyles); and
3. *Healthy urban environment and design:* a healthy city offers a physical and built environment that supports health, recreation and well-being, safety, social interaction, easy mobility, a sense of pride, and cultural identity—a city that is accessible to the needs of all its citizens

For details of the important issues and topics under each of the core themes, refer to the Phase V page on the WHO Regional Office for Europe website at http://www.euro.who.int/healthy-cities/city/20090323_1. Climate change and health literacy are included on the Phase V action list.

## CRITICAL SUCCESS FACTORS

Over twenty years, the WHO-EHCN has become a popular and effective mechanism for promoting policies and programs based on the twin concepts of health for all and human-centered sustainability. With hindsight, we can now identify five critical success factors. The first four have been required elements for membership of the WHO-EHCN in all its phases, and the fifth reflects cities' evaluation of the role of WHO.

### Municipal Leadership

Explicit political commitment to the principles and strategies of the Healthy Cities Project is needed at the highest level. At the launch of Healthy Cities in 1988, the WHO Regional Office for Europe identified municipal governments as lead partners. Since then, membership of the WHO-EHCN has been conditional upon city mayors' signing a formal commitment to the values, principles, and goals of Healthy Cities and to funding an infrastructure for developing health plans and programs. In return, the WHO-EHCN has supported city mayors in putting health high on their council's social, economic, and political agenda. Healthy Cities are political but not partisan. Commitment has not depended upon electoral fortune.

Though responsible for providing health services in only a few European states, municipalities have generally exercised a formal competence for many of the living and working conditions identified in *Targets for Health for All* (WHO Regional Office for Europe 1985) and elaborated by Dahlgren and Whitehead (1992) as key determinants of health. Municipalities have evolved as key drivers of city health development, providing both political leadership and continuity in administrative structures and processes. The trend towards devolution in European states has enhanced municipalities as powerful agents of change. Local governments can have a unique leadership position and convening power to protect and promote the health and well-being of their citizens.

### Project Infrastructure

New organizational structures are needed to manage change. A robust project organization has proved critical in determining the impact and sustainability of European Healthy Cities. From the outset in 1988 through Phase IV (2009–2013), cities applying for membership of the WHO-EHCN were required to "secure political support and adequate resources" and put in place "structures to facilitate the implementation of goals related to a healthy city" (WHO Regional

Office for Europe 2009). A key structural requirement is "a full-time identified coordinator (or the equivalent) who is fluent in English, and administrative and technical support for their healthy city initiative." A second requirement is a "steering group involving political and executive-level decision-makers."

According to city representatives, a key success factor "is a strategically located office and a well-organized team with good management and communication skills" (Lipp and Winters 2008). Cities differ regarding where the project office and staff are located: projects have been sustained in the pioneer cities of Liège and Dresden by operating from health services or public health departments; in Sandnes and Liverpool from the mayor's or chief executive's department; and in Pecs, Belfast, and Horsens via semiautonomous organizations outside the city administration (Green, Price, and others 2009). All three options are viable; a location at the heart of a city administration lends authority to consultation with external partners and facilitates contributions from many municipal departments, whereas semiautonomous organizations may better convey to citizens a degree of independence and neutrality. These qualities are also required of Healthy City coordinators in addition to diplomacy, leadership, innovation, and management skills. Many successful coordinators also hold senior positions in related organizations, for example, in Turku, directing the Baltic Healthy Cities office; in Udine, directing the provincial health authority; in Rijeka, heading the municipal health and welfare department; and in Helsingborg, heading the municipal department of sustainable development. Seniority carries authority and access to funding.

## City Partnerships

Investment in formal and informal networking and cooperation is also key. *Targets for Health for All* (WHO Regional Office for Europe 1985) highlighted social determinants of health beyond the scope of traditional health services. These prerequisites make health everybody's business. Action to improve population health requires the cooperation of decision makers in sectors responsible for shaping wider determinants. Cities applying for membership of the WHO-EHCN are required to establish an intersectoral committee for health. Technical cooperation is necessary to undertake collaborative projects and produce a strategic city-health development plan.

Key sectors are illustrated as pillars of a Parthenon on the front cover of WHO guidance on producing city health plans (WHO Regional Office for Europe 1996); these include health and social services, business, industry, transport, education, and the economic and environment sectors. In practice, partnerships within the health and social services sectors dominated earlier phases of the WHO-ECHN and still account for most collaborative partnerships (Lipp and Winters 2008). However, in Phase IV, more cities engaged with other sectors: 64 percent at the highest level with the education sector, 28 percent with the transport sector, and 42 percent with urban planning, reflecting a core theme of this phase. Cities have generally moved beyond the planning stage to implement collaborative projects and programs.

## Principles and Values

Commitment to developing a shared vision for the city is essential, with a health plan and work on specific themes. Though political perspectives differ and political cycles are often short, Healthy Cities are able to overcome the vicissitudes of electoral fortune by building upon values and principles shared by every mainstream political party. These are red threads woven into all phases of the WHO-EHCN. The Zagreb Declaration (WHO Regional Office for Europe 2008), signed by city mayors and representatives at the international conference that concluded Phase IV, committed cities in Phase V to the five principles and values of equity, empowerment, partnership, solidarity, and sustainable development.

## WHO Leadership and Support

In signing the Zagreb Declaration (WHO Regional Office for Europe 2008), mayors and senior political representatives called on WHO to provide strategic leadership and technical support for action to support the goals of Phase V (2009–2013) of the WHO European Healthy Cities Network. Essentially, the declaration affirms the role of the WHO Regional Office for Europe during the previous four phases, enacted though the democratic organization of the WHO-EHCN. In evaluations of these earlier phases, cities' responses were overwhelmingly positive about the WHO connection. The evaluation stated:

> Participation in the WHO Network is very important for promoting activity for health at the top level of legislative and executive authority, for getting progressive experience from other cities and for mutual collaboration with other cities on solving similar problems. ( Green, Price, and others 2009, 41)

Member states vest authority in WHO to discharge the five main roles summarized in *HEALTH 21*: "act as a health conscience," "function as a major information centre," "promote the Health for All policy," "provide up-to-date evidence based tools," and work as a "catalyst for action" (WHO Regional Office for Europe, 1998). The WHO-EHCN provides a forum for discharging this function at a local level of governance to complement WHO's traditional communication with national governments and international organizations. For each domain of the Healthy Cities project, the Regional Office has helped develop a conceptual framework, supplied supporting evidence, and published guidance for implementing associated policies, programs, and projects. Examples include city health development planning (CHDP), city health profiles (CHP), healthy urban planning (HUP), health impact assessment (HIA), active living, and community participation.

## SUMMARY

The WHO-EHCN has responded innovatively to the great challenges faced by European cities over the past three decades, anticipating demographic and economic trends, seizing opportunities to exploit new political priorities. The potential for municipal leadership was cemented into the EHCN in 1988, when many cities had yet to rediscover their role in public health and had yet to test new powers and competences granted by devolution in Western Europe and in the East, via dissolution of the USSR. In the economic domain, the EHCN captured the potential for relieving financial pressures on curative health services contained in both the 1978 Alma Ata Declaration on primary care and the WHO strategy on Healthy Ageing endorsed by the UN in 2002. The core themes of city health development plans, healthy urban planning, and health impact assessment are all innovative concepts and tools which address sustainable health development in a period of political pressure on public finances.

This chapter has deployed the concept of sustainability on two levels—globally and in the leadership and organization of cities. Addressing global concerns raised by the Rio Declaration, the WHO-EHCN has given the concept of environmental sustainability a human face at a local level, developing a sophisticated approach that integrates population health into urban settlement. At the city level, this chapter has demonstrated how a sustainable political and administrative infrastructure is necessary to achieve strategic health goals. The first evaluation of the WHO-EHCN indicated a ten-year timeline from Healthy Cities' project approval to population health gain. There are critical structures and processes to be deployed en route. Many of the eighteen pioneer cities that remain in the EHCN have passed through these stages, and many more entering Phases II and III have built a platform for health development.

As Sir Michael Marmot said in his inspirational speech to the Zagreb International Conference marking the end of Phase IV in 2008, though it may take a generation to close the health gap, it is a realistic aspiration. European cities and national networks are making a mark within the international community through their leadership and contribution to health and sustainable development. The principles of the WHO European Healthy Cities movement are a dynamic driving force in many

European cities, supporting politicians, public administrations, and other agencies in implementing strategies and taking action to address growing health challenges. More than twenty years on, the Healthy Cities movement in Europe is getting stronger and becoming more relevant than ever before.

# REFERENCES

Barton, H., M. Grant, C. Mitcham, and C. Tsourou. 2009. Healthy urban planning in European cities. *Health Promotion International* 24(S1):i91–i99

Dahlgren, G., and Whitehead, M. 1992. *Policies and strategies to promote equity in health* (EUR/ICP/RPD 414[2] 9866n). Copenhagen: WHO Regional Office for Europe.

Davidson, S. 1998. Spinning the wheel of empowerment. *Planning* 1262:14–15.

Dowling, B., M. Powell, and C. Glendinning. 2004. Conceptualising successful partnerships. *Health and Social Care in the Community* 12(4):309–317.

Draper, R., L. Curtice, L. Hopper, and M. Gormans. 1993. *WHO Healthy Cities Project, Review of the first five years (1987–1992): A working tool and reference framework for evaluating the project* (EUR/ICP/HSC644). Copenhagen: WHO Regional Office for Europe.

Edwards, P., and A. Tsouros. 2006. *Promoting physical activity and active living in urban environments: The role of local governments*. Copenhagen: WHO Regional Office for Europe.

Green, G. 1998. *Health and governance in European cities: A compendium of trends and responsibilities for public health in 46 member states of the WHO European Region*. Copenhagen: WHO Regional Office for Europe.

Green, G., J. Acres, C. Price, and A. Tsouros. 2009. City health development planning. *Health Promotion International* 24(S1):i72–i80.

Green, G., C. Price, A. Lipp, and R. Priestley 2009. Partnership structures in the WHO European Healthy Cities Project. *Health Promotion International* 24(S1):i37–i44.

Green, G., and A. Tsouros. 2008. City leadership for health: Summary evaluation of Phase IV of the WHO European Healthy Cities Network. Copenhagen: WHO Regional Office for Europe.

Helsingborg Department for Sustainable Development. 2009. *Plan for sustainable development in Helsingborg 2009*. Helsingborg Municipal Executive Committee's Delegation for Sustainable Development. Helsingborg, Sweden.

Heritage, Z., and M. Dooris. 2009. Community participation and empowerment in Healthy Cities. *Health Promotion International* 24(S1)i45–i55.

Ison, E. 2009. The introduction of health impact assessment in the WHO European Healthy Cities Network. *Health Promotion International* 24(S1):i64–i71.

Lafond, L. J., and Z. Heritage. 2009. National networks of healthy cities in Europe. *Health Promotion International* 24(S1):i100–i107.

Lafond, L. J., Z. Heritage, J. L. Farrington, and A. Tsouros. 2003. *National Healthy Cities networks: A powerful force for health and sustainable development in Europe*. Copenhagen: WHO Regional Office for Europe. http://www.euro.who.int/document/e82653.pdf.

Lipp, A., and T. Winters. 2008. Partnerships. In *City leadership for health: Summary evaluation of Phase IV of the WHO European Healthy Cities Network*, ed. G. Green and A. Tsouros. Copenhagen: WHO Regional Office for Europe.

Ritsatakis, A. 2009. Equity and social determinants of health at a city level. *Health Promotion International* 24(S1):i81–i90.
Ståhl, T., M. Wismar, E. Ollila, E. Lahtinen, and K. Leppo, eds. 2006. *Health in all policies: Prospects and potentials*. Helsinki: Finnish Ministry of Social Affairs.
Tsouros, A., ed. 1990. *World Health Organization Healthy Cities project: A project becomes a movement: Review of progress 1987–1990*. Copenhagen: WHO Regional Office for Europe.
Tsouros, A. 1995. WHO Healthy City projects: State of the art and future plans. *Health Promotion International* 10(2):133–141.
United Nations. 1992. *The Rio Declaration on environment and development* (U.N. Doc. A/CONF.151/5/Rev.1). United Nations: New York.
Wilkinson, R., and M. Marmot. 1998. *Social determinants of health: The solid facts*. Copenhagen: WHO Regional Office for Europe.
World Health Organization (WHO). 1946. Preamble to the constitution of the World Health Organization. Official records of the World Health Organization, No. 2: 100. http://www.who.int/about/definition/en/print.html.
World Health Organization (WHO). 1978. Declaration of Alma Ata. International Conference on Primary Health Care, Alma-Ata, USSR, 6–12 September. http://www.who.int/publications/almaata_declaration_en.pdf.
World Health Organization (WHO). 1981. *Global strategy for Health for All by the year 2000*. Geneva: WHO.
World Health Organization (WHO). 1986. *Ottawa charter for health promotion*. Geneva: WHO.
World Health Organization (WHO). 1992. Active ageing: A policy framework. Geneva: WHO.
World Health Organization (WHO), Commission on Social Determinants of Health. 2008. *Closing the gap in a generation: Health equity through action on the social determinants of health*. Geneva: WHO.
WHO Regional Office for Europe. 1985. *Targets for Health for All: Targets in support of the European regional strategy for Health for All*. Copenhagen: WHO.
WHO Regional Office for Europe. 1996. *City health planning: The framework*. Copenhagen: WHO.
WHO Regional Office for Europe. 1997. *Twenty steps for developing a Healthy Cities Project* (EUR/ICP/HSC 644(2). Copenhagen: WHO.
WHO Regional Office for Europe. 1998. *HEALTH 21: An introduction to the Health for All policy framework for the WHO European Region*. Copenhagen: WHO Regional Office for Europe.
WHO Regional Office for Europe. 2003. Phase IV (2003–2007) of the WHO Healthy Cities Network in Europe: Goals and requirements. Copenhagen: WHO Regional Office for Europe. http://www.euro.who.int/document/e81924.pdf.
WHO Regional Office for Europe. 2008. *Zagreb Declaration for Healthy Cities: Health and health equity in all local policies*. Copenhagen: WHO Regional Office for Europe.
WHO Regional Office for Europe. 2009. *Phase V (2009–2013) of the WHO European Healthy Cities Network: Goals and requirements*. Copenhagen: WHO.
Wilkinson, R., and M. Marmot. 2003. *Social determinants of health: The solid facts*. Copenhagen: World Health Organization, Regional Office for Europe.

# CHAPTER TWENTY-SEVEN

# THE HEALTHY CITY PROGRAM IN SHANGHAI

## FU HUA

### LEARNING OBJECTIVES

- Identify elements of a city health profile
- Describe an approach to starting a Healthy City program
- Identify components of a Healthy City program evaluation

THIS chapter will introduce readers to a Healthy City program, a comprehensive intervention through multisectoral cooperation and community participation to address multiple health determinants in a mega-city. We begin with presenting the background leading to a health profile that is the basis for any interventions. This includes an overview of economic development, demographic changes, epidemiology, and broad health determinants in the city. We then describe how the government addresses these urban health challenges through multisectoral cooperation and community participation under good government leadership. The Shanghai Healthy City Project, started in 2003 and now in its second three-year Action Plan, has demonstrated political commitment, leadership for intersectoral action, and benefits in terms of improved outcomes over time.

## OVERVIEW OF SHANGHAI'S HEALTH PROFILE

### Economy and Demographics

Shanghai, situated at the mouth of the Yangtze River, is one of the busiest metropolises in China. With a total area of 6,341 square kilometers and a resident population of more than 18 million (13.78 million registered population and 4.99 million floating population), Shanghai is among the world's largest and fastest growing urban areas. Rapid development has markedly increased the city's economic strength, leading to a constantly rising average per capita gross domestic product (GDP). In 1993, for the first time, Shanghai's per capita GDP exceeded $2,000 (according to the exchange rate for that year), increasing to $3,000 in 1997. Ten years later, in 2007, the per capita GDP reached $11,833 (calculated by registered population) or $8,849 (calculated by resident population).

The population pyramid for Shanghai portrays a dramatic change in its population structure. By the end of the 1970s, people over 60 years of age accounted for 10 percent of the total registered population, signifying the city's entry into the category of an aging society: it was the first city in China to achieve this. By 2000, with a modal age of 45 years old, the population over 60 years of age was 18 percent (Figure 27.1). By 2005, 11 percent of the population was 17 years and under, and 20 percent was 60 years and over. Persons aged 80 years and over accounted for 4 percent of the population. In 2005 the aging index (the number of older persons per hundred persons under the age of 15) was 134 in Shanghai's registered population. And the potential support ratio (the ratio of the population aged 15–64 years to that aged 65 years and over) was 15 in 2005.

FIGURE 27.1 The Aging of Shanghai (Native Population Excluding Migrants)

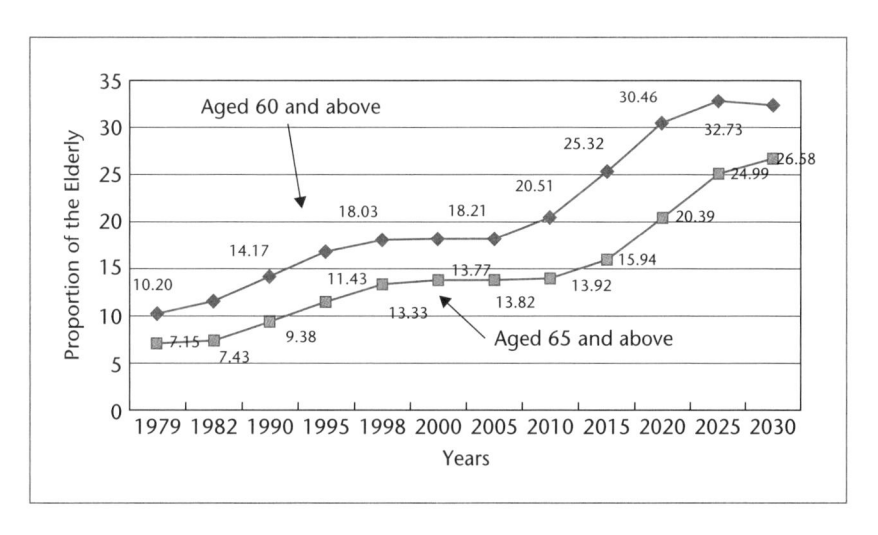

*Source:* Peng and Chen, 2005, *Demographic bonus and impact of migration: The case of Shanghai*, Kitakyushu, Japan: International Center for the Study of East Asian Development.

Several factors contribute to the demographic transition to an aging population in Shanghai. There has been a continuous increase in life expectancy of Shanghai's registered population, from 78 years old in 1998 to 81 in 2007. In 2007, the life expectancy (81 years old overall) was 79 for males and 83 for females. Life expectancy is a function of several factors, including birth rate and infant mortality rate. Before 2004, the birth rate of Shanghai declined faster than the death rate (for example, 4.5 percent and 7.7 percent, respectively, in 1998), which led to a negative natural growth rate for several decades (for example, −3 percent in 1998). In 2004, the birth rate increased to 6/1,000 (and mortality decreased to 7.2 percent) providing a balance between birth rate and natural growth rate then (−1 percent) and in 2007 (0 percent). The infant mortality rate was 10.95/1,000 and pregnant/prenatal mortality rate was 23.75/100,000 in 1990, declining to 4.01/1,000 and 8.31/100,000, respectively, in 2000, and then to 3.00/1,000 and 6.68/100,000, respectively, in 2007. While these figures contribute to understanding the expansion of life expectancy at birth, there is also a contribution due to the decrease in annual mortality among those over 65 years old. The net effect is an older population.

## Health Status of Shanghai's Population

Shanghai has experienced an epidemiologic transition (Shanghai Municipal Statistical Bureau 2008). Table 27.1 shows the leading causes of death in Shanghai over time. In 1950, the leading cause of death was contagious diseases, but the rankings declined so that by 2000, contagious diseases ranked seventh. Starting in the 1960s, diseases of the circulatory system became the leading cause of death. In 2000, diseases of the circulatory system followed by cancer, respiratory diseases, injury and poisoning, and diseases of the digestive system were the leading causes of death. In 2007, endocrine-immunity-metabolic diseases replaced the digestive disease as the fifth leading cause of death.

This pattern (that is, the change from infectious diseases and infant health problems to chronic disease) is consistent with the demographic transition to an aging population in Shanghai.

## The Health Service System in Shanghai

Shanghai has a health care service delivery system with three levels. First is the community level or primary level of health care, the community health service centers; second are the district hospitals and public health agencies; and finally are the core reference agencies, the university-affiliated or tertiary care hospitals, municipal hospitals, and the central public health agencies.

The health system is governed by health bureaus at municipal and district levels. The district health bureau is responsible for local health care service delivery at the district and community neighborhood levels. A vice-mayor and a vice-director of each district's government are designated to manage health issues, including public health and medical services. As the vice-mayor or vice-director of district government manage only two to three topics besides health in the government, some joint committees are established to oversee health policy and convene multiple agencies related to health (for example, environmental protection and education) to discuss and solve some population health problems.

In 2007, there were, on average, 3.5 doctors and 5.5 medical beds per 1,000 residents. This translates to 118,400 medical professional in 2,571 medical care institutions (534 hospitals, 232 community health service centers, and 1,719 general and specialized clinics). Shanghai also had 22 centers for disease prevention and control (CDPC) with 3,186 public health professionals, and 20 health supervision institutes with 1,254 public health professionals. The CDPCs and health supervision institutes work together for the city public health: the health supervision institutes supervise enforcement of health-related laws and regulations; the CDPC attends to other professional public health issues such as health-risk surveillance, laboratory

TABLE 27.1 The 10 Leading Causes of Death and Mortality per 100,000 for the Urban Areas of Shanghai, 1950–2007

| Rank | 1950 Cause | Rate | 1970 Cause | Rate | 1990 Cause | Rate | 2007 Cause | Rate |
|---|---|---|---|---|---|---|---|---|
| 1 | Contagious diseases | 695.8 | Diseases of the circulatory system | 160.4 | Diseases of the circulatory system | 216.1 | Diseases of the circulatory system | 257.5 |
| 2 | Diseases of the circulatory system | 71.4 | Tumors | 125.3 | Tumors | 188.3 | Tumors | 227.5 |
| 3 | Injury and poisoning | 68.9 | Respiratory diseases | 46.5 | Respiratory diseases | 115.7 | Respiratory diseases | 86.7 |
| 4 | Respiratory diseases | 62.0 | Injury and poisoning | 40.9 | Injury and poisoning | 47.6 | Injury and poisoning | 41.7 |
| 5 | Diseases of the digestive system | 53.3 | Contagious diseases | 38.5 | Disease of digestive system | 26.0 | Endocrine-Immunity-Metabolic Diseases | 30.6 |

*Sources*: Data for 1951–1990: Shanghai Academy of Social Sciences, *Shanghai Health Record*, pp. 472–473; data for 2000: Shanghai Municipal Health Bureau *Shanghai Health Yearbook*, p. 953, by the People's Health Publishing House.

tests for public health issues, response to public health emergencies, and prevention and control of communicable and noncommunicable disease. For the elderly, there were 505 nursing homes with 59,700 beds, 108 community-based daily service centers, and 233 community senior centers. The city also developed 4,345 locations (including 201 fitness gardens) embedded within communities to provide fitness equipment for residents to use.

The medical insurance system in Shanghai is the basis for paying health care. It basically covered all registered residents (more than 13 million) in 2007. Since July 1, 2009, Shanghai has also enforced a new regulation on basic medical insurance for the floating population who work temporarily in Shanghai. Under the regulation, all of the floating population can participate in the basic medical insurance program.

## Social, Economic, and Lifestyle Factors Related to Health in Shanghai

*Housing.* Dwelling area occupied by the residential population has increased continuously from 4.5 square meters per capita in 1978 to 16.5 square meters per capita in 2007. The proportion of ownership of tenement property was 39.4 percent for commercial tenements, 37.3 percent for reformed private tenements, and 20.4 percent for leasehold public tenements.

*Education.* In 2007, the rate of compulsory education was 99.99 percent, and enrollment rates were 98 percent for senior high school and 82 percent for universities. Overall, 10.8 million families have Internet service.

*Employment and income.* According to a 2007 survey, the percentage of employment per household was 54.5 percent.

In urban areas, the average disposable income per capita was 23,623 yuan (= \$3,236 [23,623/7.3]). The average consumption expenditures per capita was 17,255 yuan (= \$2,364) in 2007. Engel's coefficient was 36 percent in urban areas.

In rural areas, the average disposable income per capita was 10,222 yuan (= \$1,400), and the average consumption expenditure per capita was 8,845 yuan. Engel's coefficient was 38 percent in rural areas.

*Transportation.* Public transportation is the predominant mode of travel in the city. In urban areas, there are 991 public transportation lines with 17,000 public buses, which made 4.52 billion passenger trips in 2008. Shanghai also has nine subway lines with 262.83 kilometers of track. The subways make 2.23 million passenger trips per day. Public transportation extends to villages and it covers 75 percent of suburban areas.

*Lifestyle.* The smoking rate among Shanghai residents aged 18 years and over is 29.3 percent (61.8 percent for males and 1.2 percent for women; Xu, Li, Yao, and others 2009). Smoking among young people, especially in students of secondary vocational schools, is a problem. The smoking rates among students are 6.9 percent (10.5 percent for males and 3.2 percent for females) in junior high schools; 16.7 percent (24.2 percent for males, 9.4 percent for females) in senior high schools; and 35.2 percent (47.1 percent for males, 23.4 percent for females) in secondary vocational schools (Li, Xu, and Yao 2008).

A survey of physical activity among Shanghai residents aged 18–65 using the International Physical Activity Questionnaire (IPAQ) showed that 88.8 percent of the residents reached the standard of active physical activity (that is, moderate intensity physical activity for ≥30 min on ≥5 days/week, or vigorous intensity physical activity for ≥20 min on ≥3 days/week, equal to 600METs.min/week); 63.1 percent reached the standard of highly active physical activity (equal to 1500METs.min/week) if it included working with current paid job, transportation, family maintenance and house chores, and physical exercise during leisure time. While this is a composite measure, a breakdown of the categories shows that the amount of exercise for leisure is small. Only 19.3 percent of the population was physically active during leisure time, and 58.8 percent reported no physical activities during leisure time. Among the occupational population, only 31 percent reached an active physical activity level during leisure (Li and others 2004). Overall, 29 percent of the population aged 18 to 69 years old was overweight. Prevalence rates of self-reported hypertension, hyperlipidemia, and diabetes were 19.6 percent, 10.9 percent, and 5.6 percent, respectively (Xu, Cheng, and Li 2006).

## THE HEALTHY CITY APPROACH FOR URBAN HEALTH GOVERNANCE

According to the WHO definition (WHO Regional Office for Europe 2005), a "Healthy City" is one that is continually creating and improving the physical and social environments and expanding community resources that enable people to mutually support each other in performing all the functions of life and in developing their maximum potential. The Healthy Cities approach seeks to put health high on the political and social agenda of cities and to build a strong movement for public health at the local level. These are the four elements for action:

- Political commitment: explicit political commitment at the highest level to the principles and strategies of the Healthy Cities project
- Leadership: establishment of new organizational structures to manage change

- Institutional change: commitment to developing a shared vision for the city, with a health development plan and work on specific themes
- Intersectoral partnerships: investment in formal and informal networking and cooperation

The Shanghai Healthy City project started in 2003. It was based on the pilot of the WHO Healthy City project in Jiading District in 1996. The Shanghai municipal government initiated the program with a political commitment to implement comprehensive urban health management to achieve the goal of a healthy environment, a healthy society, and healthy people. This involved formulating and acting upon a three-year action plan for a needs assessment, policy formation, and programmatic activities. Shanghai is now in its second three-year Action Plan.

Based on the ecological health model of health determinants, the Shanghai Healthy City program adopted a comprehensive intervention approach through multisectoral cooperation and community participation. To assure effective multisectoral cooperation and involvement, the Shanghai municipal government established a multisectoral task force chaired by the vice-mayor in 2003. The task force included more than twenty municipal governmental agencies.[1] The Shanghai Municipal Institute of Health Education and an expert group from universities and institutes staffed the task force.

In 2005 (during the first three-year Action Plan), based on the work of the task force, the Shanghai municipal government approved the establishment of a Municipal Health Promotion Committee (MHPC). The vice-mayor chaired the committee, and members included representatives from the bureaus and agencies that participated in the task force. An office under the leadership of the vice-mayor was responsible for the needs assessment as well as the preparation, implementation, and evaluation of the action plan, coordination among governmental agencies, educating the public, encouraging public participation, and so on (Figure 27.2). Regular meetings with all the members of the committee were organized twice a year to assure effective implementation of the action plans for a healthy city. The office of the MHPC coordinated activities among the sectors between meetings. The MHPC produced a series of policy documents and regulations at different levels of government to support implementation of the Healthy City program.

The MHPC has been active for six years (two Action Plan periods) and has produced forty-six policy documents, and regulations related to citizens' health were developed or revised by nonhealth governmental agencies; 47 percent were developed in 2003 alone. The Office of Shanghai Municipal Health Promotion Committee also issued nine governmental documents, such as "Future Strengthening to Propagate a Healthy City," in 2005, to coordinate multisectoral work.

The city then used various forms of media to inform the public and seek their participation in the healthy city program. The television stations in Shanghai

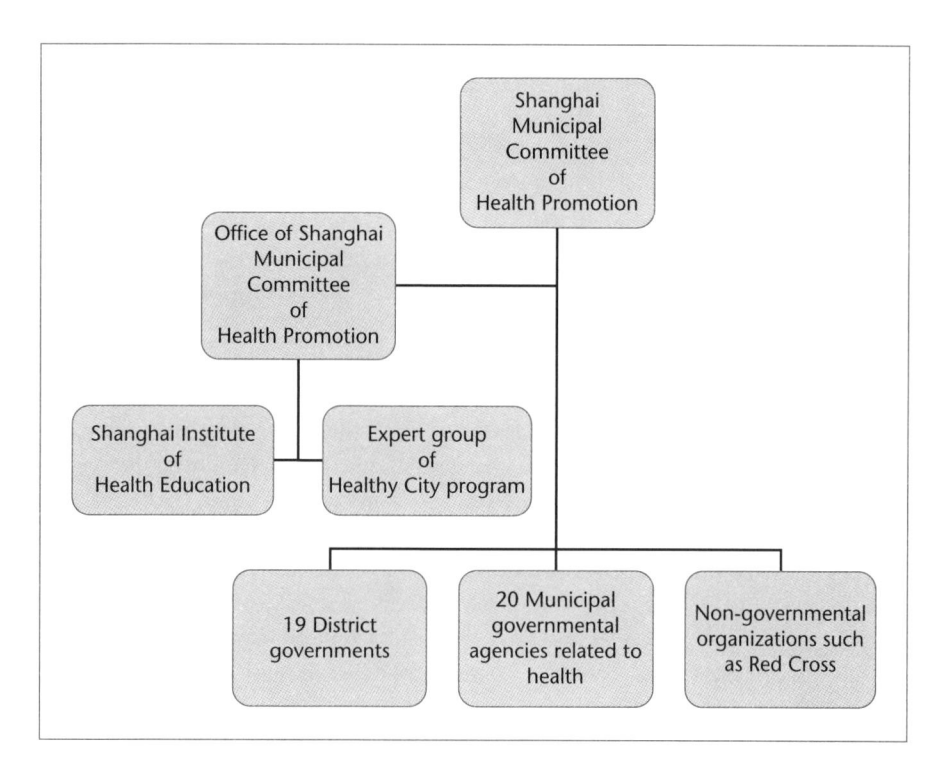

**FIGURE 27.2** Structure of Shanghai's Municipal Health Promotion Committee (MHPC)

```
                          ┌──────────────┐
                          │   Shanghai   │
                          │  Municipal   │
                          │  Committee   │
                          │      of      │
                          │Health Promotion│
                          └──────┬───────┘
         ┌──────────────────┐    │
         │Office of Shanghai│────┤
         │    Municipal     │    │
         │    Committee     │    │
         │        of        │    │
         │ Health Promotion │    │
         └────────┬─────────┘    │
    ┌────────────┴──┬────────────┤
┌────────────┐ ┌────────────┐    │
│  Shanghai  │ │Expert group│    │
│ Institute  │ │     of     │    │
│     of     │ │Healthy City│    │
│Health Educ.│ │  program   │    │
└────────────┘ └────────────┘    │
         ┌───────────────┬───────┴────────┐
    ┌─────────┐   ┌──────────────┐  ┌──────────────┐
    │19 District│  │ 20 Municipal │  │Non-governmental│
    │governments│  │ governmental │  │organizations  │
    │          │  │agencies related│ │such as Red Cross│
    │          │  │   to health  │  │               │
    └─────────┘   └──────────────┘  └──────────────┘
```

made a commitment to allocate public service advertisement time every year for the Healthy City information. The "Happy Song for a Healthy City" was created as the theme song for the project; 170,000 citizens were involved in the song project. More than 300,000 citizens attended different mass theatrical performance involving Healthy City content.

As noted above, a needs assessment was conducted with residents and governmental agencies. The results from the residents' survey showed that the most important issue for health in Shanghai was the physical environment. Residents were especially concerned about air quality, green space, and safe food. The second most important issue was social insurance, especially medical insurance from the government. The third was exposure to unhealthy behaviors of residents, especially "spitting every place" and "smoking in public places." Based on the needs assessment, the priorities for the first three-year Action Plan of the Healthy City project were focused on healthy environment, safe food, healthy behaviors, and healthy settings, including schools and communities. Eleven

Healthy City subprojects were organized and implemented, such as "protecting mother river," "creating clean air," "protecting green areas," "cleaning our city," "concerning your mental health," "physical activity by everyone," "healthy schools," and "healthy families."

In 2006, the second three-year Action Plan was implemented. The aim of this second phase was to further motivate residents' participation in the program. This phase focused on raising awareness and mastering skills of protecting the environment, enhancing confidence of safe food, and encouraging good behavior for health. There were fourteen Healthy City subprojects which focused on four kinds of healthy settings, including communities, villages, workplaces, and families. The basic message of the program was "Everybody should do five healthy things, including knowing one's own blood pressure, mastering skill for first aid, doing physical exercise, understanding safe food, and having good behaviors."

The two three-year Action Plans of the Healthy City program produced good results, based on evaluations of the Healthy City program (Gu and Fu 2009). Figure 27.3 depicts the results of an evaluation of the Healthy Cities program, which involved five dimensions—needs assessment, leadership, cooperation, resource allocation, and health policy—with each having several indicators. Ten agencies of the Shanghai government participated in constructing this evaluation. They used the Delphi process to develop the five categories, the indicator measures for each of the categories and the scales (1 to 5) on each of the dimensions. Figure 27.3 summarizes these categories and scales through depiction of five pentagons (the smallest pentagon reflecting the lowest level of the respective category and largest

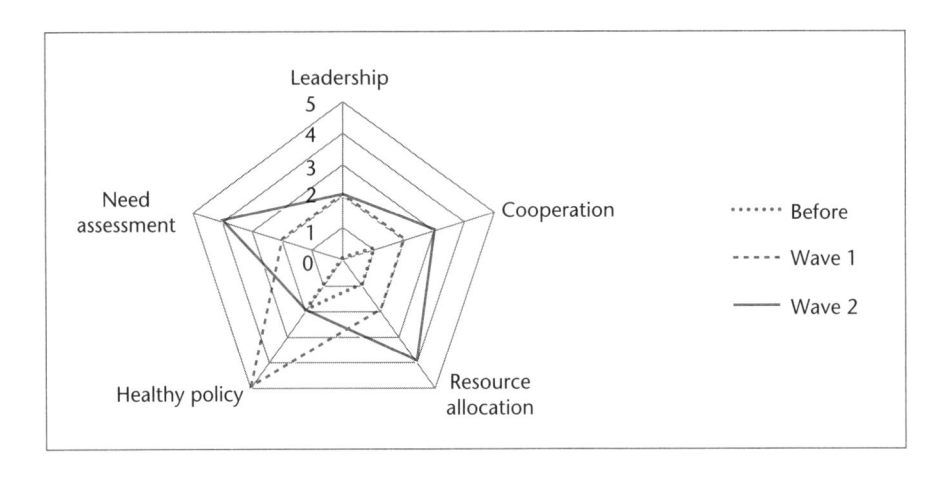

FIGURE 27.3 Political Commitment for Health Pre- and Post–Healthy City Program in Shanghai

being the highest level). The measures were taken at three time points, namely, before the implementation of the Healthy City program, at the end of the first wave of the Action Plan, and at the end of the second wave of the Action Plan. Overall, the figure demonstrates achievements in terms of more political commitment for health including leadership, multisectoral cooperation, a formal needs assessment, resource allocation, and healthy policy (Figure 27.3). While the pre-intervention evaluation showed low scores on all dimensions, the first three-year Action Plan was characterized as generating more healthy policies, and the second Action Plan focused more on programmatic issues (assessment and resource allocation).

Other visible achievements included improvements in the environment and population health in the city, as shown previously and in Tables 27.2 through 27.7. Over time, more registered residents and immigrants who moved from rural areas to Shanghai received the benefits of the healthy city program. Table 27.7 shows that the coverage rate of immunization for immigrants was nearly universal by 2008.

TABLE 27.2  Measures of Environmental Quality by Year, Before and During Healthy City Program, Shanghai

| Indicators | 2002[a] | 2005[b] | 2008[c] |
|---|---|---|---|
| Daily mean concentration of respirable particles (mg/m$^3$) | 0.108 | 0.088 | 0.088 |
| Daily mean concentration of $SO_2$ (mg/m$^3$) | 0.030 | 0.061 | 0.055 |
| Daily mean concentration of $NO_2$ (mg/m$^3$) | 0.051 | 0.061 | 0.054 |
| Average value of noise in living areas (Db) | 56.8 | 53.6 | 53.1 |
| Average value of noise in main traffic areas (Db) | 69.6 | 68.9 | 68.9 |
| Frequency of acid rain (% of days/year) | 10.9 | 40.0 | 75.6 |
| PH value of rain | 5.39 | 4.93 | 4.55 |
| Rate of sewage disposed[d] (%) | 18.8 |  | 75.5 |
| Coverage rate of natural protection areas[e] (%) | 11.8 | 11.8 | 12.1 |
| Investment for environmental protection (billion yuan) | 16.2 | 28.1 | 36.6 |

[a]The year before implementing Healthy City program in Shanghai

[b]The year of finishing first turn of three-year action plan of Healthy City program in Shanghai.

[c]The year of finishing second turn of three-year action plan of Healthy City program in Shanghai.

[d]The rate of sewage disposed is referred as percentage of disposed sewage among total sewage that should be disposed; data unavailable for 2005.

[e]The coverage rate of natural protection areas is referred as percentage of natural protection areas, including drinking water sources, scenic spots, and forest park in a city area.

TABLE 27.3  Measures of Living Environment by Year, Before and During Healthy City Program, Shanghai

| Indicators | 2002 | 2005 | 2008 |
|---|---|---|---|
| Residency area (M$^2$) | 13.1 | 15.5 | 16.5 |
| Families with gas provision (millions) | 3.5 | 4.2 | 4.7 |
| Coverage rate of water supply for urban areas (%) | 99.9 | 99.9 | 99.9 |
| Per capita water supply (M$^3$) | 89.1 | 92.2 | 133.0 |
| Facilities of physical exercise in communities | 2,318 | 4,604 | – |
| Areas of physical exercise facilities (/1000M$^2$) | 1,487 | 2,950 | – |

TABLE 27.4  Number of Outpatient Medical Visits in Millions by Year, Shanghai

|  | 2002 | 2005 | 2008 |
|---|---|---|---|
| Total outpatients | 87.83 | 106.29 | 132.18 |
| Outpatients in community health service centers | 31.59 | 36.21 | 47.40 |

TABLE 27.5  Major Indicators Related to Child (Age 0–6 Years) Health by Year, Shanghai

| Indicators | 2002 | 2005 | 2008 |
|---|---|---|---|
| Percent who received: |  |  |  |
| Any health care | 96.0 | 95.0 | 96.2 |
| Ophthalmic examination | 86.5 | 93.7 | 94.1 |
| Ear examination | 85.0 | 84.9 | 94.9 |
| Dental examination | 91.4 | 98.4 | 95.8 |
| Prevalence of anemia | 5.3 | 2.2 | 3.7 |

After six years of program implementation, surveys showed an excellent "health knowledge" score for the population. For example, 83.2 percent agreed that "the flu vaccine might protect against the flu"; 82.8 percent pointed out that a good lifestyle should emphasize "balanced diets"; 82.7 percent thought that they should "exercise more"; 81.0 percent agreed it was important to "reduce smoking,

TABLE 27.6 Morbidity or Prevalence of Selected Infectious Diseases by Year, Shanghai

|  | 2002 | 2005 | 2008 |
|---|---|---|---|
| Infectious disease incidence (/100,000) | 242.6 | 237.5 | 182.7 |
| Infectious disease mortality (/100,000) | 1.5 | 1.1 | 1.1 |
| Reported prevalence of TB (%) | 0.2 | 0.2 | 0.2 |
| Number of persons with dental examination (/1000) | 411.4 | 521.1 | 532.7 |

TABLE 27.7 Coverage Rate (%) of Immunization for Immigrants by Year, Shanghai

| Years | BCG | Polio | DTP | Measles | Hepatitis B |
|---|---|---|---|---|---|
| 2002 | 82.2 | 91.4 | 88.0 | 84.8 | 85.7 |
| 2005 | 88.3 | 90.2 | 88.6 | 92.6 | 87.2 |
| 2008 | 99.5 | 100.0 | 99.5 | 100.0 | 100.0 |

TABLE 27.8 Reported Degree to Which Shanghai Residents Felt the Healthy City Program Had Changed Health Indicators, Shanghai, 2005

| Indicators | Great improvement | Some improvement | A little change | No change | Becoming worse |
|---|---|---|---|---|---|
| Quality of environment | 33.2 | 51.4 | 9.4 | 3.3 | 2.7 |
| Availability of safe food | 17.0 | 55.1 | 18.3 | 5.7 | 3.8 |
| Healthy behaviors | 24.3 | 55.3 | 16.1 | 3.8 | 0.6 |
| Residents' participation in the Healthy City program | 31.7 | 53.1 | 11.3 | 3.2 | 0.8 |
| Good behaviors of residents | 25.3 | 53.5 | 14.0 | 5.0 | 2.2 |
| Government emphasized health issues | 34.7 | 52.1 | 9.6 | 3.3 | 0.3 |

limit liquor intake"; 80.6 percent endorsed having a "good mood every day"; 54.1 percent thought they should "control their weight."

As Table 27.8 shows, the goal of community participation was achieved. In addition, 16.2 percent of surveyed inhabitants reported that they participated more than three times in the activities related to healthy community, and almost all of the organizations in the community also participated in the Healthy City project, especially those that were government-supported organizations, such as residents' committee and mediation groups. Some nongovernmental organizations also participated in the Healthy City project, such as estate-managed companies and different kinds of sport groups. Except for providing safe food, the residents surveyed before and after the program implementation felt that the Healthy City program had improved the city's health at least somewhat (Table 27.8).

The second Action Plan adopted a focus on addressing the health issues of an aging population. As already noted, noncommunicable diseases are the leading cause of morbidity in Shanghai, due in part to its aging population. Prevention and management of chronic disease is a priority concern for Shanghai. However, the current health care system is not able to fully address this need. This is now a priority policy and programmatic area. The second Action Plan of the Healthy City program also has a focus on self-management of chronic diseases (SMCD), which has been proven to be a cost-effective strategy to tackle chronic illnesses and improve quality of life through patients' involvement, community support, and health providers' help (Dongbo and others 2003). Until the end of 2008, there were 2,394 SMCD groups that covered 41,539 patients with an average age of 65 years in all 219 administrated communities of Shanghai. The results of evaluation of the SMCD (Li and others 2009) showed that since the start of the SMCD, 75 percent of the participants had increased physical activity, reduced salty food intake, increased fruit and vegetable consumption, improved mental health, increased communication with others, scored higher on self-efficacy measures, and had higher rates of self-monitoring their blood pressure. Adherence to medications increased (54.7 percent), and 63 percent of participants talked with others about the new knowledge and skills learned from the SMCD projects. We observed that the elderly can be empowered and increase their self-efficacy for health and well-being, and we project that this can increase social capital and community empowerment.

It is difficult to disentangle the extent to which outcomes are directly attributable to the Healthy City program itself, because there was no control group for comparison. But the emphasis of multisectoral cooperation and community participation to address public health problems characterizes population health in Shanghai, which is facing the new health challenges from globalization, urbanization, and aging in the new millennium. As stated by WHO's definition of a "Healthy City," it is not one that has achieved a particular health status. Rather, it is a city that is conscious of health and striving to improve it. What is required is a commitment to health and a process and structure to achieve it. The Healthy City approach in Shanghai is practicing the strategy of new public health.

## SUMMARY

This case study provides a health profile for Shanghai, which includes demographics, mortality, birth rate, health status, the health service system, and a broad range of health-related factors. This profile of Shanghai's Healthy City program provides a useful tool by offering an empiric basis for priority-setting and action-planning. It also was used to stimulate public interest and political commitment to improve population health in the city. Based on the city health profile, the Healthy City approach addresses urban health challenges due to rapid urbanization, globalization, and an aging population. The Healthy City program in Shanghai was characterized as a political commitment demanding multisectoral cooperation. It emphasized needs assessment to incorporate public concerns in the action plans. The Shanghai Healthy City program, under the healthy promotion theory, was tailored to meet the needs of Shanghai. Two waves of Healthy City Action Plans (six years total) have increased population awareness of the Healthy Cities approach to improving public health.

## REFERENCES

Dongbo, F., F. Hua, P. McGowan, and others. 2003. Implementation and quantitative evaluation of chronic disease self-management programme in Shanghai, China: Randomized controlled trial. *Bulletin of the World Health Organization* 81(3):174–182.
Gu, S. B., and H. Fu. 2009. Evaluation of Healthy City Program in Shanghai. Doctoral thesis, Fudan University.
Li, Y., W. T. Li, B. H. Fan, and H. Fu. 2004. Study of physical activity of residents in urban Shanghai. *Chinese Journal of Labor Health and Occupational Diseases* 22:458–460.
Li, Z., G. Li, H. Fu, and others. 2009. Explore of mass prevention and control working model of hypertension in Shanghai. *Health Education and Health Promotion* 4:69–71.
Li, X. J., J. Y. Xu, and H. H. Yao. 2008. Status and influencing factors of attitudes toward tobacco control among adolescents in Shanghai. *Chinese Journal of Health Education* 24:672–674.
Shanghai Municipal Statistical Bureau. 2008. *Shanghai statistical yearbook*. Beijing: China Statistics Press.
WHO Regional Office for Europe. 2005. Introduction to healthy cities. http://www.euro.who.int/healthy-cities/introducing/20050202_1.
Xu, J. Y., Y. H. Cheng, and X. J. Li. 2006. Risk investigation on relative risk factors for chronic disease in residents of Shanghai urban areas. *Health Education and Health Promotion* 1:70–73.
Xu, J. Y., X. J. Li, H. H. Yao, and others. 2009. Smoking and passive smoking among residents in Shanghai. *Chinese Journal Prevention Control Chronic Disease* 17:234–236.

# CHAPTER TWENTY-EIGHT

# URBAN HEALTH AND GOVERNANCE MODEL IN BELO HORIZONTE, BRAZIL

WALESKA TEIXEIRA CAIAFFA

ANA LUIZA NABUCO

AMÉLIA AUGUSTA DE LIMA FRICHE

FERNANDO AUGUSTO PROIETTI

## LEARNING OBJECTIVES

- List and weigh indicators that can be used to assess determinants of the health of populations in cities
- Review the Family Health Clinic and Family Health Team model for health care
- Summarize participatory budgeting as a model of good governance, with implications for addressing the social determinants of health

THIS chapter describes Belo Horizonte City (BHC), its urban structure and health services organization, and the Democratic Governance Model the city has employed since 1994. It focuses on the use of indices of health vulnerability, quality of urban life, and environmental vulnerability as tools for government decision-making, directing interventions not necessarily at the formal health system but with health-related systems that have impact on the health of the residents of the city.

Belo Horizonte (translated as "beautiful horizon"), in southeastern Brazil, spreads over a total area of 331 square kilometers with a population of 2,412,937 and a population density of 7,290.8 inhabitants per square kilometer. BHC scores 0.839 on the Human Development Index (HDI). The GDP per capita is US$6,050.00, and its economy is based on commerce and services (80 percent) and industry (20 percent; IBGE 2007). As the population has grown, the age profile of the city has changed. Between 1970 and 2000, the proportion of the population that is at least 15 years old increased from 61.6 percent to 75.7 percent.

## A BRIEF HISTORY OF THE CITY

The city was founded in 1897 with an urban plan that emphasized a model city both in terms of its physical layout and its goal of becoming disease free (PBH 2009a). Belo Horizonte City became the political and administrative capital of the state of Minas Gerais. City growth was slow until industrialization took root in the 1950s, when new factories began to locate in the city and expanded to the periphery of the city as housing shortages for blue-collar workers became evident. Sprawling slums started to appear in the 1960s, reflecting the housing deficit and the population's need to reduce commuting distances. Growing to a million inhabitants in the 1970s, the city struggled to absorb this population influx. From 1991 to 2006, BHC was the fourth most rapidly expanding city among Brazilian cities with more than 100,000 inhabitants.

Continuous and disorderly growth was aggravated by intense construction of low-income housing developments without basic sanitary infrastructure and services. This construction, especially in proximity to existing middle- and upper-class neighborhoods, exacerbated the contrasts in the living conditions (PBH 2009a).

### The Growth of Inequalities in BHC

Although the population living in the city grew at rates below those of its metropolitan region (Brito and Souza 2005), the expansion within the city shows an uneven pace, with an annual 0.7 percent growth rate in the "formal city" and a 3.5 percent growth rate in slums or informal settlements and/or "informal city"—identified under the municipality's law on land parceling, use and occupation, known as Zones of Special Social Interest (ZEIS, the Portuguese initials). This imbalance led to the concentration of 22 percent of the overall population in just 5 percent of the city's total area (PBH 2009a).

A considerable amount of unpublished data using various indicators demonstrates a potent association between population income, spatial inequalities, and health outcomes. Health outcomes are worse in more densely populated and disadvantaged urban areas than in other better-off areas (Caiaffa and others 2005). These health inequalities are considered to be more than individual determinants, but are a function of social determinants. These social determinants include physical infrastructure and utilities (water and power supply, sewage systems, adequate housing, legal property ownership) as well as social conditions (social exclusion, poverty, income inequalities, and others related to governance such as participatory budgeting; PBH 2008; Caiaffa and others 2008; Diez-Roux 2002; Kawachi and Berkman 2001).

### The MDG Indicators for Belo Horizonte

In 2006, UN-HABITAT selected Belo Horizonte to develop a pilot program to contribute to the Millennium Development Goals (MDG) evaluation. Adopting the international treaty to eradicate extreme poverty and hunger, the city, using a multisectoral approach, has assessed, intervened, and tracked progress on indicators for eight MDGs, presented briefly in Table 28.1 (PBH 2008). The reduction of infant mortality by two-thirds as well as several MDG indicators demonstrated the municipality's strong commitment to improving health over the past few decades, despite the accelerated and unequal urbanization process.

## MAKING BHC FUNCTION TO OPTIMIZE HEALTH

### The Urban Determinants of Health in BHC

Over the past decades, mortality in Belo Horizonte has undergone an "epidemiological transition" since chronic diseases have replaced infectious diseases as the leading causes of death. Likewise, the city has undergone a demographic transition: the proportion of the population aged 65 and older has been increasing. Also, nutritional transitions, coupled with demographic transitions and globalization processes, have reshaped population health profiles (WHO 2009).

TABLE 28.1 The Performance of Eight MDG Indicators in Belo Horizonte City, from 1991 to 2007*

| MDGs | Indicator | Annual | Rates | Difference |
|---|---|---|---|---|
| Goal 1 Eradicate Extreme Poverty and Hunger | Proportion of people whose income is less than US$1 a day | 1991 18.9% | 2000 14.2% | −25.0% |
|  | Rate of hospitalization of underweight children under-five years of age (/1000) | 1998 2.1 | 2006 0.6 | −74.0% |
| Goal 2 Achieve Universal Primary Education | Net enrollment ratio in primary education | 1991 89.6% | 2000 94.3% | +5.2% |
| Goal 3 Promote Gender Equality and Empower Women | Ratios of girls to boys in secondary education (x/100) | 1991 126.0 | 2000 109.8 | −12.9 |
| Goal 4 Reduce Child Mortality | Under-five mortality rate (/1000) | 1994 47.4 | 2007 13.0 | −72.6% |
| Goal 5 Improve Maternal Health | Maternal mortality ratio | 1998 66.0 | 2007 43.0 | −34.8% |
| Goal 6 Combat HIV/AIDS, Malaria, and Other Diseases | Death rates associated with tuberculosis | 1996 2.3 | 2007 1.6 | −30.4% |
| Goal 7 Ensure Environmental Sustainability | Proportion of population using an improved sanitation facility | 1991 85.6 | 2000 93.1 | +8.8% |
|  | Proportion of population with secure ownership of housing | 1991 67.2 | 2000 80.2 | +19.3% |
| Goal 8 Develop a Global Partnership for Development | Telephone lines per 100 population | 1991 36.3 | 2000 81.4 | +124.2 |

*Depending upon data availability

As a response to such transformations and to slow the growth of chronic diseases, BHC follows the worldwide recommendations on opportunities for health promotion and prevention at the individual level. We have also acted to extend the scope of BHC health promotion beyond the main determinants of the individual's health to encompass a broader perspective of urban settings and to achieve a deeper understanding of effective urban strategies, not necessarily directly pertaining to the health sector, but which might have an impact on the health of BHC residents.

## The BHC Health System

The Brazilian Unified Health System (SUS, the Portuguese initials) intends to ensure equal and decentralized access to health services, which are managed at the municipal level. For administrative reasons, the city is subdivided uniquely into nine sanitary districts, using the census tract as the smallest geographical unit, each with multiple "planning units" that represent neighborhoods for assessment and implementation of services. Consequently, through this district system, the municipality can apply available resources in accordance to local needs and priorities. This system also makes it possible to mobilize and strengthen citizen participation in the management of health services (CONASS 2003; IBGE 2007).

Over the last two decades, BHC has been investing in the organization of its health system and in the decentralized and community-controlled implementation of the SUS. With respect to the organization of health care, the motto is "universality, integrity, and equity." In practice, the municipal efforts have focused on strengthening the network of primary care services for districts and planning units at both the individual level and the population level. Each district has approximately 250,000 inhabitants, and these services entail promotion of health, prevention, early diagnosis, treatment, and rehabilitation (PBH 2008).

To this end, the city sought to broaden access to health care through the creation and expansion of geographically dispersed (that is, among multiple neighborhood "planning units" within BHC's nine "districts" or regional administrative units) primary care health centers that would be attentive to their neighborhood, providing individual care and public health outreach. In 2002, a significant investment began with the expansion of Health Centers (CS, the Portuguese initials), through the implementation of the Family Health Program involving the formation of 176 Family Health Teams (ESF, the Portuguese initials). By 2008, this program has expanded to 146 CS with 513 ESF, which are distributed throughout the nine administrative/sanitary districts (DS, the Portuguese initials; IBGE 2007; PBH 2008).

Each CS in the regional administrative/sanitary district (DS) has a geographic coverage area, determined by a number of contiguous census tracts. Each team is responsible for a defined population area within the CS, based on a risk score calculated with the Health Vulnerability Index (IVS, the Portuguese initials) and elaborated by the BHC Health Department, as will be explained in greater detail below. By political and planners' decision, the most vulnerable areas, that is, the ones with high and medium degrees of IVS, have 100 percent of primary care coverage, guaranteeing greater equity in the provision of primary care. Three of the nine DS have 100 percent of their population covered by the ESF; one DS, with the highest socioeconomic levels, has coverage of 25 percent (PBH 2008). As a result, the Family Health Program network assists about 450,000 families living in areas with high and medium degrees of vulnerability.

# THE FOUNDATION CONCEPTS OF URBAN HEALTH IN BHC

Several elements are fundamental to BHC's urban health innovations which focus on promoting intraurban equity and addressing social determinants. They are partnership across municipality and universities, the metrics for measuring progress, and the governance model of the city (Caiaffa, Cardoso, and Proeitti 2008; Ompad and others 2007; Galea and Vlahov 2005; Vlahov and others 2007).

## The BHC Urban Health Observatory

The BHC Urban Health Observatory (OSUBH) is a partnership between the Federal University of Minas Gerais and the Belo Horizonte municipality. Founded in 2002, the OSUBH's mission is to build workforce capacity in population health research and to conduct urban-themed studies that can drive planning for improving urban health. The OSUBH is engaged in literature reviews, information gathering, and documenting interventions of programs and plans to improve the health of the city's population. This features the development of a citywide database of urban indicators and statistics to ensure the inclusion of action-oriented health data. Also, the OSUBH develops tools and conducts original data collection and analyses. The intent of these combined efforts is to provide an empirical basis for determining which urban health interventions might work best in specific contexts (Proietti and others 2002; Assunção and others 2003; UFMG 2009).

## Metrics

The municipal government of BHC has developed or incorporated a series of indexes to inform decision making about population needs, resource allocation, and program evaluation. The indicators most frequently used include (all with their Portuguese initials) the Health Vulnerability Index (IVS), the Environmental Vulnerability Index (IVA), and the Quality of Urban Life Index (IQVU). The information for these indexes is mapped according to census tract, using GIS (geographical information system) technology. The indicators and sample variables for each index are shown in Table 28.2.

**TABLE 28.2   IVS, IVA, IQVU Indicators with Their Respective Variables**

| Theme Index | Indicators | Variables |
|---|---|---|
| IVS<br>Health Vulnerability Index | Sewage | • % of permanent private households with inadequate or inexistent:<br>    supply of potable water<br>    sewage treatment services<br>    solid waste disposal services |
| | Housing | • % of improvised households in the census sector<br>• ratio of dwellers per household |
| | Education | • % of illiterate people<br>• % of household chief with <4 years of schooling |
| | Income | • % of household chief with income ≤ 2 minimum wage salaries (R$930,00)<br>• % average income of family chief (inverted) |
| | Social/health | • Death coefficient for cardiovascular diseases in people that are 20–59 years old<br>• Proportional deaths for people with <70 years of age<br>• Death coefficient for children under 5 years of age<br>• Ratio of family chief in the 10 to 19 age group |
| IVA<br>Environmental Vulnerability Index | Income | • Average income for chief of household |
| | Education | • Schooling (in years) of the chief of household |
| | Waste services | • % of households with sewage collection services |
| | Population age density | • % of households with garbage collection services |
| | Housing conditions | • Sector made up of subnormal housing conditions |

*(Continued)*

TABLE 28.2 (Continued)

| Theme Index | Indicators | Variables |
|---|---|---|
| IQVU Quality of Urban Life Index | Supply | Area in m² of:<br>  supermarkets/population<br>  butcher shops and similar establishments/population<br>  restaurants and similar establishments/population |
| | Culture | • Circulation of local publications/population × 1000 inhabitants<br>• Number of registered goods<br>• Number of cultural facilities/population × 1000 inhabitants<br>• Area in m² of bookstores and stationer shops/population × 1000 inhabitants |
| | Education | • % of students in 6 to 15 age group enlisted in primary schooling<br>• Number of students in primary schooling/number of sessions<br>• % of students in 14 to 17 age group enlisted in high school<br>• Number of students in high school/number of sessions<br>• % of promoted students |
| | Housing | • m² of adequate area/population<br>• Score for medium standard of housing in relation to the classification of Urban Building and Territorial Tax/IPTU |
| | Urban Infrastructure | • % of households with:<br>  potable water<br>  sewage system<br>  electric energy<br>  telephone line<br>• % of paved roads<br>• Number of vehicles/population<br>• Average age of the fleet of vehicles |
| | Environment | • Number of noise occurrences registered by the Military Police of Minas Gerais/population × 100 |
| | Health | • Number of:<br>  hospital beds/population × 1000<br>  health centers/population × 1000<br>  other health equipment /population × 1000<br>  dental equipment /population × 1000 |
| | Urban Services | • Number of:<br>  bank branches/population × 1000<br>  newsstands/population × 1000<br>  telephones/population × 1000 |
| | Urban Safety | • Maximum value of:<br>  homicides in the city − value of homicides in UP/ population × 1000<br>  attempted homicides in the city − value in UP/ population × 1000<br>  instances of theft or robbery in the city − value in UP/ population × 1000<br>  theft of vehicles − value in UP/population × 1000<br>  accidents in traffic − value in UP/population × 1000 |

## Health Vulnerability Index (IVS)

The BHC Health Department developed the IVS, an index composed of social, demographic, economic, and health indicators. Using multiple sources of information (including the census), the index includes the following indicators: (1) availability of water and sewage treatment, (2) community education level, (3) income, and (4) other selected social and health indicators. A specific weight is allocated to each indicator, reflecting a judgment of the relative importance for each variable contained in the indicator. The data are geo-coded by census tract and are classified according to the average score and standard deviation ($SD$) in four categories of health vulnerability: low risk (scores values lower the average); moderate risk (scores up to 0.50 $SD$ above the average); high risk (scores between 0.50 and 1 $SD$ above the average); and very high risk (scores with values of over 1 $SD$ above the average; Secretaria Municipal de Saúde de BH 2003).

## Environmental Vulnerability Risk (IVA)

The IVA is related to residential risks associated with the city's geomorphologic features. It identifies suitable areas for human dwellings in relation to vulnerability to floods and landslides stratified by socioeconomic status (as a proxy for unstable dwellings) of the resident population (Macedo and Umbelino 2008).

From this geological perspective, BHC is in a favorable region with the exception of where human dwellings have sprawled over drainage headwaters and steep slopes. The identification of such areas provides information to plan proactive and remedial interventions. The results are mapped, using GIS tools, and include (1) hypsometric and hydrographical information, (2) slope maps based upon landscape metric quotas, (3) income and education indicators, (4) health indicators, such as waste service, (5) population age density, and (6) housing conditions. The data are geo-coded by census tract, and the scores, varying from 0 to 10, are then reclassified into three priority areas for intervention: low, medium, and high vulnerability (Macedo and Umbelino 2008).

## Quality of Urban Life Index (IQVU)

Since 1996, the BHC Planning Department, in partnership with the Pontifical Catholic University of Minas Gerais, has engaged in an iterative development of the IQVU. It is an intraurban index currently composed of the following multivariable indicators: (1) food sources, (2) culture, (3) education, (4) housing, (5) urban infrastructure, (6) environment, (7) health, (8) urban services, and (9) security (see Table 28.2). This information is geo-coded into eighty homogeneous Planning Units (UP), with about 25,000 residents each. The indicators focus on the quantity and quality of public and private service provision, setting priorities (that is, weighting) for data that focus on the physical features, that is, the natural and built environment. This index measures access to the supply of goods and services in each UP correlated with spatial inequalities.

The index is expressed as a score that ranges between 0.25 and 0.81; the higher scores correspond to the UP with a better quality of urban life. Since 2000, this index has been used as a criterion for distribution of funds for assigning priorities to proposal from each UP during the Participatory Budgeting (PB) process (Nahas 2001).

## THE DEMOCRATIC GOVERNANCE MODEL OF BHC

In 1993, BHC implemented a model of democratic governance that reinforces new channels of participation through the integration of the population and organized civil society in the planning, execution, and control of public policies. The city has experimented with important advances toward the consolidation of participatory democracy, based on the principle that contemporary public institutions, regardless of the quality of their leaders and managers, cannot provide the solutions to public problems alone. Parallel to these formal instruments of representative democracy, the emerging responsibility-stimulating mechanisms emphasize the direct participation of citizens in the public policy decision-making process, through collaborative structures with deliberative powers, composed of government and organized civil society representatives.

The shared management system of municipal policies operates at different levels including the overall municipal council, the regional administrative/sanitary district councils, and more than eighty planning unit (UP) committees—all interacting with each other. There are also municipal and regional commissions of a general, thematic, or sector-specific nature. This comprehensive participation network provides transparency and accountability in the control of public policies and in proposing new initiatives.

The range of participatory public policies implemented since 1996 is extensive. Examples include childhood education, integrated health, slum upgrading, downtown revitalization without displacement of the original inhabitants, and construction of popular malls along with the phasing out of street vendors through extensive negotiations rather than police force. The regulation of transport and transit management has reduced illegal transportation. Belo Horizonte's solid waste management uses a model which incorporates social inclusion and popular participation, but perhaps the best-known example of Belo Horizonte's democratic and participatory management model is Participatory Budgeting (Azevedo and Mares Guia 2005).

## Participatory Budgeting and the Channels of Participation

With the election of a new social democratic government, the participatory budgeting (PB) process for the entire city began in 1993 as a municipal initiative; a first Directive Plan for the city was published in 1996. The planning process to develop a governance structure and system was put together through municipal offices; the plan is updated periodically with the input of the COMFORÇA (an elected set of citizen-delegates, which is described below). There is an established formula for dividing funds among administrative regions. Fifty percent of the total budget is divided equally among the nine regions; this is meant to ensure that less populated regions with a higher average income but with slums receive at least some project funding. Allocation of the other 50 percent of the participatory budget is based on a score derived from two measures: the population size and the IQVU for each of the UPs.

The participatory budgeting process is weighted toward services and infrastructure for the most vulnerable populations. To assure middle-class and upper-class involvement, 30 percent of the budget is reserved for consideration of projects that would benefit all citizens (which includes the vulnerable population). In practice, about 40 percent of projects funded fit into this category, with the other 60 percent focused on the most vulnerable populations. At the municipal level, a management board composed of representatives from all government departments and agencies that interface with participatory budgeting coordinates municipal activities related to participatory budgeting. Using the nine administrative regions, subdivided into 41 subregions, which are further divided into 80 UP, 465 discrete neighborhoods and *vilas* are identified through the IQVU, described previously. The administrative regions coordinate the priority-setting process of the planning units within their respective boundaries, and citizens apply for funds for specific projects that fit the criteria of the region.

The planning process starts with an intersectoral, municipal government committee that creates and updates the master plan for the city (Plano Plurianual de Ação Governamental [PPAG]). Representatives from five sectors (such as urban policy; urban planning; and office for disadvantaged populations—social exclusion, environment, and sanitation) meet to discuss and develop the overall city blueprint and establish citywide goals (for example, a road in one participatory budget district must connect with roads outside the district).

Though the intersectoral committee establishes the municipal master plan, the participatory budgeting process establishes priorities. The procedures for the participatory budgeting process, leading to a successfully funded project, starts with a petition of at least ten people; the municipality reviews the proposal against the PPAG. If the proposal is not consistent with the PPAG, then the proposal is rejected. A proposal that survives this step then goes to an assembly organized within the respective subregion; any citizen of the subregion can participate in the assembly. Through a vote of those present, each assembly "pre-selects" up to fifteen projects (600 overall across subregions) primarily for construction projects (roads, schools, housing, health centers, and so on) to be considered by the central planning council.

Also at the assembly, depending on the number of citizens who attend, 100–200 citizens are chosen to be delegates for the next step of the process: 20 percent of the delegates are selected by the delegates to be members of the COMFORÇA—a citizens' committee to have a voice at the municipal level in each step of the process, including selection, review, and auditing of the process and progress. Administration region-level meetings determine the final fifteen projects (for each of the nine administrative regions) that will be passed forward for implementation. As part of the process of finalizing the project list, delegates make site visits to each proposed project site (the "Priority Caravan"). Neighborhood coalitions can play a critical role in getting projects successfully through the process. Building coalitions of diverse groups that work out arrangements to be a unified bloc (where a proposal from one subgroup or faction would be put forward for one round, understanding that another proposal from another subgroup would be submitted for another round) moves proposals forward in the participatory process, providing a bloc of people to become delegates to the regional assembly and to work as a group that will "get out the vote."

The proposed projects are discussed at the regional assembly, and the final list of possible projects is slated for a general vote. Delegates from more vulnerable subregions get a higher weighted vote per person. For example, the city overall has about 202,431 slum dwellers (just under 10 percent of the population); in Barreiro DS, there are about 26,002 slum dwellers, accounting for 9.9 percent of the population, while in Centro-Sul DS there are about 38,875 slum dwellers, accounting for 14.9 percent of the population. For the former, each vote counts as 1.3 votes, and for the latter, each vote counts as 1.4 votes. This weighting provides an advantage to more vulnerable areas, but to be effective, it requires adequate voter turnout (because fewer voters with higher weighting can be cancelled out by a higher voter turnout among those from regions with lower weighting). To attract more people into the participatory process, a Web-based mechanism was implemented. To avoid biasing participation toward middle and upper classes, terminals were provided in several public places, facilitating lower-class access.

About half of the projects have been citywide for the benefit of all (infrastructure projects), one-third have been specific improvements to the *favelas*[1] (slum upgrading), ten percent have been health projects (constructing a family health center), and the rest have been split among building, schools, sports fields/physical academies, cultural centers, and the like. Since the inception of the participatory process, $300 million dollars have been committed to it, which accounts for about 3 percent of the annual municipal budget. This figure is somewhat misleading, as this estimate covers only the cost of the projects (for example, bricks and cement), while other expenses such as municipal staffing (about 100 staff) and expert consultation (such as engineers, health officials) are funded through other parts of the municipal budget.

## Redistributive Impacts of Participatory Budgeting: A Contemporary View

Between 1993 and 2008, 1,000 projects were completed (Regional PB) and more than 6,000 housing units (HPB) were approved, totaling an overall public disbursement of US$450 million. The majority of the public works of the Regional PB involved infrastructure investment (46 percent out of the total), slum upgrading (22 percent), health (11 percent) and education (10 percent). The health projects included building new health facilities (CS or others), physical academies, parks, sports, and leisure areas.

Temporal evaluation reveals that now most of the population receives the basic necessities, based on work from 1996–2008. Reflecting this, over time the percentage of approved infrastructure and urbanization undertakings has been decreasing, while that of other areas, such as health, education, culture, and sports, has been increasing (PBH 2009b).

The data of the Territorial Planning and Participatory Budgeting, URB-AL Project, reinforces the thesis that PB in Belo Horizonte is a mechanism to set priorities for resources for the neediest areas: 25 percent of the poorest areas receive 55 percent of the projects approved by the PB and 60 percent of the invested resources (PBH 2009b). Data from the 2009–2010 PB also reveal that 51.4 percent of the undertakings approved by the regional PB are located in priority areas. Simultaneously, PB undertakings are spread out in all the city's large, densely populated nuclei. Recently, data have shown that 82.9 percent of the population of BHC finds itself within a maximum radius of 500 meters from an undertaking approved by the PB (Ubirajara de Carvalho e Camargo 2007).

An analysis carried out by the Municipal Deputy Secretariat of Planning (Azevedo and others 2008), which compares the territorial distribution of the value invested in the PB through the last fifteen years with the geo-referenced data of the Health Vulnerability Index (IVS) and the IQVU also concludes that the

PB resources are essentially applied by priority in areas with the worst socioeconomic and health conditions. The regions with elevated IVS (the poorest ones) concentrate the highest number of PB works: 52.9 percent in contrast to 34 percent for the city. The value invested in the works per benefited population in the regions where the IVS is low (the richest ones) is only 21 percent of the total invested in areas where the IVS is high (see Table 28.3). Classified by the IQVU into four categories (each stratum with twenty UPs), the results show that the group of UPs with a very high IQVU (the richest ones) receive 12.5 percent of PB works and contain 22.9 percent of the total population. In the UP group with the lowest IQVU, where 13.2 percent of the city's population resides, 22.5 percent of the concluded PB works are located. The investment/population ratio shows that the UPs with the lowest IQVU received 26.9 percent of the invested value in the 1,000 works of the PB, which represents an equivalent of five times the value invested/population in areas with very high IQVU (Ferreira and others 2008; Table 28.3).

Popular participation is a key variable to understand the positive performance of the BHC in terms of social and urban indicators, especially those that are focused on reducing inequalities related to poverty. Through PB, BHC has been implementing actions that probably impact the social determinants of health, be it through the construction of housing units for the homeless population, investments in infrastructure projects, or through the construction of public facilities for health, education, sports, culture, and environment.

TABLE 28.3   Percent Distribution of the Population, the Concluded Public Works, the PB Invested Value, and Investment/Population Ratio by IVS and IQVU Categories, BHC, 1993–2008

| Indicators | | Public Works Total = 1,000 | Population Total = 2,238,288 | Investment (R$)* Total = 960,079,804.76 | Investment/ Population Average Ratio = 428.93 |
|---|---|---|---|---|---|
| IVS[a] | Elevated | 52.9 | 34.0 | 60.0 | 718.3 |
| | Medium | 35.0 | 38.0 | 32.9 | 371.6 |
| | Low | 12.1 | 28.0 | 10.01 | 155.0 |
| IQVU[b] | Low | 22.5 | 13.2 | 26.9 | 877.6 |
| | Medium | 38.1 | 34.9 | 39.0 | 479.2 |
| | High | 26.9 | 29.1 | 24.9 | 366.8 |
| | Very High | 12.5 | 22.9 | 9.2 | 172.9 |

Sources: SMAPL; SUDECAP; SMSA/PBH; *Oct. 2008.
[a] IVS = Environmental Vulnerability Index
[b] IQVU = Quality of Urban Life Index

## SUMMARY

This case study presented the development and use of quantitative measures to inform policy and programmatic planning for cities. Three different indicators were used to provide information about various dimensions of cities. Evidence showed that resources were distributed in a way that addressed the more vulnerable populations. By engaging a democratic participation of the population through participatory budgeting (PB), the initiative advanced a new model of governance and developed several interventions in the city with public health implications.

## REFERENCES

Assunção, A. A., C. D. Oliveira, E. I. de Andar, F. A. Proietti, S. A. Belisário, V. B. Oliveira, W. T. Caiaffa, M.A.S. Dias, S. G. Matos, and C. S. Rodrigues. 2003. Observatório de saúde urbana de Belo Horizonte. In *Saúde nos aglomerados urbanos: Uma visão integrada*. Brasília: Organização Pan-Americana da Saúde.

Azevedo, S., and V. Mares Guia. 2005. Reflexões sobre o orçamento participativo de Belo Horizonte: Potencialidades e desafios. In *Orçamento Participativo: Construindo a democracia*, ed. S. de Azevedo and R. Barroso, 179–196. Rio de Janeiro: Revan.

Azevedo, S., and A. L. Nabuco, eds. 2008. *Democracia participativa: A experiência de Belo Horizonte*, 89–116. Belo Horizonte: Editora Leitura.

Brito, F., and J. Souza. 2005. Expansão urbana nas grandes metrópoles: O significado das migrações intrametropolitanas e da mobilidade pendular na reprodução da pobreza. *São Paulo em Perspectiva* 19:48–63.

Caiaffa, W. T., M. C. de M. Almeida, C. D. Oliveira, A. A. de L. Friche, S. G. Matos, M.A.S. Dias, M. da C. M. Cunha, E. Pessanha, and F. A. Proietti. 2005. The urban environment from the health perspective: The case of Belo Horizonte, Minas Gerais, Brasil. *Cadernos de Saúde Pública* 21(3):958–967.

Caiaffa, W. T., C. S. Cardoso, and F. A. Proietti. 2008. Commentary: Governance: does it matter in shaping health in urban settings? How in-depth can we go? *International Journal of Epidemiology* 37:784–785.

Caiaffa, W. T., F. R. Ferreira, A. D. Ferreira, C. di L. Oliveira, V. P. Camargos, and F. A. Proeitti. 2008. Urban health: "The city is a strange lady, smiling today, devouring you tomorrow." *Ciência e Saúde Coletiva* 13(6):1785–1796.

Conselho Nacional de Secretários de Saúde (CONASS). 2003. Legislação do SUS. Brasília: CONASS. http://www.aids.gov.br/incentivo/manual/legislacao_sus.pdf.

Diez-Roux, A. V. 2002. Invited commentary: places, people, and health. *American Journal of Epidemiology* 155(6):516–519.

Ferreira, R., and others. 2008. *Resultados do orçamento participativo regional: Localização e distribuição dos recursos*. Belo Horizonte: Secretaria Municipal Adjunta de Planejamento—PBH.

Galea, S., and D. Vlahov, eds. 2005. *Handbook of urban health: Populations, methods and practices*. New York: Springer.

Instituto Brasileiro de Geografia e Estatística (IBGE). 2007. Cidades @2007. http://www.ibge .gov.br/cidadesat/topwindow.htm?1.

Kawachi, I., and L. F. Berkman. 2001. Social ties and mental health. *Journal of Urban Health* 78(3):458–467.

Macedo, D. R., and G. Umbelino. 2008. *Mapeamento da vulnerabilidade ambiental em Belo Horizonte.* Secretaria de Planejamento de Belo Horizonte. *Revista do Observatório do Milênio* 1(1):107–117.

Nahas, M.I.P. 2001. Metodologia de construção de índices e indicadores sociais, como instrumentos balizadores da gestão municipal da qualidade de vida urbana: Uma síntese da experiência de Belo Horizonte. In *Migração e ambiente nas aglomerações urbanas*, ed. Hogan and others, 461–487. São Paulo: Núcleo de Estudos de População/UNICAMP.

Ompad, D. C., and others. 2007. Social determinants of the health of urban populations: Methodologic considerations. *Journal of Urban Health* 84:i42–i53.

Prefeitura Municipal de Belo Horizonte (PBH). 2008. *Relatório de acompanhamento dos Objetivos de Desenvolvimento do Milênio—2008. Belo Horizonte.* Observatório do Milênio. Secretaria Municipal de Planejamento, Orçamentro e Informação—2008.

Prefeitura Municipal de Belo Horizonte (PBH). 2009a. BH 100 anos: Uma lição de história. 2001–2004. http://portalpbh.pbh.gov.br/pbh/ecp/comunidade.do?evento=portlet&pIdPlc=ecp%20TaxonomiaMenuPortal&app=historia&tax=11794&lang=pt_BR&pg=5780&taxp=0&.

Prefeitura de Belo Horizonte (PBH). 2009b. *Relatório de monitoramento do Orçamento Participativo.* Belo Horizonte: Secretaria Municipal Adjunta de Planejamento.

Proietti, F. A., W. T. Caiaffa, V. B. Oliveira, E. Andrade, C. S. Rodrigues, M.A.S. Dias, S. G. Matos, and C. D. Oliveira. 2002. A saúde das cidades: o observatório de saúde urbana da região metropolitana de Belo Horizonte. *PensarBH/Política Social* 3:33–36.

Secretaria Municipal de Saúde de Belo Horizonte, Gerência de Epidemiologia e Informação. 2003. Índice de vulnerabilidade à saúde, 2003. http://www.pbh.gov.br/smsa/biblioteca/gabinete/risco2003.pdf.

Ubirajara de Carvalho e Camargo, M. 2007. Instrumentos de articulación entre planificación territorial y presupuesto participativo. URBAL R9-A6-04. Manual Metodológico. Prefeitura Municipal de Belo Horizonte.

Universidade Federal de Minas Gerais (UFMG). 2009. Observatório de saúde urbana de Belo Horizonte. http://www.medicina.ufmg.br/osubh.

Vlahov, D., and others. 2007. Urban as a determinant of health. *Journal of Urban Health* 84 (3 Suppl):16–26.

World Health Organization (WHO). 2009. Cardiovascular diseases. http://www.who.int/cardiovascular_diseases/en.

# CHAPTER TWENTY-NINE

# IMPROVING POPULATION HEALTH IN A RAPIDLY URBANIZING WORLD

NICOLE VOLAVKA-CLOSE

ELLIOTT D. SCLAR

## LEARNING OBJECTIVES

- Understand the nature of urbanization and the connection between urbanization and urban population health
- Understand the underlying determinants of health outcomes for the urban poor
- Understand why addressing poverty is the most efficient way to address urban population health problems and to achieve health equity
- Understand why improving urban governance is important to addressing poverty and urban population health and how improvements in urban governance can be made

## THE DIMENSIONS OF THE URBANIZATION CHALLENGE TO HEALTH

In 2008, for the first time in history, more than half of the world's population (over 3.3 billion people) was classified as living in urbanized places, as distinct from rural areas. By 2025, 57 percent of the population will live in urban settings. By 2050, the urban population will be an estimated 6.4 billion people—or almost 70 percent of the world's predicted total population of approximately 9 billion. The urbanizing areas in the developing world[1] will absorb almost all of this growth. Over the next four decades, the urban population of these places is expected to increase by more than 120 percent (from 2.4 billion in 2007 to 5.3 billion in 2050).[2] Urban population growth is expected to be most rapid in Africa and Asia, which are currently only about 40 percent urban (United Nations Population Division 2008). Unless measures are taken to reduce gaping inequalities accompanying this global urban transformation and its rapid advance in the least developed portions of the world, much of the urban population growth will result in a significant increase of the number of urban poor; many will live in slums.

About one billion people already live in slums today. These are places of concentrated extreme disadvantage, which concentrates health risks. The health of populations on our rapidly urbanizing planet depends to a large extent on how we address the issue of urban poverty to achieve health equity. To begin, we need to more fully understand the ways that urban life aggravates or mitigates threats to population health.

## THE CONTEXT OF URBANIZATION

### The Evolution of Urbanization

Urbanization—or the increase in the proportion of the population living in towns or cities—is not a new phenomenon. From the late eighteenth through the early twentieth centuries, it was associated with industrialization. Industrialization made many urban places magnets for massive rural-to-urban migrations to cities in the Global North. As with the older pattern, so too with the present one: cities in the Global South are having a difficult time providing the necessary urban infrastructure and services to accommodate this rapid population

---

The authors would like to thank Jonathan Chanin for his assistance.

expansion. The social dislocations are also similar. What is new about this current wave of urbanization is that the fast pace of urban growth in the low- and middle-income countries of the Global South is not associated with a clear pattern of industrialization.

A second difference is time frames. There has been a vast compression in the amount of time that it takes for urban populations to expand. The scale of change is perhaps best conceptualized by considering the increasingly compressed time span that it takes to add one billion urban residents to the world's population (see Table 29.1). This compression makes it more difficult to deal with the problems that can arise with rapid, unplanned urban growth.

Urbanization implies a qualitative change in the way residents relate to one another, to the formal institutions of government, and their means of livelihood (Writh 1938). While cities in the Global North struggled to provide necessary infrastructure and institutions to support growing urban populations during the nineteenth and early twentieth centuries, the time frame during which these places adapted was longer. Though the rates of urbanization then and now are similar, the absolute increase in population size and rapid advances in technology and globalization are among the factors that are compressing the time during which cities must react to growing urban populations. People are literally straddling centuries; they may have access to cell phones but not to clean water or decent sanitation.

As mentioned above, one of the principal differences between the present urbanization process and the nineteenth-century variant is that the contemporary one is occurring without the benefit of an easily identifiable process of industrialization with a strong, explicit demand for more urban-based labor. However, this should not be mistaken for the absence of a vibrant urban economy; it is simply

TABLE 29.1  The Declining Time Needed for One Billion Additional Urban Dwellers

| World Population of Urban Dwellers | Number of Years |
| --- | --- |
| 0 to 1 billion urban dwellers | 10,000 years (c. 8000 BC–1961) |
| 1 to 2 billion urban dwellers | 25 years (1961–1986) |
| 2 to 3 billion urban dwellers | 17 years (1986–2003) |
| 3 to 4 billion urban dwellers | 15 years (2003–2018) |

*Source:* Adapted from D. Satterthwaite, 2007, The transition to a predominantly urban world and its underpinnings, Human Settlements Discussion Paper Series, Urban Change-4, p. 1, International Institute for Environment and Development. Data from United Nations Population Division, 2006, World urbanization prospects: The 2005 revision.

less visible because it is heavily informal. Many of the contemporary economies in the urbanizing locations of the Global South are organized largely around the production and exchange of labor-intensive services. It is not unusual for urban slum dwellers and enterprises to be engaged in informal work directly connected to the needs of enterprises of the formal global economy (Perlman 1976). The challenge for urban policy makers is to recognize its value and better account for its economic contribution.

## Urbanization: Opportunities and Challenges

The attraction of urban life has always rested on the expanded array of opportunities that population concentration and population diversity afford. No country classified as "high income" has attained that living standard without also attaining a high level of urbanization. That said, the economic attraction of cities is also the source of its greatest problem—population density. When sizable numbers of people from diverse backgrounds live in close proximity, it energizes human tendencies of innovation, creativity, and increased productivity (Jacobs 1969). But close proximity also creates social tensions that tend to fracture along lines of ethnicity and social class. The greater the degree of inequality along these lines, the worse the social tension. If nothing is done via social policy, social tension becomes manifest in acts of violence and injury across racial and ethnic lines, criminal and health-destroying behavior. In terms of communicable disease, density facilitates the rapid transmission of pathogens among large, concentrated populations, particularly where adequate water, sanitation, and health services are not accessible (for example, in slums).

We tolerate the density and its concomitant problems because, as an economic phenomenon, this proximity or co-location is extremely valuable. It significantly lowers the time and money costs ("transaction costs") of the production of goods and services. This economic gain is a major reason why it is almost impossible to halt the urbanization process, though attempts to do so are made repeatedly on the assumption that if rural life were better, people would not move to urban places. Therefore, the urban challenge is to create institutions that permit us to capture the economic gains of efficiency, innovation, and creativity that urban life fosters while diminishing the social costs of this same proximity and diversity. Urban population health policy becomes an important instrument for meeting this challenge, as the gains should include widespread improvement in the living standards of the entire urban population.

Widespread improvement in living conditions is presently not the case among specific urban populations and across all urban populations. The photographic juxtapositions of modern, high-rise buildings and slum settlements that are the iconic images of the rapidly growing cities of the Global South show the extreme inequality and the relationship between unmanaged rapid urban growth, poverty, and ill health (WHO 2008). Anna K. Tibaijuka, under-secretary general of the United Nations and executive director of UN-HABITAT, succinctly expresses the simultaneous threat and promise of urbanization: "Cities present an unparalleled opportunity for the simultaneous attainment of most, if not all of the internationally agreed [Millennium] development goals.... However, unless such concerted action is taken to redress urban inequalities, cities may well become the predominant sites of deprivation, social exclusion and instability worldwide" (UN-HABITAT 2007, iv).

## THE CHALLENGES OF POVERTY, HEALTH, AND SLUMS IN THE TWENTY-FIRST CENTURY

In 2005, one in three urban dwellers in the world's low- and middle-income countries lived in slums (UN-HABITAT 2008, 74). As mentioned earlier, the overwhelming majority of population growth in the next four decades will take place in the rapidly urbanizing Global South. Figure 29.1 illustrates by region the proportion

FIGURE 29.1 Proportion of Urban Populations Living in Slums, by Region, 2005

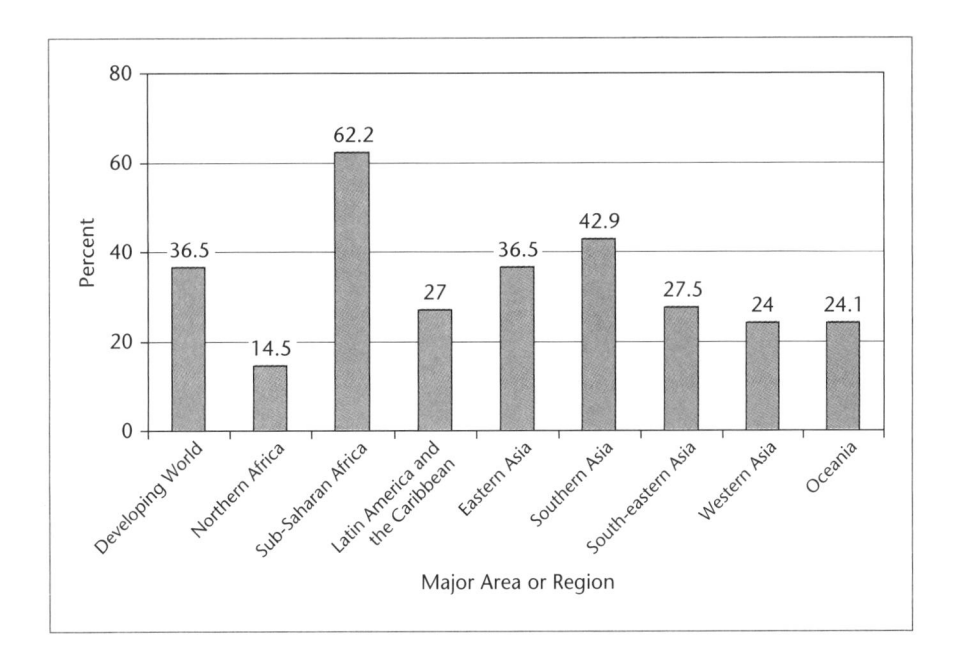

| Major Area or Region | Percent |
|---|---|
| Developing World | 36.5 |
| Northern Africa | 14.5 |
| Sub-Saharan Africa | 62.2 |
| Latin America and the Caribbean | 27 |
| Eastern Asia | 36.5 |
| Southern Asia | 42.9 |
| South-eastern Asia | 27.5 |
| Western Asia | 24 |
| Oceania | 24.1 |

of the urban population living in slums, and Figure 29.2 illustrates the absolute number of slum dwellers by region. If nothing is done to intervene, a large part of future urban growth will be made up of poor people who will live in slums (Garau, Sclar, and Carolini 2005).

This is not to say that population growth in cities is what causes slums. Urban growth is often accompanied by a rapid expansion in unplanned and underserved neighborhoods with high populations of poor people, but this is due in large part to a lack of attention to the needs of the poor rather than to urbanization per se. Issues of governance and a lack of vision for urban growth are underlying problems (UNFPA 2007, 37).

UN-HABITAT (2008, 92) uses five indicators to determine whether a shelter is a slum: lack of access to improved water, lack of access to sanitation, nondurable housing, insufficient living area (overcrowding), and insecure tenure. If a dwelling exhibits any one of these characteristics, it is considered a slum.[3] Additionally, slum dwellings often lack sunlight and are poorly ventilated. Slums are often situated on land that is not suitable for development—on land that is vulnerable to hazards, such as low-lying flood-prone areas, areas prone to mudslides, and areas along railway lines or near industries, waste sites, or traffic.

Not surprisingly, these living conditions and deprivations present a number of health risks. These risks, as discussed in previous chapters, lead to drastically higher

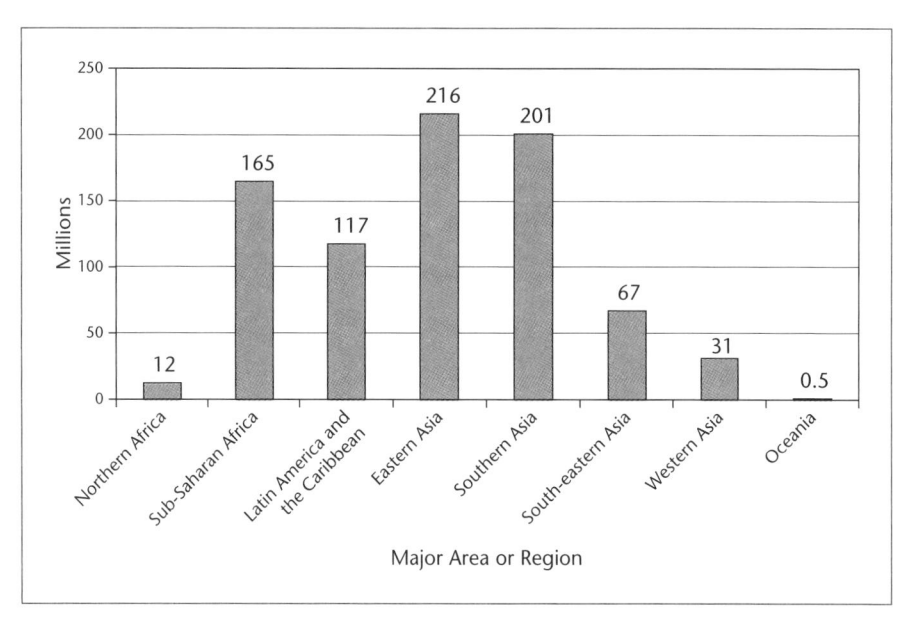

FIGURE 29.2 Slum Population by Region, 2005

| Region | Millions |
|---|---|
| Northern Africa | 12 |
| Sub-Saharan Africa | 165 |
| Latin America and the Caribbean | 117 |
| Eastern Asia | 216 |
| Southern Asia | 201 |
| South-eastern Asia | 67 |
| Western Asia | 31 |
| Oceania | 0.5 |

incidences of communicable diseases which translate into much higher mortality rates, particularly for infants and children under the age of five. Slum dwellers are also particularly at risk to effects of climate change, mental illness, injuries, and violence. As health burdens shift from communicable to noncommunicable diseases, it is anticipated that the populations most at risk to communicable diseases will also be at high risk to noncommunicable ones, such as obesity and heart disease.

Health risks faced by most people living in slums extend far beyond the physical characteristics of their living situation. While many of these living conditions might lead to manifestations of ill health that may be attributable to immediate/ environmental health causes, it must be kept in mind that the incidence of diseases (emergent and reemergent) among the urban poor is inextricably linked to the upstream or social determinants of health, mainly in the form of social exclusion—a form of impoverishment that goes beyond the single dimension of per capita income.[4] The UN Millennium Project's Task Force Report on Improving the Lives of Slum Dwellers notes, "There is a high degree of exclusion in cities. Slum dwellers are excluded from many of the attributes of urban life that are critical to full citizenship but that remain a monopoly of a privileged minority: political voice, secure and good quality housing, safety and the rule of law, good education, affordable health services, decent transport, adequate incomes, and access to economic activity and credit" (Garau, Sclar, and Carolini 2005, 1). Taken together, all these indicate that the major public health challenge of the coming decades is to address the underlying, or upstream, causes and pathways that lead to ill health and health inequities.

## MEASURING INEQUALITY IN THE HEALTH OUTCOMES OF THE URBAN POOR

Health status measures are much more telling than economic measures as indicators of the overall social well-being of populations, because they reflect the degree of equity with which a society treats its members. One way to think about these two sets of measurements of social well-being is to consider the economic indicators, such as income per capita, as reflections of a society's ability to meet the needs of its population, that is, as "inputs." But if our concern is with how well society is serving all its residents, given its income, then we need "output" indicators that reflect how equitably all members of society are treated. Population health status is a relatively clear measure of how well society is doing in meeting the needs of its entire population. Economic indicators account only for items with market value. They do not account for social assets and transactions that have no market or exchange value but real social value. Health status indicators more often capture these vital "intangibles."

While health indicators are better measures of social well-being, they too have to be carefully interpreted for this purpose. In looking at health indicators, it is always important to understand how they are constructed. Urban residents in developing countries typically have, on average, better health outcomes than their rural counterparts. Results from Demographic and Health Survey (DHS) data indicate that infant and child mortality rates in urban areas are lower than those in rural areas in most of Africa, Asia, and Latin America (Montgomery and others 2003, 127). However, urban averages do not often include health data from slums, and when they do, they hide significant intraurban disparities in disease and injury burdens and premature deaths. In considering urban population health, it is important to break out the data to account for the impacts of social inequality that are camouflaged by spatial location. This is especially the case when we are considering the urban condition in the Global South.

Because urbanization is a double-edged sword—the promise of economic and social advantage versus the harsh conditions of life for the urban poor—there is a large literature that debates where the poverty problem is worse: rural versus urban. It is an important one to the extent that it shapes poverty reduction policies and subsequent allocation of resources. The debate is also important because it has spilled over into the question of population health. Although the overall urban-advantage/urban-penalty debate may not yet be resolved, it is clear that health inequities within cities are vast and that attention must be targeted towards reducing these inequities and improving the health/lives of the urban poor (Harpham 2007).

A striking example of extreme health inequalities between countries and within them is a comparison of health status within Nairobi and among Kenya, Sweden, and Japan (see Table 29.2). Average infant and child mortality rates are lower in Nairobi than in rural Kenyan areas, but within Nairobi, rates vary between low- and high-income areas. In Nairobi's informal settlements in general and in the slums of Kibera and Embakasi in particular, infant and child mortality rates are much worse than in rural areas. A child living in these slums, as opposed to other areas of Nairobi, is three to four times more likely to die before the age of five (APHRC 2002, 87; WHO 2008).

# THE FUTURE OF URBAN POPULATION HEALTH

## The Importance of a Pro-Poor Approach to Urban Health

The strongest social correlate with virtually all urban population health problems is poverty. Therefore, addressing poverty in its urban context must be the central strategic element in any policy and planning initiative to improve urban

TABLE 29.2    Infant and Under-5 Mortality Rates in Nairobi, Kenya, Sweden, and Japan

| Location | Infant Mortality Rate (IMR) | Under-5 Mortality Rate (U5M) |
|---|---|---|
| Sweden | 5 | 5 |
| Japan | 4 | 5 |
| Kenya (rural and urban) | 74 | 112 |
| Rural | 76 | 113 |
| Urban (excluding Nairobi) | 57 | 84 |
| Nairobi | 39 | 62 |
| High-income area, Nairobi (estimate) | likely < 10 | likely < 15 |
| Informal settlements, Nairobi (average) | 91 | 151 |
| Kibera slum in Nairobi | 106 | 187 |
| Embakasi slum in Nairobi | 164 | 254 |

Source: African Population and Health Research Center (APHRC), 2002, *Population and Health Dynamics in Nairobi's Informal Settlements*, cited in WHO Centre for Health Development, 2008, *Our Cities, Our Health, Our Future*.

IMR = deaths per 1,000 newborns; U5M = deaths per 1,000 children under 5.

health (Laflamme and others 2009). We will not get measurable improvement in overall urban population health unless we place a significant emphasis on addressing health risks from the perspective of the poorest urban residents. The aggregate social and demographic statistics make this abundantly clear. Approximately one-third of all the world's urban residents, or one billion people, presently live in slums. By 2030, if nothing is done, that proportion will reach approximately two-fifths (1.7 billion people; Garau, Sclar, and Carolini 2005). Addressing urban poverty then is the most efficient way to improve urban health.

The metric for successfully addressing urban health should be health equity—the absence of systematic disparities in the health status of urban populations or in the social determinants of health between groups with different levels of underlying social advantage/disadvantage (Pridmore and others 2007; Barten and others 2007). The elimination of social disparities in health outcomes has always been important as a matter of social justice and equity. But it is also important as a matter of long-term viability on an increasingly urban planet. The dense nature of urbanization cannot fulfill its promise of a better life for all if much of society's resources are invested in absorbing the social costs that are caused by excluding urban residents living in poverty and therefore suffering disproportionately from the stresses and diseases of urban life. Resources would be invested more efficiently in efforts to establish processes of social inclusion that can help to vanquish the now-global scourge of urban poverty.

## Improving Urban Governance

The key to successfully addressing urban poverty in terms of the sophisticated and coordinated strategy called for by a pro-poor policy and planning approach is to improve the quality of urban governance. The term *governance* is used in distinction from the word *government* because governance is something significantly more than the formal exercise of governmental power. *Governance* refers to the relationship between civil society and the agencies of government (particularly local governments; Mitlin 2004; Montgomery and others 2003). Good governance, or a positive and cooperative working relationship, is the key to overcoming the social exclusion and inequality that are at the root of so many of the urbanized risks to population health. Getting to good governance requires the existence of institutions (both formal and informal) that provide the framework for enabling broad-based civic participation and therefore social inclusion. But how can we achieve this shift in the relations of power between those that govern and those who are governed? More specifically, how can we improve the dialogue between the city and state governments that are responsible for supplying services and safety and the urban poor who are dependent on the actions of government?

Any solution must entail "the expansion of assets and capabilities of poor people to participate in, negotiate with, influence, control, and hold accountable institutions that affect their lives" (Narayan 2002, 14; Sheuya 2008). In other words, we are seeking actions that build capacity. But capacity building is a two-part exercise. It must improve the ability of both government and civil society to do their own work and also to work with one another.

## Improving Local Governments

Although there are important actions (discussed in the next section) that community-based groups can take to improve their situation, ultimately it is government that must embody society's responsibility for improving the lives of the urban poor. The best of community-based organizations can facilitate improvements, but only when these improvements are institutionalized in government processes and actions do they become sustainable changes in governance and thus in the quality of urban life. It is important to remember that the urban poor—no matter how well organized—cannot and should not be expected to solve what is, in the final analysis, society's problem. Many local governments are not prepared to tackle the challenges that rapid urban growth has brought. Making matters more difficult in many countries is the reality that these local governments are imbedded in nations where the stated policy is to discourage and prevent urbanization. Such a context makes the necessary planning almost impossible to achieve. At the same time, local governments, as opposed to state and national ones, are closest to the communities and are in the most suitable position to understand, represent, and respond to their interests/issues (Satterthwaite 2001; Garau, Sclar, and Carolini 2005). Many urban planning and management decisions, including land use, infrastructure, and provision of services, are decided at the local level, and the outcomes of these decisions either empower or further marginalize the position of slum dwellers. Local governments need training to fulfill their roles, as well as resources to carry them out. First steps then are to focus on improving the proficiency of local government and making resources available to them.

## The Role of Communities in Building Social Capital

Strengthening social capital within and among communities and bridging it to influential actors and institutions in the policy arena who decide, for example, how resources are distributed can influence urban governance and improve health equity (Mercado and others 2007; Pridmore and others 2007; Montgomery and others 2003). Social capital can be defined as "networks and local associations . . . that might support collective action, enforce norms, generate expectations of reciprocity or foster feelings of mutual trust" (Montgomery and others 2003, 40). Linked to empowerment and participation, it is a critical means of changing power relations and local governance processes in cities.

Along with building social capital within and among communities, enhancing the capacity of local governments to engage in dialogue with their constituents is also crucial. This interaction creates the good governance which is so vital to the entire enterprise.

One of the most powerful governmental functions is the allocation of the public budget. Participatory budgeting, or sharing the decision making with the community, is a highly successful way to create a meaningful dialogue between civil society and local government. Begun in the southern Brazilian city of Porto Alegre in 1989 (which has a population of over 1.3 million today), participatory budgeting involves working from the grassroots up each year as the capital budget is constructed. The process in Porto Alegre is based on the work of sixteen regional forums and five thematic forums addressing education, health and social services, transportation, city organization, and economic development. Representatives from the regional and thematic forums take part in a municipal budget council (Montgomery and others 2003; Cabannes 2004; Satterthwaite

2007a). The Porto Alegre example is a case of participatory governance, in which changes in government processes have allowed for or created more pro-poor outcomes (Satterthwaite 2007a; Mitlin 2004). Evidence suggests that the system is very effective at mildly redistributing services to the poorest residents even as it improves municipal performance for all residents (Serageldin, Solloso, and Valenzuela 2003).

Participatory budgeting is a government-initiated effort. There are also many examples of community-initiated efforts to achieve the same dialogue. An example of such community-initiated change is the role of alliances of the urban poor in India. In this case, a three-organization alliance is particularly noteworthy. SPARC (Society for Promotion of Area Resources), Mahila Milan (cooperatives formed by women slum and pavement dwellers), and the National Slum Dwellers Federation (NSDF) compose an alliance that works on issues such as access to transport and electricity as well as slum upgrading, resettlement, and new housing development programs. This alliance works closely with local authorities and provides over half a million slum dwellers with improved sanitation via community-designed, -built, and -managed toilet blocks, as well as facilities for hand washing (Burra, Patel, and Kerr 2003). Notably, these groups create bridges within communities and across communities with other federations of the urban poor and with governments (often local and sometimes central) and other actors with whom they partner and/or engage and have effectively linked these groups to outside resources.[5]

## The Role of Urban Professionals

Urban professionals—public health specialists, urban planners, and others—can play a major role in shaping the pro-poor good governance that is so essential to improving the health status of urban populations. These professionals can make a major contribution to capacity building and to the establishment of institutions of good governance that are central to the institutionalization of the urban services that lead to improved population health. They can play this role via ways that they apply their expertise to improve dialogue between government agencies and civil society organizations. But they, too, need to improve their capacity for this work, which includes both a technical component and a process component. The need to work directly with communities during training is now well recognized and acted upon.[6] Training and a range of employment opportunities in government, NGOs, and international agencies are increasingly placing urban professionals in positions where they can use their skills to not only address immediate problems but also help to create the institutions that can sustain a pattern of infrastructure development and service delivery that will meet the needs of all urban residents.

Consider this example: the Orangi Pilot Project (OPP) and Research Training Institute (RTI) is an NGO working in Karachi, Pakistan. OPP-RTI has worked with the residents of the Orangi community since 1980 to provide sanitation for about 100,000 households and has also supervised smaller sanitation projects in about 250 other locations (Hasan 2006). OPP-RTI has contributed to the capacity of Orangi residents through lectures by planners, sociologists, economists, and educators and also through training provided to almost 1,000 visiting groups (Hasan 2004, cited in Garau, Sclar, and Carolini 2005).

Overall, if planners, public health professionals, and others are to help create an inclusive city, they (as well as other actors in the urban arena) need to be aware of local processes and use local knowledge in their work. This will enable a necessary shift in the traditional source of legitimization for these professionals from state-centered government to people-centered governance. The goal is to work with governments and help them to evolve in ways that are functional in terms of addressing the complex interconnections among poverty, the physical environment, and the local economy to improve the health status of urban populations.

## Conclusion

The most significant determinant of population health is the condition of social exclusion and its resulting impact upon the physical environment where the rapidly growing urban population lives. When we focus our attention specifically on the health status of urban populations, the condition of both the social and physical environment is framed by the complex interconnected challenges discussed in this chapter. Success in overcoming the challenges of the urban environment hinges on our ability to broaden our perspectives concerning linkages among the direct transmission of pathogens, social behavior, infrastructure, public services, and governance. We will fail in our task if we do not embrace both the complexity of the issue as well as the individual pieces.

For some, the answer to the challenge of the rapid pace of urbanization is to try to stop it or at least slow it down. This has always proven to be a fruitless policy direction. In simplest terms, the history of human civilization has always been a history of the continual evolution of society from a rural to an urban existence. The future of the world for better or worse is going to be determined by how well we handle this strong pull inherent in the human condition. We believe that the key to success rests upon the degree to which we emphasize meeting the needs of the poor in our policy and planning efforts and the degree to which we succeed in creating good urban governance. Taken together, these provide a context that maximizes the chances for specific health or planning interventions to be successful.

## SUMMARY

Urbanization is a double-edged sword. Cities are places where challenges such as threats to urban population health are concentrated, yet they also present the best opportunities to overcome them.

The urban poor are largely excluded from the potential benefits of urban life. They lack access to secure and good quality housing, to health, and other basic services such as clean water, decent sanitation, and transportation. They lack political voice and are more vulnerable to economic risks and violence. These underlying factors lead to poor health outcomes for the urban poor.

Improving urban population health rests largely on addressing the challenges faced by the urban poor. For example, slum conditions lead to higher incidences of communicable diseases. While it is important to treat these diseases, it is far more efficient to prevent them by addressing their causes. They are rooted in urban poverty, the definition of which encompasses social exclusion. This will help eliminate the social disparities in health outcomes of urban populations.

Addressing social exclusion and inequality requires improvements in governance, or the relationship between civil society and the (mainly local) government agencies that are responsible for the quality of their citizens' lives. Broad-based civic participation is key to inclusive societies and cities.

## REFERENCES

African Population and Health Research Center (APHRC). 2002. *Population and health dynamics in Nairobi's informal settlements: Report of the Nairobi cross-sectional slums survey 2000.* Nairobi: African Population and Health Research Center.

Barten, F., and others. 2007. Integrated approaches to address the social determinants of health for reducing health inequity. *Journal of Urban Health* 84(3):164–173.

Burra, S., S. Patel, and T. Kerr. 2003. Community-designed, built and managed toilet blocks in Indian cities. *Environment and Urbanization* 16(1):1–32.

Cabannes, Y. 2004. Participatory Budgeting: A significant contribution to participatory democracy. *Environment and Urbanization* 16(1):27–46.

Garau, P., E. Sclar, and G. Y. Carolini. 2005. *A home in the city*. Task Force on Improving the Lives of Slum Dwellers, United Nations Millennium Project. London: Earthscan.

Harpham, T. 2007. Background paper on improving urban population health. Paper prepared for the Rockefeller Foundation's Global Urban Summit, July.

Hasan, A. 2006. Orangi pilot project: The expansion of work beyond Orangi and the mapping of informal settlements and infrastructure. *Environment and Urbanization* 18(2):451–480.

Jacobs, J. 1969. *The economy of cities*. New York: Random House.

Laflamme, L., and others. 2009. Addressing the socioeconomic safety divide: A policy briefing. Copenhagen: WHO Regional Office for Europe.

Mercado, S., K. Havemann, M. Sami, and H. Ueda. 2007. Urban poverty: An urgent public health issue. *Journal of Urban Health* 84(1):7–15.
Mitlin, D. 2004. Reshaping local democracy. *Environment and Urbanization* 16(1)):3–8.
Montgomery, M., and others. 2003. *Cities transformed: Demographic change and its implications in the developing world*. Washington, DC: National Academies Press.
Narayan, D., ed. 2002. *Empowerment and poverty reduction: A sourcebook*. Washington, DC: World Bank.
Perlman, J. 1976. *The myth of marginality: Urban poverty and politics in Rio de Janeiro*. Berkeley: University of California Press.
Pridmore, P., and others. 2007. Social capital and healthy urbanization in a globalized world. *Journal of Urban Health* 84(3):130–143.
Satterthwaite, D. 2001. From professionally driven to people-driven poverty reduction: Reflections on the role of shack dwellers international. *Environment and Urbanization* 13(2):135–138.
Satterthwaite, D. 2007a. In pursuit of a healthy urban environment in low- and middle-income nations. In *Scaling urban environmental challenges: From local to global and back*, ed. P. J. Marcotullio and G. McGranahan. London: Earthscan.
Satterthwaite, D. 2007b. The transition to a predominantly urban world and its underpinnings. Human Settlements Discussion Paper Series, Urban Change-4, September, International Institute for Environment and Development.
Serageldin, M., E. Solloso, and L. Valenzuela. 2003. Local authority-driven interventions and processes. Background report prepared for UN Millennium Project Task Force 8. Cambridge: Harvard University, Centre for Urban Development Studies.
Sheuya, S. 2008. Improving the health and lives of people living in slums. *Annals of the New York Academy of Sciences* 1136:298–306.
UN-HABITAT. 2007. *State of the world's cities 2006/2007*. London: Earthscan.
UN-HABITAT. 2008. *State of the world's cities 2008/2009: Harmonious cities*. Sterling, VA: Earthscan.
UN-HABITAT, Global Urban Observatory. 2008. The global urban observatory databases. http://ww2.unhabitat.org/programmes/guo/guo_databases.asp.
United Nations Population Division. 2006. *World urbanization prospects: The 2005 revision*. CD-ROM edition (POP/DB/WUP/Rev.2005). New York: United Nations.
United Nations Population Division. 2008. *World urbanization prospects: The 2008 revision*. New York: United Nations.
United Nations Population Fund (UNFPA). 2007. *The state of the world population 2007: Unleashing the potential of urban growth*. New York: UNFPA.
WHO Centre for Health Development. 2008. Our cities, our health, our future: Acting on social determinants for health equity in urban settings. Report to the WHO Commission on Social Determinants of Health from the Knowledge Network on Urban Settings. Kobe: WHO.
Writh, L. 1938. Urbanism as a way of life. *American Journal of Sociology* 44:1–24.

# CHAPTER THIRTY

# FUTURE DIRECTIONS

## JACOB KUMARESAN

### LEARNING OBJECTIVES

- Understand and be able to describe the main urban health challenges communities face that affect health equity
- Describe some opportunities for the future
- Articulate concepts for a way forward
- Consider the actions suggested in the chapter and others that could be added

LOOKING twenty to fifty years into the future to model what our urban communities will look like is a matter of great conjecture. We know that if we continue at our present pace, almost two-thirds of the world's population will be urban dwellers by 2030. With this global trend currently under way, we can consider not only the two polarized absolute ways (good and bad) that cities might emerge, but also the shades of grey in between (getting better and getting worse). Broadly speaking, municipalities will either be urban areas where the health of the population has been very well cultivated and planned for, or urban areas where public health has been ignored and left to languish. Most cities will fall in the gray spectrum in the middle, acting on their capacity to meet the health needs of citizens in some areas but perhaps not as much as they could to maintain and promote optimal health.

As cities grow, the health inequities inherent to them are likely to proliferate. In order to create a community where health is a priority, one must look at the current problems that cities face, troubleshoot the problems that are on the rise, and attempt to predict what will emerge out of current behavior patterns. Once the problems and challenges have been identified, the work of combating and preventing them can begin.

This chapter will summarize the challenges to health equity for growing cities and look at the way forward. The topics covered include current urban health challenges, opportunities for the future, and actions for reducing urban health inequities and a proposed way forward. All these concepts can be combined to develop plans for creating urban areas where the health of the population has been well planned for and cultivated.

## URBAN HEALTH CHALLENGES

There are many reasons why an urban community may not be as healthy as it could be. Many of the health challenges facing urban areas are similar to those of rural communities, but several are unique to urban landscapes. As urban landscapes expand, their health challenges and inequities will expand with them. This section will examine these challenges and how they underscore the plan of action moving forward.

### Access to Care

One of the primary factors preventing an urban population from attaining good health is access to care. There are several reasons why it might be difficult for people to get the health care that they need. The proximity of appropriate health care facilities and resources is frequently regarded as a rural problem, but this is one of the critical barriers to health for many urban dwellers, especially the poor. Too often hospitals, clinics, and private providers are in inconvenient locations or they are understaffed and overutilized. In general, the health infrastructure is unable to keep pace with the growth of urban dwellers. One example of this barrier and its serious negative health effects is the lack of urban services for maternal and child health care. This includes not only the physical lack of services but also the quality of care that individuals receive. The inability of pregnant mothers in urban locations to get prenatal treatment explodes into a host of subsequent health problems such as premature birth, high infant mortality rates, and elevated maternal mortality rates. Service delivery reforms are needed to fix the problem of availability and access to quality care (WHO 2008).

Another factor in promoting people's access to care is to ensure the availability of appropriate medicines. In Cuba, the ratio of doctors per person is very high, but there is a serious shortage of medicines and supplies. The cost of care and medicines can also be a barrier for urban populations—out of reach for a population that subsists day to day. Examples are the HIV positive mother who cannot afford AZT to prevent the transmission of HIV to her unborn baby, the heart patient who cannot afford cardiac surgery, and the worker who is injured on the job and cannot afford treatment to become fully functional and therefore loses employment.

## Social Determinants for Healthy Living

There are a number of key building blocks that are essential for creating a healthy urban community (Vlahov and others 2007). These are the social determinants of health which are often taken for granted by communities. In this section we describe three of the building blocks.

1. **Socioeconomic factors.** Access to financial resources is possibly the most important social determinant of health affecting urban populations today. Insufficient income affects all the choices an urban dweller makes. First, it affects living conditions. Urban dwellers without solid financial resources often live in dangerous, unhealthy slums or shanty towns. According to UN-HABITAT (2008), one in three urban dwellers lives in a slum or a shanty town, and one in every six people on earth lives in a slum (UN Millennium Project 2005).

Income also determines food choices—not only how much but also the type of calorie intake: nutritional foods or the often cheaper higher-fat foods. This can result in gastrointestinal illness, obesity, starvation, parasites, malnutrition, vitamin deficiencies, and other health problems. Financial resources correlate directly to the amount of health care and preventive care a person receives.

Many of the people who live in slums or shanty towns are able-bodied enough to be eligible for work but have limited resources to seek such opportunities. Similarly, the elderly who are economically vulnerable are often unable to provide for themselves financially and require social service assistance as well. The number of elderly in developing countries is expected to rise sixteenfold in the next fifty or so years (Commission on Social Determinants of Health 2008). This population group is especially susceptible to health inequities, especially as cities grow at the same rate as the elderly population.

2. **Environment.** The most basic human need is clean air, followed closely by clean water. Environmental contamination of either element results in ill health. These determinants are often difficult to obtain, and as cities expand, problems usually worsen.

Air pollution in urban centers is most often caused by human actions, but there are also natural causes. Human-made causes include industrial pollutants, smog, and fires as well as unprecedented events such as the 9/11 disaster that New York City experienced. Natural causes of air pollution range from volcanoes to pollen. Despite the fact that human-made causes of air pollution are generally more detrimental to health, such factors are so entrenched in the way that a city functions that they can take years to reverse or change. Improving air quality requires systemic societal change and significant political will from the government.

Clean water is a problem for up to one of every five people in the world. Clean water is vitally important for drinking but also for cooking, bathing and washing. Diarrheal diseases are the number-one killer of children in the world, the majority of which can be prevented by access to clean water. One of the main problems facing policy makers is how to ensure and distribute clean water to an ever-growing population in a city that is rapidly expanding. The development of unplanned settlements or shanty towns is often too fast for municipal services to keep pace with.

3. **Crime.** Crime is an important and debilitating social determinant of health, especially for women (Commission on Social Determinants of Health 2008). In addition to physical injury, crime perpetrates fear and anxiety in communities and mental trauma. All people are vulnerable to crime, and it is not necessarily something that always takes place outside the home or direct living environment. This specific social determinant of health is difficult to combat because the victims or target population for services are not always obvious or ready to receive assistance.

## Education for Communicable Diseases, STDs, and Preventable Chronic Conditions

Knowing the path to a healthy life is not always easy, especially when confronted with many choices in an urban environment. The lack of health education and knowledge are a significant threat to individuals and communities. Cities need to empower their citizens with the right education so that they can build healthier lives.

In urban communities without centralized health education campaigns, there is often misinformation about how communicable diseases, especially sexually transmitted diseases (STDs) are acquired. Prevalent myths include "You can't get an STD if you are a virgin," "HIV only affects certain people," and "He or she looks healthy so he or she must not have an STD." Additionally, the mechanisms and vectors of parasitic diseases are not well understood. In several coastal communities, cost-free mosquito nets provided to prevent malaria transmission end up being used for fishing nets.

Furthermore, there can also be a tremendous lack of knowledge about what constitutes good health choices in an urban environment when it comes to chronic conditions. As the habits of industrialized countries are adopted in less-developed nations, chronic conditions that were once rare in those urban populations are on the rise. Misinformed choices about what to eat and how much to eat have led to a "nutrition transition" in many cities and spiraling rates of obesity (Dixon and others 2007). Lifestyle choices such as how much to exercise, whether to smoke tobacco, and whether to use alcohol and drugs can all lead to chronic diseases that are preventable. These include diabetes, cardiac problems, pulmonary problems, some types of cancer, and drug- and alcohol-related problems.

## OPPORTUNITIES FOR THE FUTURE

Some urban communities are on the right track either by promoting health or reversing a downward trend of ill health. These communities have achieved success over several years and are models for other communities that wish to create healthier and more vibrant urban environments. A healthy city is not a destination but a continual journey. Two illustrations of this journey are presented here.

### WHO European National Healthy Cities

In Europe over 1,200 towns and cities have joined together under the WHO National Healthy Cities initiative to foster and promote public health policy and programs to obtain a healthier lifestyle for their inhabitants. These cities have not necessarily achieved optimal health for their residents but have recognized good health as a priority and have committed to working towards it. The 1,200 cities come from the countries of Austria, Croatia, the Czech Republic, Denmark,

Finland, France, Greece, Hungary, Israel, Italy, Kazakhstan, Norway, Poland, Portugal, Russia, Slovakia, Slovenia, Spain, Sweden, and Turkey.

The Healthy Cities approach encompasses four main tenets (WHO 2006):

1. Explicit political commitment at the highest level to the principles and strategies of the Healthy Cities project
2. Establishment of new organizational structures to manage change
3. Commitment to developing a shared vision for the city, with a health development plan and work on specific themes
4. Investment in formal and informal networking and cooperation

This journey began over twenty years ago and has built momentum along the way. The Healthy Cities approach seeks to put health high on the political and social agenda of cities and to build a strong movement for public health at the local level. The program has evolved over five-year phases, each giving special attention to a number of priority themes. For example, in Phase IV, cities focus on healthy aging, healthy urban planning, health impact assessment, physical activity, and active living.

City health profiles have been developed and published as an indispensable tool for informing citizens, policy makers, and politicians about health and for using as an evidence base for city health planning.

This initiative helps local governments in networking, exchanging experiences, and learning lessons to apply in their own contexts through annual meetings. The Healthy Cities Conference offers a meeting point for more than three hundred mayors and experts from all over Europe.

### New York City

New York City has demonstrated successful interventions that relate to health determinants and health outcomes in the face of urbanization. It has introduced laws and regulations such as taxes on cigarettes and a policy on smoke-free workplaces; more recently, under the New York City health code, chain restaurants are now required to post calorie counts for food items on menus and menu boards. It was also the first city in the United States to eliminate trans-fats from restaurants.

New York City estimates that the tax increases on tobacco in 2002 contributed in five years to a 21 percent drop in adult smoking and a 52 percent drop in smoking among public high school students. The poor and the young are the most susceptible to price changes, so tax increases have a greater impact on those vulnerable groups. Overall, the drop in smoking equates to an estimated

300,000 fewer smokers in New York since 2002, which can prevent 100,000 premature deaths.

The city has also taken action to target individual health outcomes. In 2004 New York City implemented a program called Take Care New York (NYC DOHMH 2009). It is a list of ten things every individual in New York should do to protect his or her health. The New York City Department of Health and Mental Hygiene established this program based on 2002 data and set its goals to be achieved by 2008. One of the promotable facets of the program is the Passport for Health, a booklet that an individual can use to record and monitor personal health information such as blood pressure, cholesterol level, body mass index, and vaccinations.

The ten things people can do to protect their health are these:

1. Have a regular doctor or other health care provider
2. Be tobacco-free
3. Keep your heart healthy
4. Know your HIV status
5. Get help for depression
6. Live free of dependence on alcohol and drugs
7. Get checked for cancer
8. Get the immunizations that you need
9. Make your home safe and healthy
10. Have a healthy baby

Each of the ten items has one or more specific indicators for which the city set targets. Here is a summary of the progress made on various indicators between 2002 and 2007:

- 364,000 more New Yorkers have a regular doctor
- 300,000 fewer adult New Yorkers smoke
- 598 fewer deaths from HIV
- 143 fewer deaths from alcohol
- 73 fewer drug-related deaths
- 48 percent increase in colonoscopy screening rates
- 319 fewer children were newly identified with lead poisoning
- 20 percent reduction in women killed by intimate partners
- 10 percent decrease in infant deaths

In the global arena, not all cities have the authority to introduce laws and regulations such as those in New York City. However, cities can launch campaigns targeted to individuals and approach health from an advocacy perspective, as demonstrated here. New York City is a good example of implementing a multifaceted approach to integrate better health among residents. Specific health issues were targeted based on good data assessments, and a systematic approach was implemented to tackle determinants affecting those health outcomes, followed by an aggressive advocacy campaign to ensure that city dwellers were part of their own health solution. Finally, surveillance and monitoring continues to measure impact on health outcomes.

# THE WAY FORWARD: REDUCING URBAN HEALTH INEQUITIES

What is the path forward? How can urban health inequities be reduced as cities continue to rapidly grow? What concepts need to be evaluated and put into action? Answers to these questions are based on lessons learned from successful initiatives and form the basis to move ahead.

### Gather Political Will

It is very difficult for change to occur in a vacuum. Sometimes change can move from the people up to government, but more often and especially with change in health patterns, the impetus must be from government to the people (Blas and others 2008). Gathering the political will to make change is the first and most important step toward reducing urban health inequities and establishing healthier lives for urban dwellers. While political will is necessary to initiate change, collaboration with stakeholders is crucial in making it a success.

### Universalize Health Care

The provision of urban health care includes public and private sectors, academic institutions, and civil society. The lack of coordination among service providers and the fragmentation of services has left thousands of people without basic health care and exposed to avoidable ill health. Those seeking care in these settings must pay at the time of service or are forced to accumulate catastrophic health care bills. The people who need the most care are often neglected. The consequence is unequal health outcomes, a by-product of socioeconomic conditions. Establishing a universalized system of care, or at the very least primary care, is critical to ensuring good health for urban populations (WHO 2008).

## Encourage Community Participation

Many urban dwellers lack the opportunity to become decision makers about their lives. People who have a stake in the process of how a community establishes and sustains its health will be more likely to promote and protect it. Achieving the buy-in of urban dwellers affected by health inequities is a critical step in creating and maintaining a healthy community (Israel and others 2006). Municipal leaders must engage the public through open and honest two-way communication. If urban residents are given the opportunity to be involved in the development of programs, provide feedback, and communicate with the government, programs will succeed with high participation and compliance rates.

## Engage Local Non-Governmental Organizations

While governments have a key stewardship role, non-governmental organizations (NGOs) function as major service providers in many situations. Engaging and challenging local NGOs to develop programs that reduce urban health inequities is critical for achieving a healthier population. Often NGOs are able to focus on the vulnerable and underserved sections of an urban population that the government is unable to reach. They can be a viable, nonthreatening service provider complementing local government providers.

In addition to city-specific NGOs, who serve locally, there are many civil society organizations both within and outside the country whose experiences should be utilized to build a healthier community. When considering external resources, focus should be broad in scope and not be limited to those already in the health field. For example, the success of economic micro-loan programs to disadvantaged community groups has created a great deal of change locally with minimal capital outlay.

## Influence the Business Community

The business community is an integral part of the whole of society. In recent decades and years, it has been viewed positively by other stakeholders with regard to its role as a partner with governments and the civil society in addressing a multitude of global and local health issues and concerns.

In an ever-changing environment threatened by climate change, emerging and reemerging infections, rapid urbanization, and demographic change, the context for understanding business risk and opportunity is being redefined. Business stakeholders now more than ever before are sensitized to the impact of their business on society, the environment and ultimately the bio-psycho-social well-being of individuals and communities they cater to. As key stakeholders, they need to proactively think through and decide if and when, and how far they should go in helping to address a wide range of social issues beyond their fence line of economic benefits.

The business community can be influenced to play a supporting role in ensuring that governments and the civil society have the resources to carry out required actions. Thus, it can assist governments in (1) being a provider or guarantor of human rights and essential services, (2) being a facilitator of policy frameworks that provide the basis for equitable health improvement, and (3) being a gatherer or monitor of data and information on health outcomes and health equity. The business community can also support civil society actors who are powerful drivers for positive social, political, and economic changes that affect health equity. It can finance informal community groups, formal civil society organizations, and large-scale social movements.

Finally, business stakeholders can support good practices by providing incentives for local governments to work effectively with communities. It can be the bridge for establishing and strengthening trust among different sectors to ensure that reduction of health inequity remains a priority on an intersectoral agenda.

# A FRAMEWORK FOR ACTION

The WHO Center for Health Development in Kobe, Japan, is working with partners and municipalities to develop key actions that policy makers can undertake to reduce health inequities. Three actions are proposed for the future.

## 1. Identifying Priorities and Interventions

There are many challenges to health in urban communities, but some are more pressing than others. To avoid duplication of effort and the ineffective use of resources, systematic research should be conducted to identify priorities. This research need not be costly or take years to develop and implement. A preliminary report on what challenges are top priorities and what needs have to be met is not only important to begin the process of change but also to measure progress and eventually evaluate program success.

The Urban Health Equity And Response Tool (HEART) can measure health inequities and determine appropriate responses for intervention (WHO 2009). The Urban HEART initiative was launched by the World Health Organization in April 2008 and was field tested in seventeen cities in ten countries worldwide. The tool is intended for decision makers and policy makers at country and local levels to prioritize actions toward eliminating health inequities. It will identify disparities in health determinants and outcomes within and between cities among different socioeconomic classes and recommend interventions that eliminate those disparities. The tool has two components: health equity assessment and health equity response. The health equity assessment is a checklist that helps decision makers determine what health inequities are present, where they are present, and what determinants of health need priority attention. The health equity response component is a group of strategic interventions that allows the selection of customized solutions specific to the urban context.

## 2. Advocacy and Implementation

In implementing an urban health equity program, it is imperative to advocate for it. An advocacy campaign explaining the problem and educating the public on the solution and the program is crucial for gaining the buy-in and active participation of community that the program will need in order to succeed. Goals, targets, and key indicators of success must be defined so that the program can be properly measured and evaluated. Building these specifics in the beginning ensures that milestones are met and goals are achieved within a reasonable time frame. Getting the word out that the program is operational and successful is critical for attracting the target population. Sadly, many services are available to urban dwellers, but they are not aware that the services exist.

## 3. Monitoring Progress Toward MDGs

A business adage states, "What gets measured gets done." This applies equally to the realm of public health. It may sound simple and obvious, but the more we are able to acquire and analyze data, the more informed our policies and the more obvious the impact on outcomes. Resources flow where data can prove interventions work.

By looking at the metrics of cities, we know where the problems are, what they are, and how to address them. Monitoring the ongoing status of a program helps to keep things moving in the right direction and allows for the possible amendment of program implementation if the goals are not being met. Such flexibility will encourage community participation and increase success rates.

Figure 30.1 illustrates the movement towards reducing health inequity. It includes prioritizing the interventions that work through such tools as Urban HEART, advocating for health policies at the municipal level, and documenting successes through evidence-based reports. The key to success is the engagement of different stakeholders in taking intersectoral actions. To gather political will, it would be essential to develop a policy commitment and a framework to assess progress toward the goal of reducing urban health inequities.

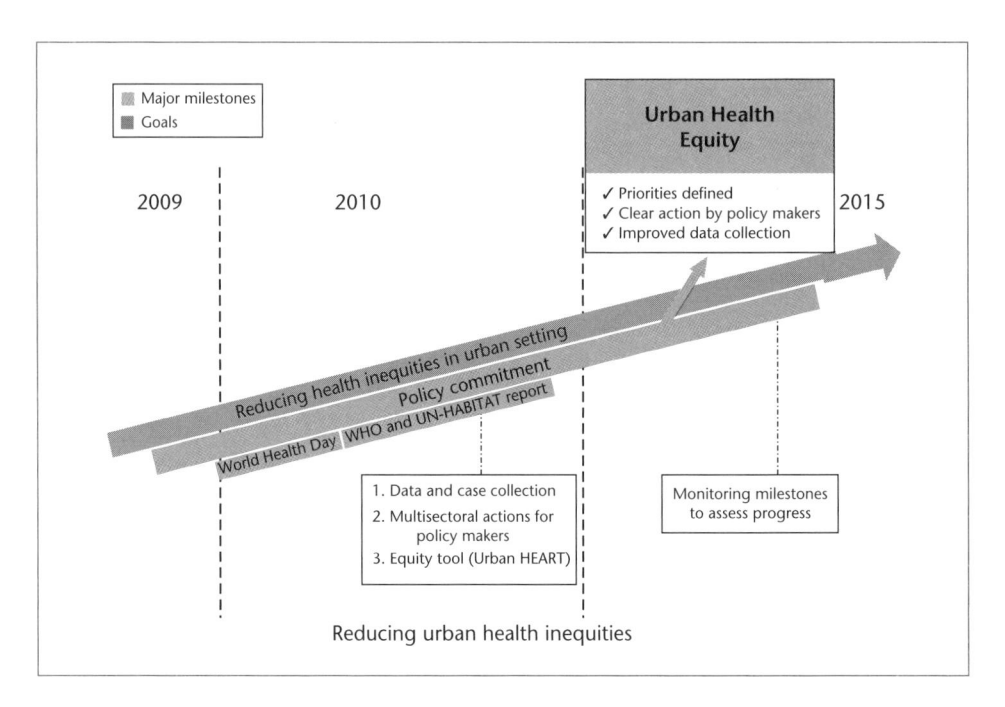

### FIGURE 30.1 Reducing Urban Health Inequities

- Major milestones
- Goals

2009 | 2010 | 2015

**Urban Health Equity**
- ✓ Priorities defined
- ✓ Clear action by policy makers
- ✓ Improved data collection

Reducing health inequities in urban setting
Policy commitment
World Health Day — WHO and UN-HABITAT report

1. Data and case collection
2. Multisectoral actions for policy makers
3. Equity tool (Urban HEART)

Monitoring milestones to assess progress

Reducing urban health inequities

## SUMMARY

Cities and countries face many challenges in the near future to prepare themselves for the imminent population growth that they will experience. Some of the health equity challenges that urban areas face include access to care, affordability of services and medicines, stabilized social determinants for healthy living, and appropriate health education. Cities must be especially mindful of the fact that as the population expands, it is very likely that urban health inequities will grow as well. Working toward a healthier community is not an absolute destination but a continual progression requiring adequate planning of infrastructure that supports population growth, improves urban living conditions—especially for the slum dwellers—and ensures that communities are engaged in decision making and participation of the services to promote healthy behaviors.

Promoting and maintaining urban health equity needs to be a priority task for all governments in the coming years. As more and more of the world's population gravitates toward cities, creating healthy environments for living should not be considered an alternative; it should be considered the only alternative.

# REFERENCES

Blas, E., L. Gilson, M. P. Kelly, R. Labonté, J. Lapitan, C. Muntaner, P. Ostlin, J. Popay, R. Sadana, G. Sen, T. Schrecker, and Z. Vaghri. 2008. Addressing social determinants of health inequities: What can the state and civil society do? *Lancet* 372(9650):1684–1689.

Commission on Social Determinants of Health. 2008. *Closing the gap in a generation: Health equity through action on the social determinants of health.* Final Report of the Commission on Social Determinants of Health. Geneva: World Health Organization.

Dixon, J., A. Omwega, S. Friel, C. Burns, K. Donati, and R. Carlisle. 2007. The health equity dimensions of urban food systems. *Journal of Urban Health* 84(Suppl 1):118–129.

Israel, B., A. Schulz, L. Estrada-Martinez, S. Zenk, E. Viruell-Fuentes, A. Villarruel, and C. Stokes. 2006. Engaging urban residents in assessing neighborhood environments and their implications for health. *Journal of Urban Health* 83(3):523–539.

New York City Department of Health and Mental Hygiene (NYC DOHMH). 2009. Take care New York. http://www.nyc.gov/html/doh/html/tcny/index.shtml] February 2009.

UN-HABITAT. 2008. *The state of the world's cities 2008–2009: Harmonious cities.* London: Earthscan/James & James.

United Nations Millennium Project. 2005. *A home in the city.* Task Force on Improving the Lives of Slum Dwellers. London: Earthscan.

Vlahov, D., N. Freudenberg, F. Proietti, D. Ompad, A. Quinn, V. Nandi, and S. Galea. 2007. Urban as a determinant of health. *Journal of Urban Health* 84(Suppl 1):16–26.

World Health Organization (WHO). 2006. Healthy Cities and Urban Governance. http://www.euro.who.int/healthy-cities/introducing/20050202_2.

World Health Organization (WHO). 2008. The world health report 2008: Primary health care now more than ever. Geneva: World Health Organization.

World Health Organization (WHO). 2009. Urban health equity assessment and response tool (Urban HEART). http://www.who.or.jp/urbanheart/index.html.

# NOTES

## CHAPTER THREE

1. See http://uhrc.in/module-ContentExpress-display-ceid-4.html for an account of the Urban Health Resource Centre's research in Indore, India, which began with 225 slum communities identified in the government's lists and, in consultation with local NGOs and a range of officials, uncovered a further 314 slums (African Population and Health Research Center 2002).

## CHAPTER TEN

1. The ethical ramifications of conducting such a study in a setting where poverty is rampant and health services not easily accessible or affordable pushed APHRC to consider cost-effective ways of managing these conditions in the study communities.

## CHAPTER ELEVEN

1. There are three general types of crimes—personal (contact) crimes, property crimes, and crimes against the public order, and there are many definitions of what constitutes a crime within each category, depending on jurisdiction and locale. See the *Global Report on Human Settlements 2007*, pp. 51–52 (UN-HABITAT 2007).
2. See the *World Report on Violence and Health* (WHO 2002), pp. 5–7 for definitions and typologies of violence.
3. For example, in some poor Jakarta neighborhoods, crime rates are low. Behavior is guided and constrained by the local mosque and by the all-enveloping embrace of religion and associated traditional social norms. See *Planning the Megacity: Jakarta in the Twentieth Century* (Silver 2008).
4. The connection between community infrastructure and health has been documented since at least 1854, when Dr. John Snow used geographic analysis of community well locations to identify the water-borne source of a cholera outbreak in London. See *The Ghost Map* (Johnson 2006).

## CHAPTER TWENTY-SEVEN

1. The municipal agencies included in the multisectoral task force included the Shanghai Municipal Development and Reform Commission; the Shanghai Municipal Economic Commission; the Shanghai Municipal Education Commission; the Shanghai Municipal Agriculture Commission; the Shanghai Municipal Population and Family Planning Commission; the Shanghai Municipal Culture, Radio Broadcasting, Film and Television Administration; the Shanghai Municipal Finance Bureau; the Shanghai Municipal Bureau of Public Security; the Shanghai Administration of Sports; the Shanghai Municipal Health Bureau; the Shanghai Municipal Water Affairs Bureau; the Shanghai Urban Construction & Communications Bureau; the Shanghai Municipal Environmental Protection Bureau; the Shanghai Municipal Administration of Industry and Commerce; the Shanghai Municipal Food and Drug Supervision Administration; the Shanghai Municipal Tourism Administrative Commission; the Shanghai Municipal City Planning Administration; the Shanghai Municipal Housing, Land and Resources Administration; the Shanghai Municipal Urban Communications Administration Bureau; the Shanghai City Appearance & Environmental Sanitation Administration Bureau; and nineteen district governments.

## CHAPTER TWENTY-EIGHT

1. In Belo Horizonte *favela* is a term that is considered stigmatized and considered interchangeable with *vila*. In other areas of Brazil, *vilas* are areas without roads connecting to the other parts of the city, while *favelas* have connecting roads.

## CHAPTER TWENTY-NINE

1. By "developing world," we mean those countries classified as low- or middle-income by the World Bank. These countries are often referred to as the "Global South" and distinguished from the "Global North," which comprises the world's high-income countries, the bulk being in the northern hemisphere. We use the terminology of Global North and South in this chapter.
2. These projections come with a word of caution—there is no standard definition for urban areas across countries. While this definitional heterogeneity applies mainly to smaller settlements, these settlements are numerous and, therefore, can strongly impact urban totals reported at national levels (Montgomery and others 2003).
3. The magnitude, type, and number of shelter deprivations experienced vary within and between cities.
4. There have been attempts to redefine and expand the more traditional definition of poverty (for example, UN-HABITAT, 1996; Chambers, 1995), and it has now been expanded to include broader social and economic factors, such as an inadequate, unstable, or risky asset base; limited or no safety net; inadequate protection of poor groups' rights through the operation of the law; and

poor groups' voicelessness and powerlessness within political systems and bureaucratic structures (Satterthwaite 2004; Sheuya, Howden-Chapman, and Patel 2007; Sheuya 2008).
5. The foundation of Shack/Slum Dwellers International, composed of federations of the urban poor from twenty-three countries in the Global South, is evidence of their extensive reach.
6. For example, Global Studio is an action-oriented research program that brings together international students from multiple disciplines, academics, and urban professionals to collaborate on community-based projects (The Global Studio 2009, http://www.theglobalstudio.com/).

# INDEX

Page references followed by *fig* indicate an illustrated figure; followed by *t* indicate a table.

## A

Abuja master plan (Nigeria), 309
Access to care: as health care system pillar, 226–228; migrant health and, 55–56; universal health care providing, 476; as urban health challenges, 470–471. *See also* Health care systems
Activism. *See* Urban poor activism
*Aedes albopictus*, 113
*Aedes egyptii*, 113
Aesthetics: brief history of health, urban planning, and, 346–349; current state of urban, 349–351; definition of, 340; factors shaping public health and urban, 342–346; interrelation of health, urban form and, 340–342
*Aesthetics, Well-Being and Health: Essays within Architecture and Environmental Aesthetics* (Cold), 342
African Population & Health Research Center (APHRC), 150, 152
Aga Khan Health Services, 234
Age differences: Shanghai's aging of native population, 423*fig*; vulnerability to small arms violence and, 165*fig*
Age-friendly cities: *Global Age-Friendly Cities: A Guide* (WHO) on, 96; New York City Age-friendly Cities (AFC NYC) project, 96–102; WHO Ageing and Life Course program on, 95–96
AIDS. *See* HIV/AIDS
Air pollutants: air toxics, 323*t*, 330; biological, 79, 324*t*; carbon dioxide ($CO_2$), 292, 322*t*, 328–329; climate change and greenhouse gas (GHG) emissions, 291–292; lead, 322*t*, 329–330; nitrogen dioxide ($NO_2$), 327; nitrogen oxides ($NO_x$), 323*t*, 327; PM (particulate matter), 323*t*, 324–326; sources, health effects, and regulations of major, 322*t*–324; sulfur dioxide ($SO_2$), 322*t*, 326–327; tropospheric ozone, 323*t*, 328; urban microenvironment sources of, 321*t*; VOCs (volatile organic compounds), 324*t*, 329; WHO guidelines on target levels for, 334
Air pollution: climate change impact on, 291–292; health risks associated with urban, 322*t*–331; history of, 318–319; increasing temperatures impact on, 78–79; motor vehicles and, 290; pollen allergies, 79; public health implications for, 330–331; urban environments and exposure to, 320–321*t*; weekly mortality/sulfur dioxide levels of London Fog (1952), 318*fig*
Air quality: EPA's Air Quality Index on, 332; global mega-cities and annual ambient, 319, 320*t*, 334; London Congestion Charging Scheme (2003) to manage, 332–333; management in urban environments, 331–334; public health litigation in Delhi over, 333
Air toxics, 323*t*, 330
Alma-Ata Declaration of Primary Health Care, 406
American Public Transportation Association (APTA), 286
Amsterdam: characteristics of, 60–61; ethnic diversity in, 61; health promotion in multicultural population, 64–66; health status of population, 61–62; migrant health educators in, 65–66; public health policies in, 62–66
Animal importation, 111
*Anopheles* vectors, 114

Anthrax terrorism (2001), 193
Antibiotic-resistant bacteria, 117–118
Antimicrobial resistance, 119–120
Argentine *villa miseria*, 307
Asia: inadequate water/sanitation infrastructure in, 272–276; informal settlements found in, 308

## B

Bastee Basheer Odhikar Surakha Committee (BOSC), 394
Beijing Olympic Games (2008), 18, 20
Belfast Healthy Cities initiative, 351
Belo Horizonte (Brazil): Brazilian Unified Health System (BHC) of, 441–450; brief history of, 438–439; MDG (Millennium Development Goals) indicators for, 439, 440*t*; urban determinants of health in, 439, 441; ZEIS (Zones of Special Social Interest) in, 439
Berlin International Building Exhibition (IBA), 348
Bicycling transportation, 296
Biological air pollutants, 79, 324*t*
Bogotá public transportation, 333
Brain drain: long-term solutions, 53; migration and resulting, 51–52
Brazil: Brazilian Unified Health System (BHC) of, 441–450; bus rapid transit system in, 296–299*fig*; crime rates and near collapse of health system in, 165; CRRU (Concession of the Real Right to Use) in, 314; determinants to vulnerability to small arms violence in, 165*fig*; *favelas* of, 307; NHCP (National Health Card Project) of, 245, 246; S[box198]o Paulo's integrated public health system in, 245–247; urban health and governance model in Belo Horizonte in, 438–451; ZEIs (zones of "special interest") in, 314. *See also* Latin America
Brazilian Unified Health System (BHC): COMFORÇA of, 447–448; democratic governance model of the, 446–450*t*; IQVU (Quality of Urban Life Index) of the, 445–446; IVA (Environmental vulnerability Risk) of the, 445; IVS (Health Vulnerability Index) of the, 445; metrics of the, 443*t*–444*t*; overview and goals of the, 441–442; Urban Health observatory (OSUBH) and, 442
"Broken windows theory," 159
Built environment: CPTED (crime prevention through environmental design), 159, 166–169; influencing disasters and their consequences, 179–180, 183; influencing disease transmission, 273*t*; interrelation of health, form, and aesthetics of, 340–342; London Plan (GLA) for, 261; macro, meso, and micro levels of crime and, 166–168; policy interventions to promote health, 135; urban crime and associated design of, 166; urban health framework on, 7–8*fig*. *See also* Environment; Urban physical environment
Bus Rapid Transit (BRT) systems, 296–299*fig*
Business sector: governance of, 361–362; how health is impacted by, 372–374*t*; how public health professionals influence health impact of, 382–385; reducing urban health inequities through efforts of, 477–478; strategies to influence health-related practices of, 379–382. *See also* Employment; Multinational corporations

## C

*Campylobacter*, 112
*Can Our Cities Survive?* (Sert), 347
Canada: crime prevention strategies used in, 169; Health Infoway system of, 239; welfare reforms recommended by IMF, 21
Carbon dioxide ($CO_2$): as air pollutant, 322*t*, 328–329; motor vehicles emissions of, 292
Carboxyhemoglobin (COHb), 329
Centers for Disease Control and Prevention (CDC), 295
*The Challenge of Slums* report (2003), 18, 19, 306
Chemical exposures, 79
Child Protection Centre Zagreb survey (2003), 210
Children: Croatian programs for prevention of violence among, 215; infant and under-5 mortality rates, 461*t*; malnutrition in rural and urban India, 39*fig*–40
Chilean *callampa*, 307
*Chlamydia trachomatis* (CT), 62
Cholera, 346
Chronic disease: "causes behind the causes" of, 131*t*; increasing risk of, 126–127; magnitude and scope of, 129–133; multiple sclerosis (MS), 82; myths about, 127–128; providing public education on preventable, 472–473; taking action on, 134–136; what cities are doing to counter risk of, 135. *See also* Diseases
CIAM movement (1920s and 1930s), 347
Cities: Amsterdam, 60–66; Belo Horizonte (Brazil), 438–450; climate change trends impacting, 70–73; cultural of peace against

## INDEX

violence in Zagreb, 208–218; Delhi (India), 72*fig*, 77*fig*–78, 290, 333; disaster preparedness of, 185–186; disaster response and recovery of, 186–187; documented/potential health threats of climate change to, 73–82; growth of mega-cities, 223; health-relevant exposures/effects of climate change on, 74*fig*; Healthy Cities project (WHO), 10, 135, 208, 408–418; impact of climate change on "fully workable days" in Delhi, 77*fig*–78; infectious diseases spread and temperature change in, 111–112; policies to counter chronic disease risk, 135; policies to reduce health impacts of climate change, 82–85; rapid growth of, 109, 126; risk of chronic disease in, 126–127; summary of temperature change in selected, 71*t*; UN-HABITAT's Safer Cities Program, 168; WHO definition of healthy, 427. *See also* Community; Healthy Cities project (WHO); Informal settlements; Nairobi City (Kenya); New York City; Urbanization

"Cities without slums" initiative (UN), 306

Citybike Wien program (Vienna), 296, 297*fig*

Civil society: governance role of, 357–358; informal settlements and involvement of, 312–314; role in solving Luka Ritz's homicide, 214–215. *See also* NGOs (nongovernmental organizations)

Clean Air Act, 291, 327

Clientelism, 395

Climate change: city policies to reduce health impacts of, 82–85; documented and potential health threats of, 73–82; global and regional trends in, 70–73; greenhouse gas (GHG) emissions and, 291–292; health threat of, 70, 291–292; health-relevant exposures/effects of, 74*fig*; summary of temperature change in selected cities, 71*t*; as twenty-first century health trend, 5. *See also* Environment

*Clostridium difficile*, 118

*Clostridium perfringens*, 81

Colombia: air quality management through public transportation n, 333; Medellín Metrocable system of, 300–301

COMFORÇA (Brazilian Unified Health System), 447–448

Commission on Social Determinants of Health (WHO), 2, 22, 48

Communicable diseases. *See* Infectious diseases

Communication systems: e-health, 239–244; New York City's PCIP, 100, 241–242; S[box198]o Paulo's integrated public health system and, 245–247. *See also* Information flow

Community: e-health system development and role of, 248; microgovernance and networks of, 363–364; need to belong to, 223; reducing urban health inequities through efforts of, 477; role in building social capital and urban health, 463–464; urban aesthetics and walkability enhancing the, 349–350. *See also* Cities

Community Organizations Development Institute (CODI), 361

Competition state, 19–20

Composite International Diagnostic Interview (CIDI), 62

Contraceptive use, 41*t*

Copernicus theory, 127

Corporate average Fuel Economy (CAFE) standards, 286–287

Costa Rican workforce, 79*t*

Crime fear, 165–166

Crime prevention through environmental design (CPTED), 159, 166–169

Crime. *See* Urban crime

Criminal gangs terrorism: criminal-based terrorism response to, 202–203; description and rise of, 197–198

Croatia: Croatian War of Independence (1991-1995) of, 209–210; "Golden Generation" of, 211; government anti-violence programs in, 215–217; history of violence in, 209; Program of Activities for the Prevention of Violence Among Children and Adolescents of, 215. *See also* Yugoslavian civil war; Zagreb (Croatia)

Croatian Football Association (FA), 213

Culture: as individual health factor, 63*fig*; migrant health and role of, 50; as urban crime variable, 159–161

## D

*The Death and Life of Great American Cities* (Jacobs), 341

Death rates. *See* Mortality rates

Delhi: hourly air temperatures in, 72*fig*; impact of climate change on "fully workable days" in, 77*fig*–78; motor vehicle emissions in, 290; public health litigation over air quality in, 333. *See also* India

Demographic and Health Surveys (DHS), 37

**490 INDEX**

Demographic shifts: definition of, 3–4; as twenty-first century health trend, 3–5. *See also* Urban demographic transformation
Dengue, 107, 113
Developed countries: e-health systems in, 239–240; integrated e-health systems in, 240–242; urban terrorism responses by, 203–204. *See also* Global North
Developing countries: brain drain depleting, 51–52, 53; creating good practices addressing migrant health issues in, 49; "double job schedules" of women in, 76–77; e-health systems in, 242–244; growth rates of total urban population in, 32*fig*; resource constraints of, 52; total urban population by region in, 31*fig*; urban terrorism responses by, 203–204; water and sanitation services in urban areas of, 268–280. *See also* Global South
Diarrheal diseases: inadequate water/sanitation and, 271–272; water and sanitation interventions to reduce, 278–279
Disaster management: mitigation as, 183–185; preparedness as, 185–186; response and recovery as, 186–187
Disasters: early warning systems for, 185; examining the health and economic costs of, 176; health effects of, 177–178; Hurricane Katrina, 164, 181; interaction between physical and social environments during, 183; natural versus humanmade, 176; social environment influencing effects of, 180–183; in urban areas, 178; urban physical environment influencing effects of, 179–180
Disease spread factors: international travel, 108; urbanization, 108–109
Disease transmission: epidemiology of, 272–276; fecal-oral pathogen transmission routes, 275*fig*; inadequate water/sanitation and, 271–276; physical factors influencing, 273*t*; vector-borne, 81*t*, 107, 113–114
Diseases: climate change impact on, 81*t*–82; factors affecting microbial spread of, 108–109; Global Burden of Disease (GBD) study on, 130, 331; globalization and infectious, 106; inadequate water/sanitation and, 271–276; migration and, 50–51; recommendations for preventing emerging/resurgent, 118–120; vector-borne, 81*t*, 107, 113–114. *See also* Chronic disease; Infectious diseases
DOHMH (NYC Department of Health and Mental Hygiene): on population health, 92–93; public health interventions by, 93–94

**E**
*E. Coli*, 112
*E. coli* O157:H7, 112
E-health systems: current status in the developed world, 239–240; in the developing world, 242–244; integrated developed world, 240–242; lessons learned from efforts of, 247–249; S[box198]o Paulo's public health, 245–247
Early warning systems: as disaster preparedness, 185; Los Angeles Terrorism Early Warning (TEW) Group model of, 202
Economic inequalities: disaster vulnerability impact of, 181; shaping urban aesthetics and health, 345–346; susceptibility to disease related to, 274, 276; urban life and, 17–18. *See also* Family income
Education levels (Shanghai), 426
Electronic health records (EHR): used in the developed world, 239–240; in the developing world, 242–244; integrating systems in developed world, 240–242; lessons learned from experience with, 247–249; S[box198]o Paulo's public health use of, 245–247
Emerging infectious diseases: overview of, 107–108; recommendations for prevention of, 118–120
Employment: impact of inadequate water/sanitation on, 271–272; New York City, 99; as Shanghai health factor, 426. *See also* Business sector
Entrepreneurship governance, 361–362
Environment: air quality management in urban, 331–334; as individual health factor, 63*fig*; New York City accessibility and physical, 99–100; as social determinant for healthy living, 471–472; syndemic situation created from hazards of, 270–271; urban health and social, 8*fig*, 9; urban health and urban physical, 7–8*fig*. *See also* Built environment; Climate change; Social environment
Epidemiological Intelligence (Epi-Intel) Cell, 202
European Healthy Cities Network (WHO-EHCN): content and themes of the phases of the, 411–413*fig*; critical success factors of the, 414–417; organizational structure of the, 410–411; origins of the, 406–409; *Social Determinants of Health* published by, 411. *See also* Healthy Cities project (WHO)
The European School survey Project on Alcohol and Other Drugs, 210
Extreme weather incidents, 80

## F

Family income: relatives murdered by minimum wage and, 162*fig*; as Shanghai health factor, 426; urban crime association with inequalities of, 163*fig*–164. *See also* Economic inequalities

Fatah (the PLO), 194

*Favelas* (Brazil), 307

Firearm manufacturers/sales, 377–379

Food supply: food and beverage industry impact on healthy, 375–377; infectious diseases spread through transported, 112

"Football" War (Zagreb, Croatia), 212–213

Freetown (Sierra Leone): inadequate water services in, 269*fig*; latrines in urban slum in, 270*fig*

Freight road transportation, 289

Fuel efficiency: CAFE standards for, 286–287; green auto technologies and, 294

Fuel quality: air pollution and, 290; green auto technologies and, 294

Fuels: alternative, 294; hazardous material spills of, 291; health effects of additives to, 291; reducing use of, 293–294; types of, 290

*Fumifugium or the Aer and Smoake of London Dissipated* (Evelyn), 318

## G

Gender differences: Costa Rican workers exposed to sunlight during work, 79*t*; as determinant of vulnerability to small arms violence, 165*fig*; sensitivity to heat and, 76–77

Ghana: age and sex structure of urban relative to rural, 37*fig*; health and urban poor of, 36–38

*Global Age-Friendly Cities: A Guide* (WHO), 96

Global Burden of Disease (GBD) study, 130, 331

Global demography: changes in the, 128–129; percentage of population in low-, middle-, and high-income countries, 129*t*; shifts in twenty-first century, 3–5; three leading causes of death by income group, 131*t*

Global economy: inequalities of, 17–18, 181, 274, 276, 345–346; SDH (social determinants of health) balanced with, 21–23; the state role in the, 19–20

Global financial crisis (GFC): fragility revealed through, 133; poverty increase due to, 133

Global North: e-health in the, 243–244; health care system fragmentation in the, 245; informal settlements in the, 307; links between Global South and, 197; threat of terrorism in the, 195. *See also* Developed countries

Global South: e-health in the, 243; health care system challenges in the, 246, 249; informal settlements in the, 307–315; lack of PTSD treatment following terrorism in, 201; links between Global North and, 197; poverty concentration in rural areas of, 373; terrorist attacks in the, 195, 197. *See also* Developing countries

Global Strategy for Health for All, 406

Global urban terrorism: distribution of, 194–198; impact of, 198–201; incidents of terrorism by year (1998-2007), 196*t*; response strategies to, 201–204

Globalization: definition of, 2; "disequalizing" nature of, 14–17; HIV/AIDS spread and, 114–115; infectious diseases and, 106; migration impacted by, 47–49; state role in creating barriers to, 20–21; as twenty-first century health trend, 2–3

Globalization and World Cities study group, 16

Governance: Belo Horizonte (Brazil) model of urban health and, 438–451; civil society role in, 357–358; definition of, 356; good governance versus, 358–359; health-related business decisions driven by, 381; healthy city approach for urban health in Shanghai, 427–435; healthy urban, 356–366; improving health by improving urban, 462; informal settlements, 312–314; Nairobi City (Kenya), 141–144; for NYC public health interventions, 93–94; public affairs and, 359; shaping urban aesthetics and health, 344–345; three main elements of, 356–357; Zagreb (Croatia) anti-violence programs, 215–217. *See also* Public health policies; The state

Gram-negative bacilli, 118

Greater London Authority (GLA): establishment of, 254, 257; healthy urban development strategy of, 257–263; HIA (health impact assessment) tool used by, 259–262

Greenhouse gas (GHG) emissions, 291–292

Greenway Project (South Bronx), 295

## H

H1N1 influenza strain, 117, 119

H5N1 influenza strain, 117, 119

Hamas, 194

Hazards: climate change and chemical exposures, 79; fuel spills, 291; syndemic situation created from environmental, 270–271; UN ISDR definition of, 177; WHO on inadequate water/sanitation, 270

**492** INDEX

*HEALTH 21:* (WHO regional Office for Europe), 416–417

Health care services: innovations in delivery of, 230–232; KEPH (Kenya Essential Package of Health), 144–145*t*; Nairobit City (Kenya), 141–154; New York City's, 100; urban health framework on, 8*fig*, 9

Health care systems: Brazilian Unified Health System (BHC), 441–450; financial support of, 229–230; Mexican health care reform of, 226–228, 232–233; opportunities to strengthen urban, 233–234; shortage of health care workers in, 249; as spread of infectious diseases factor, 110; three pillar of urban, 225–232; universal, 476. *See also* Access to care; Participatory budgeting

Health effects: air pollutants and, 322*t*–324; climate change, 74*fig*; disasters and, 177–183; how business decisions impact, 372–374*t*; of inadequate water/sanitation infrastructure, 272–276; migration and, 49–51; urban terrorism, 198–199. *See also* Mental health effects; Urban health

Health Effects Institute, 331

Health impact assessment (HIA): evidence-based policy changes based on, 261–262; as urban development tool, 259–261

Health inequalities: addressing London, 255, 262–263; definition of, 6; disequalizing globalization impact on, 14–17; measuring urban poor, 459–460; as twenty-first century trend, 5–7

Health inequities: definition of, 6; framework for action in reducing, 478–480*fig*; reducing urban, 476–478; as twenty-first century trend, 5–7; Urban Heart tool for measuring, 478–479

Health inequities reduction: advocacy and implementation for, 479; framework for reducing, 478–480*fig*; identifying priorities and interventions for, 478–479; monitoring progress toward MDGs, 479

Health promotion: Amsterdam population and, 64–66; as health care system pillar, 228–229; providing public health education as, 472–473

Health-related business practices: government responses to drive, 381; market responses to drive, 380–381; moral and political responses to drive, 381–382; reducing urban health inequities through, 477–478

Healthy Cities project (WHO): creation of the, 406–409; description of, 10, 135; four elements for action, 409; on qualities of a healthy city, 407–408; in Shanghai, 422–435; six strategic goals of, 408–409; Zagreb (Croatia) membership in, 208. *See also* Cities; European Healthy Cities Network (WHO-EHCN)

Healthy Migrants for Healthy Thailand, 49

Healthy urban government: definition of, 356; elements and examples of, 360–364; governance versus good and, 358–359; importance to health, 359–360; limits of, 364–365; non-government contributions to, 357–358; public affairs importance of, 359; Shanghai adoption of, 427–435; three main elements of, 356–357. *See also* Urban health

Helsingborg Plan for Sustainable Development, 413*fig*

High-income countries: percentage of population in, 129*t*; three leading causes of death in, 131*t*

HIV/AIDS: Amsterdam population health risks for, 62, 63; globalization impact on spread of, 114–115; health promotion in Amsterdam to prevent, 64–65; injecting drug use (IDU) and, 115; morbidity and mortality in Nairobi City, 149; providing public education on, 472–473; Sonagachi Project as prevention intervention to, 364; trend toward being leading cause of death, 130; urbanization and growth of, 106, 107. *See also* Infectious diseases; Sexually transmitted infections (STIs)

Hodood Ordinances (Pakistan), 159

Homicides: Croatian civil society role in solving Luka Ritz, 214–215; family income, minimum wage, and relatives victim of, 162*fig*; macro, meso, and micro levels of analysis of urban design and, 166–168

Housing: healthy urban governance role in, 360–361; as Shanghai health factor, 426; United Nations Special Rapporteur on, 20

Human rights: migrant health, access to care, and, 55–56; United Nations Special Rapporteur on housing as, 20

Humanmade disasters: definition of, 176; interaction between physical and social environments during, 183; social environment influencing effects of, 180–183; urban physical environment influencing effects of, 179–180

Hurricane Katrina: economic inequalities impacting effects of, 181; violence following, 164

Hygiene promotion, 279–280

## I

Immigrant criminal gangs, 197–198
India: child malnutrition in, 39*fig*–40; measuring urban and rural living standards, 38–41; National Slum Dwellers Federation activism in, 396–398, 464; prenatal care in urban and rural, 38*fig*; Sonagachi Project to reduce HIV rates among sex workers, 364. *See also* Delhi
Indiana University School of Medicine (IUSM), 241
Indianapolis Network for Patient Care and Research (INPCR), 241
Indonesia: population data gathered from, 35–36; population exposed to seaward hazards in, 35*fig*
Inequalities: "disequalizing" nature of globalization, 14–17; economic, 17–18, 181, 274, 276, 345–346; family income, 162*fig*, 163*fig*–164, 426; health, 5–7, 14–17, 255, 262–263, 459–460; London and existing, 254–255; urban crime association with income, 163*fig*–164
Infant and under-5 mortality rates, 461*t*
Infectious diseases: antibiotic-resistant bacteria and, 117–118; cholera, 346; climate change impact on, 81*t*; dengue, 107, 113; emerging, 107–108; globalization and, 106; malaria, 113–114, 243; migration and, 50–51; multiple-drug-resistant tuberculosis (TB), 106, 107; pandemic influenza, 117, 119–120; providing public education on, 472–473; recommendations for prevention of, 118–120; SARS (severe acute respiratory virus), 106, 107, 115–117, 357; Shanghai and morbidity or prevalence of selected, 433*t*; urbanization and the growth of, 106–107, 109–112. *See also* Diseases; HIV/AIDS; Sexually transmitted infections (STIs)
Influenza, 117, 119
Informal settlements: definitions of, 306–307; formation and persistence of, 308–310; government strategies on, 312–314; Kayamandi Zone F (Cape Town), 311*t*; living in an, 311–312; scale, location, and trends of, 307–308. *See also* Cities; Slums
Information flow: Canadian Helath Infoway system for, 239; e-health systems and, 239–244; PCIP (Primary Care Information Project) [NYC], 100, 241–242. *See also* Communication systems
Injecting drug use (IDU), 115
Injury risk, 224
International arms trade, 377–379
*International Compendium of Crime Prevention Practices*, 169
International Monetary Fund (IMF): asymmetries of decision making by the, 15; Canadian welfare reforms recommended by, 21; SAPs (structural adjustment programs) mandated by, 19
International Organization for Migration's (IOM) Migration Health Dialogue, 49
International Physical Activity Questionnaire (IPAQ), 427
International Sanitary Conferences, 346
International travel: infectious disease spread through, 111; microbial spread through, 108

## J

Japan: infant and under-5 mortality rates in, 461*t*; Kobe earthquake (1995) response and recovery in, 186; murder and property crime rates in, 161*fig*

## K

Kenya: Aga Khan Health Services working on e-health system in, 243; infant and under-5 mortality rates in, 461*t*; Kenya Diabetes Management and Information Centre (DMI), 151; KEPH (Kenya Essential Package of Health) in, 144–145*t*; service provision for noncommunicable diseases (NCD) in, 144–145. *See also* Nairobi City (Kenya); Sub-Saharan Africa
KidsWalk-to-School program (CDC), 295

## L

Language/migrant health link, 50
Latin America: Colombia, 300–301, 333; informal settlements found in, 308. *See also* Brazil
Lead, 322*t*, 329–330
Leadership. *See* Governance
Less developed (LDC) countries, 30*fig*
Lifestyle (Shanghai), 426–427
London: addressing health inequalities in, 255, 262–263; Congestion Charging Scheme (2003) to manage air pollution in, 332–333; GLA's healthy urban development strategy for, 257–263; using health impact assessment tool for urban development in, 259–261; LHC (London Health Commission) of, 258; London subway bombings (2005), 195, 197; overview of, 254–255; SDH (social determinants of health) in, 255–257; SmokeFree London forum, 262. *See also* United Kingdom
London Fog (1952), 318*fig*

**494  INDEX**

Los Angeles Terrorism Early Warning (TEW) Group model, 202
Low-income countries: percentage of population in, 129*t*; three leading causes of death in, 131*t*; water and sanitation services in urban areas of, 268–280

**M**
Madrid train bombings (2004), 195, 200
Mahila Milan, 464
Malaria: health effects of, 113–114; Tamil Nadu urban malaria control, 243
Maldevelopment, 222
Malnutrition, climate change and increased, 80
Mara Salvatrucha-13 (MS-13), 197–198
Mayors Against Illegal Guns, 379
Medellín Metrocable system (Colombia), 300–301
Mega-cities: air quality of, 319, 320*t*, 334; global locations of, 32; increase of, 223; UN forecasts on, 32–33
Men having sex with men (MSM) health risk, 62
Mental health effects: PTSD (post-traumatic stress disorder), 199–201; urban terrorism, 199–201. *See also* Health effects
Menu labeling laws, 135
Methicillin-resistant *S. aureus* (MRSA), 118
Mexican Mafia (La Eme), 197
Mexico: bus rapid transit system in, 299; health care reform in, 226–233; leading causes of death in, 224; Mexico City earthquake, 182; NAFTA between U.S. and, 376; Popular Health Insurance (*Seguro Popular*) of, 227–228, 230; System of Social Protection in Health (SSPH) law in, 227
Middle-income countries: percentage of population in, 129*t*; three leading causes of death in, 131*t*
Migrant health: Amsterdam public health education for, 65–66; communicable diseases and, 50–51; human rights, access to care, and, 55–56; living conditions and, 50; noncommunicable diseases and, 51; reproductive health, 51; role of language and culture in, 50; ways to improve, 56–57; working conditions and, 50
Migration: globalization impact on, 47–49; health impact of, 49; health impact on receiving countries, 49–51; impact on countries of origin, 51–52; increasing rate of, 225; microbial spread through, 109; perspectives and solutions to problems of, 52–55; significance to urban growth through, 46–47; urban demographic transformation due to, 33–34

Millennium Development Goals (MDGs) [UN]: Belo Horizaonte City and performance of eight indicators of, 440*t*; burden of human diseases reduction as, 118; e-health value to achieving, 247; as human rights issue for migrants, 55; on improving lives of slum dwellers, 308, 314; international community commitment to, 23, 233; monitoring progress toward, 479. *See also* United Nations
*Mini-manual of the Urban Guerrila* (1969), 193–194
Mitigation of disaster, 183–185
More developed (MDCs) countries, 30*fig*
Mortality rates: HIV/AIDS trend as being leading cause of death, 130; infant and under-5 mortality in selected countries, 461*t*; leading causes of death in Mexico, 224; London Fog (1952) and, 318*fig*; ten leading causes of death/mortality in Shanghai, 425*t*; three leading causes of death by income group, 131
Motor vehicles: fuel efficiency of, 286–287, 290–291, 293–294; global trends in ownership of, 288*t*–289; greenhouse gas (GHG) emissions of, 291–292; injuries due to accidents, 224; vehicle miles of travel (VMT), 286. *See also* Road transportation
MRSA (methicillin-resistant *S. aureus*), 118
Multinational corporations: food and beverage industry, 375–377; impact on urban health by, 375–379; international arms trade by, 377–379; reducing urban health inequities through efforts of, 477–478; strategies to influence health-related practices of, 379–382. *See also* Business sector
Multiple Indicator Cluster Surveys (MICS), 37
Multiple sclerosis (MS), 82
Multiple-drug-resistant tuberculosis (TB), 106, 107

**N**
Nairobi City (Kenya): APHRC health promotion partnership with, 152; APHRC survey on health facilities in, 143–144; CCN (City Council of Nairobi) governance and health service provision in, 141–144; comparison of child mortality rates rural areas and, 42*fig*; CVD clinics project in two slums of, 145–152; diabetes/hypertension outcomes among adult slum residents (2008-2009), 147*t*; future plans and policy implications in, 154; HIV/AIDS morbidity and mortality in, 149; infant and under-5 mortality rates in, 461*t*; interim outputs and improved clinical outcomes in, 152–154; Kenya Diabetes Management and

Information Centre (DMI), 151; KEPH (Kenya Essential Package of Health) in, 144–145*t*; overview of city of, 140–141; selected health and demographic indicators in slums of, 141*t*; slum dwellers and urban poor of, 41–42. *See also* Cities; Kenya

National Debt Reduction Strategy Paper, 52

National Slum Dwellers Federation (India), 396–398, 464

National Transit Database (2007), 289

Natural disasters: definition of, 176; Hurricane Katrina, 164, 181; interaction between physical and social environments during, 183; social environment influencing effects of, 180–183; urban physical environment influencing effects of, 179–180

Network of European National Healthy Cities Networks, 410–411

New Urbanism movement, 348–349

New York Academy of Medicine (NYAM), 97

New York City: anthrax terrorism (2001) disruption in, 193; demographics and overview of, 92–93; governance and range of public health interventions in, 93–94; moving toward implementing findings on, 100–101; older population in, 94–95; PCIP (Primary Care Information Project) for information flow, 100, 241–242; population aging and urbanization planning in, 95–96; September 11, 2001 attacks on, 194–195; tobacco control strategy used in, 135; *Toward an Age-Friendly New York City: A Findings Report* on, 98–101; urban intervention policies of, 94–98. *See also* Cities

New York City Age-friendly Cities (AFC NYC) project: assessment of city agencies for, 96–97; assessment of community needs for, 97–98; engaging political leadership in, 96; lessons learned from, 101–102; origins and development of, 95–96; *Toward an Age-Friendly New York City: A Findings Report* on, 98–101

NGOs (nongovernmental organizations): African Population & Health Research Center (APHRC), 150, 152; Bastee Basheer Odhikar Surakha Committee (BOSC), 394; governance role of, 357–358; Mahila Milan, 464; National Slum Dwellers Federation (India), 396–397, 464; OrangiPilot Project Research and Training Institute (OPP-RTI), 393, 465; reducing urban health inequities through efforts of, 477; role in reducing urban poverty, 400–401; SDI (Slum/Shack Dwellers International), 398; SPARC (Society for Promotion of Area Resources), 464; urban health improvement role of, 463–465. *See also* Civil society; Social services; Urban poor activism

NHCP (National Health Card Project) [Brazil], 245, 246

Nigerian Abuja master plan, 309

Nitrogen dioxide (NO$_2$), 327

Nitrogen oxides (NO$_x$), 323*t*, 327

Noncommunicable diseases. *See* Diseases

North American Free Trade Agreement (NAFTA), 376

## O

Obesity: food and beverage industry contributing to, 375–377; as heat disorder risk factor, 82; HIA (health impact assessment) used to reduce, 262; menu labeling laws to fight, 135

OECD countries' brain drain, 51–52, 53

OrangiPilot Project Research and Training Institute (OPP-RTI), 393, 465

Ottawa Charter for Health Promotion, 406

Ovations (United HealthCare Group) chronic disease initiative, 136

Oxford Health Alliance Syndey Summit, 135–136

## P

Pakistan: e-health system developed in, 243; Hodood Ordinances of, 159

Pandemic influenza, 117, 119–120

Panel on Urban Population Dynamics (2003), 37–38

Participatory budgeting: Brazilian Unified Health System (BHC) model of, 447–450*t*; PREM (Participatory Public Expenditure Management), 363; public spending through, 363, 447–450, 464. *See also* Health care systems

Particulate matter (PM), 323*t*, 324–326

Pathogens: *Campylobacter*, 112; *Chlamydia trachomatis* (CT), 62; *Clostridium difficile*, 118; *Clostridium perfringens*, 81; *E. Coli*, 112; *E. coli* O157:H7, 112; factors affecting concentrations of environment, 272–273; fecal-oral pathogen transmission routes, 275*fig*; methicillin-resistant *S. aureus* (MRSA), 118; *Salmonella*, 81, 112; *Shigella*, 112; *Staphylococcus aureus*, 81

PCIP (Primary Care Information Project) [NYC], 241–242

Personal Responsibility and Work Opportunity Reconciliation Act, 21
Physical activity: International Physical Activity Questionnaire (IPAQ), 427; as Shanghai health factor, 426–427
Physical environment. *See* Urban physical environment
*Planet of Slums* (Davis), 23
Political-based terrorism responses, 201–202
Pollen allergies pollution, 79, 324*t*
Pollutants. *See* Air pollutants
Popular Health Insurance (*Seguro Popular*) [Mexico], 227–228, 230
Population: demographic shifts of, 3–5; demographics associated with urban crime, 164–165*fig*; estimates on future African urban, 46; exposed to seaward hazards in Indonesia, 35*fig*; Indonesian, 35–36; as spread of infectious diseases factor, 109–110; UN estimates on urban, 300; UN forecasts on growth, 29–30*fig*, 32–34; urban demographic transformation, 29–36
Poverty. *See* Urban poverty
PREM (Participatory Public Expenditure Management), 363
Preparedness of disaster, 185–186
Prison gangs, 197–198
Program of Activities for the Prevention of Violence Among Children and Adolescents (Croatia), 215
PTSD (post-traumatic stress disorder): description and symptoms of, 199; DSM-IV criteria for, 201; September 11, 2001 and, 200; urban terrorism and, 199–201
Public health: Amsterdam policies on, 62–66; balancing global politics with needs of, 21–23; connections between crime prevention and, 169–170; connections between urban planning, aesthetics, and, 340–351; health-related business practices influenced by, 382–385; NYC governance and interventions, 93–94; NYC health and human services, 100; S[box198]o Paulo's integrated system of, 245–247; social model of, 256*fig*; urban air pollution implications for, 330–331; violence prevention as priority of, 158–159
Public health policies: Amsterdam, 62–66; e-health system development and role of, 248–249; reducing climate change health impacts, 82–85. *See also* Governance
Public spending: Brazilian Unified Health System (BHC) model of, 447–450*t*; participatory budgeting approach to, 363, 447–450, 464; PREM (Participatory Public Expenditure Management), 363
PulseNet, 118

R
Rail transit: improvements and growth of, 299–300; trends in, 289–290
Rape victims, 159
Reproductive health: contraceptive use by residence/poverty status, 41*t*; migration and, 51
Resource constraints, 52
Rio Declaration, 406
Road transportation: alternative fuels for, 294; global trends in vehicle ownership for, 288*t*–289; green auto technologies for, 294; health and safety risks associated with, 290–293; increasing fuel efficiency for, 293–294; promoting transit instead of, 296–300; promoting walking or bicycling instead of, 294–296; trends for, 286–288; trends in freight, 289. *See also* Motor vehicles
"Rough City" (Maric), 214

S
Safer Cities Program (UN-HABITAT), 168
Safety risks: transit security and, 293; transit system and related, 292–293; transportation and associated health and, 290–293
*Salmonella*, 81, 112
SALTRA (Salud y Trabajo en América Central) program, 78
Sanitation services: epidemiology of disease transmission and, 272–276; health benefits of interventions for, 278–280; impact on livelihoods of inadequate, 271–272; in low-income urban settlements, 268–271; perceptions of ill health and demands for improved, 276–278
S[box198]o Paulo public health system, 245–247
SARS (severe acute respiratory virus), 106, 107, 115–117, 357
SARS-CoV, 115
SDI (Slum/Shack Dwellers International), 398
Security issues: governance role in policing and, 362; transit system, 293
September 11, 2001, 194–195, 200
Sexually transmitted infections (STIs): Amsterdam population health risks for, 62, 63; globalization and spread of, 114–115; health promotion in Amsterdam to prevent, 64–65; providing public

education on, 472–473. *See also* HIV/AIDS; Infectious diseases
Shanghai (China): aging of native population, 423*fig*; economy and demographics of, 422–423; health service system in, 424, 426; health status of population, 424; social, economic, and lifestyle factors related to health in, 426–427; ten leading causes of death/mortality in, 425*t*
Shanghai Healthy City project: "Happy Song for a Healthy City" theme song of, 429; major indicators related to children, 432*t*; measures of environmental quality during, 431*t*–432*t*; morbidity or prevalence of selected infectious diseases, 433*t*; number of outpatient medical visits in, 432*t*; origins and development of, 428–435; political commitment to, 430*fig*; reported degree on changed health indicators by residents, 433*t*; structure of MHPC (Municipal Health Promotion Committee), 429*fig*
*Shigella*, 112
Sierra Leone: inadequate water services in, 269*fig*; latrines in urban slum in, 270*fig*
Slow Cities movement, 351
Slums: aesthetic neglect of, 347–348; *The Challenge of Slums* report (2003) on, 18, 19, 306; CVD clinics project in two Nairobi, 145–152; health challenges in, 457–459; health impact of inadequate water/sanitation infrastructure in, 272–276; of Nairobi, 41–42; population by region (2005), 458*fig*; proportion of urban populations living in, 457*fig*; risk factors for chronic disease in, 132; selected health and demographic indicators in Nairobi, 141*t*; as spread of infectious diseases factor, 110; urban poor activism by inhabitants of, 396–399. *See also* Informal settlements; Urban poverty
Small-arms production, 377–379
SmokeFree London forum, 262
Soccer War (Zagreb, Croatia), 212–213
Social capital: advantages of, 182; influencing relocation following disasters, 182–183
*Social Determinants of Health* (WHO-EHCN), 411
Social determinates of health (SDH): balancing global economy with, 21–23; as cause behind the causes of chronic disease, 131*t*; Commission on Social Determinants of Health (WHO) on, 2, 22, 48; importance of, 14; London and, 255–257; socioeconomic, environment, and crime as, 471–472; as urban health challenge, 471–472

Social environment: influencing disasters and their consequences, 180–183; shaping urban aesthetics and health, 345–346; urban health framework on, 8*fig*, 9. *See also* Environment
Social model of public health, 256*fig*
Social services: social model of public health and, 256*fig*; urban health framework on, 8*fig*, 9. *See also* NGOs (nongovernmental organizations)
Socioeconomic health factors, 471–472
Sonagachi Project, 364
South Africa: Kayamandi Zone F (Cape Town) informal settlement in, 311*t*; World Cup (2010) held in, 18. *See also* Sub-Saharan Africa
South Asia: inadequate water/sanitation infrastructure in, 272–276; informal settlements found in, 308
SPARC (Society for Promotion of Area Resources), 464
Squatter settlements, 306
*Staphylococcus aureus*, 81, 118
The state: "competition," 19–20; global economy role of, 19–20; globalization barriers created by, 20–21. *See also* Governance
*State of World Population 2007*, 33
Structural adjustment programs (SAPs), 19
Sub-Saharan Africa: Abuja master plan (Nigeria), 309; estimates on future urban population of, 46; health impact of inadequate water/sanitation infrastructure in, 272–276; informal settlements found in, 308, 310, 311*t*; migration issues for, 54–55; Sierra Leone, 269*fig*, 270*fig*; UN-HABITAT's Safer Cities Program in, 168. *See also* Kenya; South Africa
Substance abuse/violence link, 210–211
Sulfur dioxide ($SO_2$), 322*t*, 326–327
Swedish infant/under-5 morality rates, 461*t*
Syndey Summit of Oxford Health Alliance, 135–136

## T

Tamil Nadu urban malaria control, 243
*Targets for Health for all* (WHO Regional Office for Europe), 415
Technological health factor, 343–344
Temperature: hourly air temperatures in Delhi, 72*fig*; impact on air pollution by rising, 78–79; infectious diseases spread and change in, 111–112; summary of change in selected cities, 71*t*; Wet Bulb Globe Temperature (WBGT), 75–76*fig*

Terrorism: anthrax (2001), 193; global incidents by year (1998-2007), 196*t*; as major modern issue, 192; by region (1998-2008), 196*t*; September 11, 2001, 194–195, 200. *See also* Urban terrorism

Tobacco use: HIA (health impact assessment) used to reduce, 262; NYC's tobacco control strategy, 135

*Toward an Age-Friendly New York City: A Findings Report*, 98–101

Transit system: Bogotá air quality management through use of, 333; Bus Rapid Transit (BRT), 296–299*fig*; health and safety risks associated with, 290–293; improving the, 293–300; Medellín's Metrocable, 300–301; promoting use of public, 296–300; rail, 289, 299–300; security issues of, 293; as Shanghai health factor, 426; TOD (transit-oriented developments) and, 348–349; trends in, 289–290

Transportation. *See* Urban transportation

Tropospheric ozone, 323*t*, 328

*Twenty Steps for Developing a Health Cities Project* (WHO), 408

*2007 Global Report on Human Settlements* (UN-HABITAT), 158

**U**

UN Millennium Development Goals, 2

UN-HABITAT: *The Challenge of Slums* report (2003), 18, 19, 306; Safer Cities Program of, 168; *2007 Global Report on Human Settlements* by, 158; "What is Adequate Shelter?" on, 313

UNICEF studies: on SAPs (structural adjustment programs), 19; on violence in schools, 210–211

United Kingdom: Black report on health divide in, 255; Crime and Disorder Act (1998) of, 169; crime and violence prevention policies in, 168–169; murder and property crime rates in, 161*fig*. *See also* London

United Nations: "cities without slums" initiative of, 306; estimates on urban populations by, 300; global population growth forecasts by, 29–30*fig*, 34; mega-cities forecast by, 32–33. *See also* Millennium Development Goals (MDGs) [UN]

United Nations Office on Drugs and Crime (UNODC), 161

United Nations Population Fund Report (2007), 3

United Nations Special Rapporteur, 20

United States: murder and property crime rates in, 161*fig*; NAFTA between Mexico and, 376; September 11, 2001 attacks on the, 194–195, 200; "stealth urban policies" in the, 22; transportation infrastructure in the, 284–286*t*. *See also* U.S. legislation

Universal health care, 476

Urban crime: age, gender, and employment status related to, 164–165; "broken windows theory" of, 159; comparison of recorded homicide per population, 160*fig*; environmental design characteristics associated with, 166; family income and relatives murdered by minimum wage, 162*fig*; fear of, 165–166; governance role in policing to control, 362; Hurricane Katrina and increased, 164; macro, meso, and micro levels of analysis of urban design and, 166–168; poverty association with, 161–163; as social determinant for healthy living, 472; sociocultural and economic variables of, 159–164; as sociopathology, 158. *See also* Violence

Urban crime prevention: connections between public health and, 169–170; CPTED (crime prevention through environmental design), 159, 166–169; interventions for, 168–169

Urban demographic transformation: examining the process of, 29; forecasting urban and city growth, 34; mapping urban data on, 34–36; migration versus natural increase, 33–34, 46–57, 225; sketch of urban growth and, 29–33. *See also* Demographic shifts; Urbanization

Urban design/development: CPTED (crime prevention through environmental design), 159, 166–169; disasters and role of, 179–180; GLA (Greater London Authority) strategy for healthy, 257–263; HIA (health impact assessment) as tool in, 259–262; interrelation of health, form, and aesthetics of, 340–342; macro, meso, and micro levels of analysis of crime and, 166–168; outcomes of healthy development and, 27. *See also* Built environment; Urban planning

Urban health: challenges of, 222–225, 454, 470–473; conceptual framework for, 7–9; disaggregated approach to, 28–29; disaster impact on, 177–178; documented and potential climate change threats to, 73–82; governance importance to, 359–360; how business decision affect, 372–374*t*; importance of pro-poor approach to, 460–462; improving local governments to improve, 462–463; improving urban governance to improve, 462; inequalities of, 5–7, 14–17, 255, 262–263, 459–460; inequities of, 5–7, 476–480*fig*; interrelation of form, aesthetics, and, 340–342;

# INDEX

issues and concerns of, 48; maldevelopment concept of, 222; meeting challenges and opportunities in, 9–10; megatrends in 21st century, 2–7; migration impact on, 49, 50–57; multinational corporation impact on, 375–379; opportunities for the future of, 473–476; role of communities in building social capital and, 463–464; role of urban professionals in, 464–465; SDH (social determinates of health) and, 2, 14, 21–23, 48, 131*t*, 255–257; socioeconomic, cultural, and environmental conditions for, 63*fig*; transportation and associated risks of safety and, 290–293; urban form, aesthetics, and, 340–351; urbanization impact on, 48. *See also* Health effects; Healthy urban government; Urbanization

Urban health challenges: access to care as, 470–471; dimensions of the, 454; education for communicable diseases, STDs, and preventable chronic conditions, 472–473; overview of global, 222–225; SDH (social determinates of health) which are, 471–472

Urban health framework: health and social services, 8*fig*, 9; social environment, 8*fig*, 9; urban physical environment, 7–8*fig*

Urban health trends: climate change as, 5; demographic shifts as, 3–5; globalization as, 2–3; health inequalities and inequities as, 6–7; urbanization as, 5–6

Urban Heart initiative, 478–479

Urban infrastructure: demands for improved water/sanitation, 276–278; health benefits of water/sanitation interventions, 278–280; health effects of inadequate water/sanitation, 272–276; impact on livelihoods by inadequate water/sanitation, 271–272; low-income areas and water/sanitation, 268–271; as spread of infectious diseases factor, 110; U.S. transportation, 284–286*t*

Urban physical environment: influencing disasters and their consequences, 179–180, 183; influencing disease transmission, 273*t*; shaping urban aesthetics and health, 342–343; urban health framework on, 7–8*fig*. *See also* Built environment

Urban planning: factors shaping public health and aesthetics of, 342–346; Helsingborg Plan for Sustainable Development, 413*fig*; New Urbanism movement of, 348–349; for urban retrofitting, 350–351. *See also* Urban design/development

Urban poor: child malnutrition among Indian rural and, 39*fig*–40; comparison of child mortality rates in Nairobi and Kenya, 42*fig*; comparisons of rural households, urban nonpoor, and, 40*t*–41; contraceptive use by women by residence and poverty status, 41*t*; Demographic and Health Surveys (DHS) on, 37; examining health status of the, 36–42; measuring health inequalities of the, 459–460; Multiple Indicator Cluster Surveys (MICS) on, 37; Panel on Urban Population Dynamics (2003) on, 37–38; relative poverty of Indian, 38*fig*–39; slum dwellers and the, 41–42

Urban poor activism: clientelism role in, 395; to get needs addressed, 393–396; from protest to coproduction, 396–399; role of international agencies in, 400–401. *See also* NGOs (nongovernmental organizations)

Urban poverty: conventional approaches to reduction of, 390–391; role of international agencies in reducing, 400–401; 21st century challenges of, 457*fig*–459; urban crime association with, 161–163; urbanization context of, 391–393. *See also* Slums

Urban terrorism: criminal gangs form of, 197–198; definition of, 192–193; global distribution of, 194–198; Los Angeles Terrorism Early Warning (TEW) Group model, 202; Madrid train bombings (2004), 195, 200; mental health issues of, 199–201; *Mini-manual of the Urban Guerilla* (1969) in, 193–194; physical health issues of, 198–199; roots of, 193–194; September 11, 2001, 194–195, 200. *See also* Terrorism

Urban terrorism responses: criminal-based, 202–203; developed world and developing world differences in, 203–204; political-based, 201–202

Urban transportation: aggregate trends in U.S., 287*fig*; characteristics of U.S. infrastructure, 284–286*t*; global trends in vehicle ownership for, 288*t*–289; health and safety risks associated with, 290–293; improving the system, 293–301; as Shanghai health factor, 426; trends in road, freight, and transit, 286–290

Urbanization: as context of poverty, 391–393; definition of, 5; evolution of, 454–456; growth of infectious diseases and, 106–107; increased risk of injuries and, 224; microbial spread and, 108–109; opportunities and challenges of, 456–457; as twenty-first century trend, 5–6. *See also* Cities; Urban demographic transformation; Urban health

U.S. Department of Energy (DOE), 292

U.S. Department of Homeland Security (DHS), 202

U.S. Department of Transportation (DOT), 286, 291, 292

U.S. Environmental Protection Agency (EPA): Air Quality Index of, 332; fuel standards of, 290

U.S. legislation: Clean Air Act, 291, 327; Personal Responsibility and Work Opportunity Reconciliation Act, 21. *See also* United States

## V

Vector-borne diseases: climate change impact on, 81; dengue, 107, 113; emerging, 107; malaria, 113–114; by vector and pathogen types, 81*t*

Vehicle miles of travel (VMT), 286

Violence: criminal gangs, 197–198; cultural of peace against Zagreb, 208–218; fear of crime-related, 165–166; gender/age as determinants to vulnerability to small arms, 165*fig*; multinational corporations selling firearms, 377–379; public health priority of prevention of, 158–159; as sociopathology, 158; substance abuse association with, 210–211. *See also* Urban crime

Volatile organic compounds (VOCs), 329

## W

Walkability, 349–350

Walking transportation, 294–295

Water services: disease transmission through contamination of, 271–276; epidemiology of disease transmission and, 272–276; health benefits of interventions for, 278–280; impact on livelihoods of inadequate, 271–272; in low-income urban settlements, 268–271; perceptions of ill health and demands for improved, 276–278

Web sites: Belfast Healthy Cities initiative, 351; British crime prevention strategies, 169; Canada's crime prevention strategies, 169; Globalization and World Cities study group, 16; *International Compendium of Crime Prevention Practices*, 169; London Congestion Charging Scheme, 332; Oxford Health Alliance Syndey Summit, 135; United Nations Special Rapporteur, 20

West Nile virus, 107

Wet Bulb Globe Temperature (WBGT), 75–76*fig*, 78

"What is Adequate Shelter?" (UN Millennium Project), 313

WHO (World Health Organization): collaborative study on SARS headed by, 116, 357; Commission on Social Determinants of Health of, 2, 22, 48; *Global Age-Friendly Cities: A Guide* by, 96; on global disease burden due to inadequate water/sanitation services, 270; *HEALTH 21:* (WHO regional Office for Europe), 416–417; healthy city definition by, 427; Healthy City projects, 10, 135, 208, 406–418; influenza classifications by, 117; OECD countries' brain drain estimated by, 52; Ottawa Charter for Health Promotion, 406; *Social Determinants of Health* (WHO-EHCN), 411; on target levels for air pollutants, 334; *Targets for Health for all* (WHO Regional Office for Europe), 415; *Twenty Steps for Developing a Health Cities Project*, 408; Urban Heart initiative of, 478–479; *World Report on Violence and Health* by, 213–214

Women: contraceptive use by residence and poverty status, 41*t*; "double job schedules" of developing countries, 76–77; Pakistan's Hodood Ordinances on rape victims, 159; reproductive health of, 41*t*, 51

World Bank: asymmetries of decision making by the, 15; SAPs (structural adjustment programs) mandated by, 19; on Tanzanian health system reports, 244

World Health Assembly, 158

*World Report on Violence and Health* (WHO), 213–214

## Y

Yugoslavian civil war, 212–213. *See also* Croatia

## Z

Zagreb (Croatia): Child Protection Centre Zagreb survey (2003), 210; civil society role in solving Luka Ritz murder, 214–215; "football" war in, 212–213; government programs against violence in, 215–217; Healthy Cities movement membership by, 208; history of violence in, 209–213; international programs against violence applied in, 213–214; overview of, 208–209; positive signs of progress in, 217–218. *See also* Croatia

Zagreb Declaration, 416

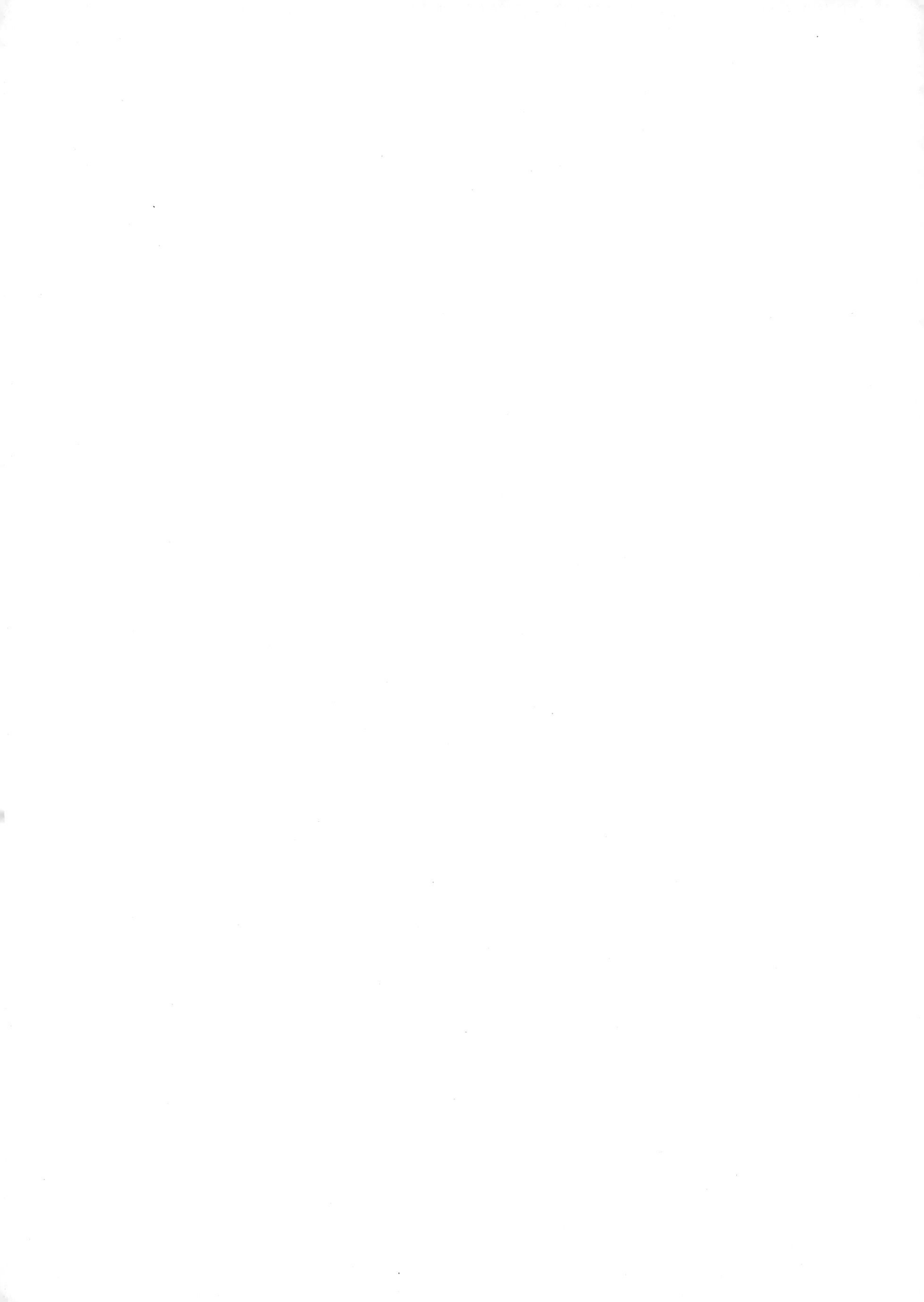